Child Health in the Community

Child Health in the Community

Edited by
Ross G. Mitchell
MD(Edin) FRCP(Edin) DCH
James Mackenzie Professor of Child Health,
University of Dundee

Foreword by
S. D. M. Court
CBE MD FRCP(Lond) FCST
Emeritus Professor of Child Health,
University of Newcastle upon Tyne

SECOND EDITION

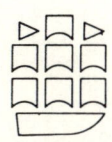

CHURCHILL LIVINGSTONE
EDINBURGH LONDON MELBOURNE AND NEW YORK 1980

CHURCHILL LIVINGSTONE
Medical Division of the Longman Group Limited

Distributed in the United States of America by
Churchill Livingstone Inc., 19 West 44th Street,
New York, NY 10036, and by associated companies,
branches and representatives throughout the world.

© Longman Group Limited 1977, 1980

All rights reserved. No part of this publication may
be reproduced, stored in a retrieval system, or
transmitted in any form or by any means, electronic,
mechanical, photocopying, recording or otherwise,
without the prior permission of the publishers
(Churchill Livingstone, Robert Stevenson House,
1–3 Baxter's Place, Leith Walk, Edinburgh,
EH1 3AF).

First published 1977
Second edition 1980

ISBN 0 443 02195 3

British Library Cataloguing in Publication Data
Child health in the community.–2nd ed.
   1. Community health services for children–Great Britain
   I. Mitchell, Ross Galbraith
362.7'8'10941   RJ103.G7   80–40314

Printed in Great Britain by Butler & Tanner Ltd, Frome and London

Foreword

I said in the first edition that this was an important and timely book; and a second edition within three years confirms that conviction. The central theme is unchanged: 'Health is determined by the interaction between the child, his environment, and the society in which he lives, and is not a measurable quantity independent of this relationship.' Within this context, a company of experienced authors consider the nature of childhood, the contemporary needs of children and families, the epidemiology of childhood illness, the prevention of disease and the promotion of health, and the varied services which society and the professions provide.

The child is their centre of reference: the child from fetus to adolescent—in the antenatal clinic, at home, in the playgroup, school, games field, health centre, youth club, family court, accident department, outpatient clinic and hospital ward; this is a child's 'community' and the ground of this book's exploring.

The authors take a positive approach, but all too frequently they are confronted with the negative attitudes of government and administration, which regard the child not as a person in his own right, a full citizen whatever his age, but as a number in a social class, an ethnic group, or a problem category. Child health in the United Kingdom is a story of contrasts and contradictions; much that is commendable and much that is unacceptable in a civilized society. And when we are willing to look, the explanation is not difficult to find. It is a remarkable fact that, from its beginning in 1948 until 1972, services for children were never identified separately in the planning or finance of the National Health Service. And if we accept that health care for children is a basic human right and also highly cost effective, since handicapping illness is better prevented or treated early than managed for a lifetime, then the lack of rational purpose in this approach is as surprising as it is unacceptable. However, the tide of inattention is turning. The first signs were detailed examinations of the health needs of children, the structure and quality of their health services, and the special educational needs of the handicapped, by joint parent and inter-professional committees—Brotherston (1973), Court (1976) and Warnock (1978). The relevance of these three reports to the wider purpose of this book is considered in appropriate chapters. I have referred to them here because they point to the need for an increase in the study and practice of social paediatrics.

As expected, the response at first was cautious or rejecting but a wider debate and a greater impetus to change have followed. Government has committed itself to the central concept—the progressive development of a single, comprehensive health service for children—and has stressed the need for 'the integration of preventive and therapeutic care and of hospital and community services' (Health Circular, 1978, 5). The way forward will not be easy. Nowhere are need and uncertainty more evident than in 'prevention'; and those who use the word most readily are often least aware of their ignorance of how to achieve it. Apart from the infectious diseases and certain specific disorders such as haemolytic disease of the newborn, little progress has been made in preventing the present hazards for children—low birth weight, malformations, respiratory infection, accidents, mental handicap, psychiatric disorders and child abuse—and the damaging and lethal diseases of adult life which have their origins in childhood.

The second edition of this necessary book is addressed to the same readership as the first—general practitioners, particularly those with a special interest in children, paediatricians, paediatric nurses, health visitors, social workers, teachers, health administrators and those who decide priorities in local and central government. Used with guidance it will also be useful to students in all these disciplines. I hope that it will be widely read.

Newcastle upon Tyne,   S. D. M. C.
1980

Preface

Throughout the world, resources for the medical care of children are largely committed to the urgent problems presented by malnutrition, infection and other acute disorders of childhood. In the more technically developed areas, however, advances in medical science have virtually eradicated some conditions and rendered the treatment of others rapid and effective. With this easing of the pressure from life-threatening disease have come a new appreciation of the importance of preventive paediatrics, greater commitment to the care of handicapped children in and out of hospital, and realization that health care must reach those who require it most.

Interest in the planning of health services has been growing in many countries, and not least in the United Kingdom where recent reorganization offered the prospect of a unified child health service attuned to children's needs. Unfortunately, financial difficulties and entrenched attitudes have so far prevented full exploitation of the opportunities afforded, while changes in political thought have made the prospects for disadvantaged children less promising. Nevertheless, as Professor Court has said in his Foreword, the seeds have been sown by the Court and Brotherston Reports and we can but hope that they will germinate in time and ultimately produce new and better patterns of health care for children.

This book is concerned with the health of infants and children in the community as a whole. It considers the background to the maintenance of health in childhood, the nature of the work undertaken in a child health service, and the resources and organization required. The contributors are drawn from a wide range of disciplines—general practice, paediatrics, psychiatry, community medicine and the social sciences. They include specialists in child health and paediatrics, health education, educational medicine and various aspects of sociology and social work.

To doctors embarking on a career in paediatrics, this book offers information and guidance about what to expect, what will be expected of them and how to go about their work. It provides a ready source of reference for all doctors responsible for the health of children, whether in general or specialist practice. The contents should also be of interest to those in other professions whose work involves the care of the young.

Dundee,   R. G. M.
1980

Contributors

Frank N. Bamford, MD, MRCP, DPH, DCH, MFCM, Reader and Honorary Consultant in Developmental Paediatrics, University of Manchester.

J. H. Barber, MD, FRCGP, MRCP(Glas), DRCOG, Norie-Miller Professor of General Practice, University of Glasgow.

Terence J. R. Bruce, MA, MB, BChir, MRC Psych, DPM, Consultant Child Psychiatrist, St Bartholomew's Hospital, London.

George Cust, MB, ChB, DPH, DTM&H, FFCM, Chief Medical Officer, Health Education Council, London.

Donald Houston, BA, Senior Lecturer in Social Work, University of Glasgow.

David R. May, BA, PhD, Dip Crim, Lecturer in Sociology, Department of Psychiatry, University of Dundee.

Ross G. Mitchell, MD, FRCP(Edin), DCH, James Mackenzie Professor of Child Health, University of Dundee.

Phyllida Parsloe, BA, PhD, Dip Soc Sci, Cert Ment Hlth, MBASW, Professor of Social Work, University of Bristol.

Philip Pinkerton, MD, FRC Psych, DPM, Director of Studies in Behavioural Paediatrics, University of Liverpool.

I. D. Gerald Richards, MD, PhD, FRCP(Glas), Professor of Community Medicine, University of Leeds.

Michael G. H. Rogers, MA, MB, BChir, DPH, DCH, Senior Clinical Medical Officer, West Berkshire Health District, Reading.

Werner H. Schutt, MB, BCh, FRCP(Edin), DCH, Consultant Neuropaediatrician, United Bristol Hospitals.

Philip M. Strong, BA, MA, Research Officer, Department of Social and Community Medicine, University of Oxford.

C. Eric Stroud, BSc, MB, BCh, FRCP(Lond), DCH, Professor of Child Health, King's College Hospital Medical School, London.

J. K. G. Webb, OBE, MA, BM, BCh, FRCP(Lond), James Spence Professor of Child Health, University of Newcastle upon Tyne.

Kingsley Whitmore, MRCS, LRCP, DCH, Research Community Paediatrician, Thomas Coram Research Unit, Institute of Education, University of London.

Contents

Part One: **Introduction**
Social and community paediatrics ... 3

Part Two: **The Social Background**
1. Childhood as an estate ... 19
2. The social and physical environment ... 37
3. The child in his family ... 48
4. The adolescent years ... 70
5. Troubled and troublesome children ... 89

Part Three: **The Foundations of Child Health**
6. Health education ... 107
7. The epidemiology of disease in childhood ... 126
8. Nutrition and nutritional disorders of children ... 147

Part Four: **Health and Social Services**
9. Community child health services ... 161
10. Preventive aspects of child health practice ... 185
11. Primary paediatric care ... 209
12. Hospital services for children ... 233
13. Handicapped children ... 246
14. Social work services for children ... 261

Part Five: **Health and School**
15. The School Health Service: organization ... 289
16. The School Health Service: methods ... 299
17. The handicapped child in school ... 313

Index ... 343

Part One: Introduction

Ross G. Mitchell

Social and community paediatrics

Social paediatrics is not a separate branch of paediatric medicine but rather a concept that focuses attention on the social and cultural background of the child as well as the interaction between his inborn characteristics and the effects of his physical environment. There has always been a strong sociological flavour to the practice of paediatrics, for few doctors can treat ill children without being aware of the malign influence of adverse social circumstances. The extent to which clinicians take this into consideration has varied greatly and has tended to diminish with increases in medical knowledge and a rising standard of living, especially in technically advanced countries. This decline in interest has been associated with a loss of knowledge, so that today paediatricians skilled in technical investigations and the use of powerful therapeutic agents may lack corresponding understanding of the sociology of childhood. Yet the social processes involved in the aetiology of disease are at least as complex as the biochemical ones and require the same systematic scientific study (Stacey, 1979). Moreover, in recent years the social sciences have been rapidly developing new concepts and a new methodology directly applicable to the biosocial problems of paediatrics (Badgley & Bloom, 1973).

The isolation of the social and medical sciences from one another, with practically no sharing of educational experience and little communication, has been a major obstacle to mutual understanding (Richardson, 1970). As a result, paediatricians have often failed to recognize that health is determined by interaction between the child, his environment and the society in which he lives, and is not a measurable quantity independent of this relationship. The term 'social paediatrics' can therefore be justified as a means of reasserting the importance of the social milieu without suggesting that this is a new specialty. Similar considerations apply to developmental paediatrics, which is not a new concept but serves to remind us that disordered development is a concomitant of childhood malformation and disease, and that the study of normal and abnormal development in all its aspects—social, intellectual, emotional and physical—is an integral part of paediatric practice.

Community medicine is concerned with the health of groups of people rather than with individual clinical care. Community paediatrics should therefore mean paediatrics as it applies to a population of children. In recent years the word 'community' has been abused and has been taken to mean the antithesis of 'hospital', so that in Britain community paediatrics has come to imply the practice of paediatrics outside the hospital. This is unfortunate since hospitals should be considered simply as one of the resources of the community, just as are schools, health centres and residential homes. It would be preferable to drop the terms 'community paediatrics' and 'hospital paediatrics' and to consider paediatrics whether in or out of hospital as 'general paediatrics', differentiating only one or two real subdivisions like perinatal paediatrics and a number of specialties such as paediatric cardiology or paediatric neurology. Nevertheless, the term 'community paediatrics' is useful since it emphasizes the importance of paediatric practice outside the hospital at a time when major changes are taking place in the child health services. It may be expected that eventually the need for the terms 'developmental paediatrics' and 'social paediatrics' will also lessen as the balance of general paediatrics is restored and the need to stress these aspects passes. At present, however, the central role in child health played by social factors deserves to be restated. This is especially important in affluent countries where the misconception has gained hold that poverty, malnutrition and other manifestations of social deprivation no longer exist or are so unimportant that they no longer warrant attention.

There are two main areas of study in social and community paediatrics:
1. The health of the child population in relation to its social environment.
2. The effects of particular combinations of social advantage and disadvantage on the health of individual children.

The first constitutes a branch of the larger subjects of social medicine and medical sociology and uses the methods of the epidemiologist, the sociologist and the statistician. The second is part of clinical paediatrics. Both are of concern to the practising doctor, for understanding of the place of children in society and the cultural, economic and educational pressures which bear on all children is essential if the problems of one child are to be seen in perspective, while it is in the medical care of the ill or abnormal child that the need to restate the importance of social factors is most cogent.

Children in society

As a society develops, its power structure and value systems undergo continuous change. New demands require modification of educational patterns so that order in communities at various stages of adaptation will be maintained and needs arising out of reorientation will be satisfied. Attitudes to children and adolescents change correspondingly and often constitute a delicate indicator of the stage of evolution of the society and the stresses imposed by its struggles to readjust to new circumstances. The child in a pre-industrial society, with its high birth and infant mortality rates, large numbers of children, and continuing deaths in childhood, has a lower status than one in a technically advanced country with an ageing population and few children, where each child has a high life expectancy and is in consequence greatly valued from an early age. At the same time, the quality of child life, which should be improved by community affluence, may be eroded by the pressures and increasingly complex relationships of an industrial society. The elaborate stratification of such a society leads to increasing divergence in attitudes towards children in different social categories. The consequent disparity in child-rearing practices, affording varying opportunities for social and psychological experiences in infancy, is reflected in differing patterns of child health.

Childhood is a time of life to be enjoyed for its own sake and has its own rights and responsibilities. It is also a time of preparation for adulthood. This status is achieved by a process of socialization, through which the child learns what is expected of him and becomes familiar with the cultural characteristics and system of social relationships of his environment. The fundamental aims of socialization are the same in all societies, but there are wide differences in what must be learned and the way in which it is taught. The result is that the child acquires a pattern of behaviour which indelibly stamps him as a member of his own community.

While there is thus pronounced variation between and within societies in attitudes towards children and in the behaviour expected of children, the child is always in a state of dependency, subject to restrictions and penalties and only accorded limited privileges.

Role of social factors in child health
The many determinants of health in childhood—biological, physical, epidemiological, economic and social—must all be considered in the ecology of disease occurring at this time. The age structure of the population, birth- and death-rates, parental age at marriage and childbearing, and size and spacing of families are but a few of the demographic features which profoundly influence the pattern of child health in the community.

In underprivileged communities, many women grow up ill-nourished and of short stature. They have poor health, inadequate education and low incomes. They are likely to bear children early and frequently. Infants of such mothers are smaller at birth, die more readily, and have more illnesses than those of mothers from more affluent backgrounds. In the United Kingdom, perinatal and infant death rates are inversely related to socio-economic status, with mortality lowest in the professional classes and highest among the offspring of the least skilled labourers, whose wives at every age and parity experience a greater risk of reproductive failure than do the wives of professional men (Baird, 1975). Thus, for example, the perinatal mortality rate for Scotland in 1977 was 18.3, but 23.5 in social class V and only 10.9 in social class I. The number of infants dying after the neonatal period is relatively small but of these at least one third die suddenly and unexpectedly—nearly 2000 every year in the United Kingdom. There is an excess of such 'cot deaths' among infants of underprivileged families and mothers of affected infants tend to be younger and of higher parity than those of controls: many other factors, such as the type of feeding, the pattern of infection and the immunological status of the infant may also be important (Froggatt et al, 1971; Working Party, 1977). The causes of cot deaths thus appear to be multiple and their interaction complex. Nevertheless there are social implications which cannot be ignored in the struggle to reduce infant mortality, for there is evidence that many of the factors leading to death in infancy are avoidable (Richards & McIntosh, 1972; McWeeny & Emery, 1975).

Malnutrition

Malnutrition is another major threat to children who survive the perinatal period. It not only causes overt deficiency diseases but also affects growth and development and undermines resistance to infection (see Ch. 8). The work of Field & Baber (1974) in Hong Kong has shown that the nutritional state of children commonly suffers at the time of weaning. When the food intake of children is evaluated, consideration should be given not only to joules and balanced diets, but also to the origins of malnutrition in poverty, poor housing, disease, parental ignorance and family disorganization. Such adverse environmental conditions exist in every society, and result in an increase in childhood disease, especially respiratory infections and parasitic infestations. Even when material standards are adequate, ignorance of the principles of nutrition may affect the health of children. A mother who ignores instructions and makes up too concentrated a milk feed for her infant can unwittingly cause hypernatraemia leading to brain damage or death (Finberg, 1969). The increase in rickets among Glasgow children reported in the 1960s was largely due to the mothers' erroneous belief that fresh cow's milk, with its low content of vitamin D, was better than dried milk fortified with the vitamin (Arneil et al, 1965). Rickets still occurring in Asian immigrants is attributable to traditional dietary habits unsuitable for British conditions and to language barriers which prevent communication (Singleton & Tucker, 1978; Goel, 1979).

Severe undernutrition in infancy may affect mental as well as physical development, for there is evidence that it can reduce the size and number of brain cells and retard the process of myelination in the central nervous system (Martin, 1973). This is reflected in the poor performance of schoolchildren who were severely malnourished in the first year of life (Richardson et al, 1973; Cravioto, 1979).

Birth weight and social class

The mean intelligence of children is also affected by birth weight and social class, being lower in children of low weight at birth compared with their heavier peers and lower for each birth-weight category in children born to mothers of lower socio-economic status (Illsley, 1966). The reasons are complex, for intelligence depends not only on genetic endowment, intrauterine environment and perinatal events, but also on social and cultural influences in infancy and childhood, which are likely to be similar to those which affected the mother's reproductive functioning.

Effects of improving circumstances

One of the priority aims of the child health services is to identify and help families rendered especially vulnerable by adverse environmental circumstances. At the same time, it must be realized that improving the quality of life for the whole population will eliminate some paediatric problems and reduce the importance of others (Tizard, 1975). In large parts of the developing world, one quarter to one half of all the children die before the age of five years, largely as a result of malnutrition, intestinal infection and excess fertility, all of which are socially determined and eminently preventable. Rising social and economic standards and more efficient medical care should result in increased survival rates, and a reduction in the incidence of many types of disease in childhood. In some wealthy countries illness due to infection and malnutrition is now numerically less important than developmental disorders and educational or social maladjustment. Indeed, it has been reported from the United States that among children in the poorer areas of some cities, obesity is a greater problem than undernutrition (Stunkard et al, 1972). In this context poverty is a relative term and not comparable with the extreme privation experienced by children in many other countries, though even in the United States there is malnutrition among some very poor children of African or Mexican origin, particularly in the southern States (American Academy of Pediatrics, 1973).

The effect of an improving economy on the health of children is influenced by the cultural characteristics of the community concerned. The value placed on child life by the community will largely determine the resources allocated to child health. The way money is spent sometimes depends on factors other than the real needs of children, which are at times subordinated to the desire for prestige or for visible signs of technical progress. Distribution is often markedly uneven and in many countries the health status of large numbers of underprivileged children in rural areas and urban shanty towns is deteriorating while at the same time the health of the minority of urban elite is close to the level in the most developed countries. In Africa, where more than 40 per cent of the population are under the age of 15 years and where child mortality is up to 50 times as great as in Europe, the most pressing requirements are not large modern hospitals but better nutrition and sanitation, control of malaria and immunization against specific infections (Hendrickse, 1972).

Attitudes to disease
Folklore and custom shape attitudes, so that a condition accepted fatalistically as 'normal' in one society will elicit a vigorous response in another. Even in the same community the reaction to, for example, parasitic infestation may differ widely from one social class to another.

The roles assumed by different children with the same illness, and the reactions of their environments to their condition, vary enormously and depend to a considerable extent on socio-economic factors. These may also play a direct part in the genesis of disease in the individual child and influence the duration and severity of illness and the child's response to it. Thus, for example, asthma is likely to be more severe in a child from the large family of a manual worker than in the child of professional parents with a small family (Mitchell & Dawson, 1973). Illness may be induced by changes in the psychosocial environment, such as starting a new school, loss of a close relative or some other family crisis. Failure to adjust to such life events may cause disturbed behaviour and can result in physical or mental disease (Heisel et al, 1973). It has also been shown that social stress can result in an increase in the inappropriate use of health services (Haggerty, 1980).

Educational difficulties
Learning disorders and other educational problems are often the result of a complex interaction of adverse influences, both at home and in school, including

the far-reaching effects of prenatal and early postnatal deprivation as well as inadequate educational opportunity. Thus Rutter et al (1970) found an association between social class and specific reading retardation and concluded that the variation in reading ability was determined partly by biological factors and partly by different patterns of family life and communication.

The acquisition of speech may be slow when contact with adults in the early years is limited, as may happen in very large families: the resulting retardation of development of thought, which seems to depend on language, may affect educational achievement. This will also be influenced by physical factors such as illness, fatigue, or hunger, especially if the child comes from an underprivileged home. Many studies have shown that adverse social conditions militate against success at school. The education system itself is biased towards socially advantaged children, in that the language used, the behaviour expected and the teachers themselves reflect the same standards. Hence some of the failure of disadvantaged children is attributable to differences between their own language, values and experiences of life and those explicitly or implicitly put forward by the school. When we add to these the adverse effects of cultural deprivation in the home, and of the associated overcrowding, poverty, malnutrition and disease, it is small wonder that they experience educational difficulties far more often than do other children.

The belief that severe mental subnormality renders a child ineducable is widely held and until recently children below a certain level of intelligence were rigidly excluded from our educational system. However, the view has gained ground that every child should be considered capable of some achievement, no matter how small. As the Warnock Report (1978) states, all human beings are entitled to education and therefore there is a clear obligation to educate the most severely disabled, if for no other reason than that they are human. Educational authorities in Britain now have responsibility for the education of all children, including those formerly described as ineducable or untrainable. Children with behaviour disorders, whatever their level of intelligence, frequently have educational difficulties arising out of their emotional disturbance, and they too require special educational provision.

Family care

Despite suggestions that family life inhibits spontaneity and crushes children into conformity, an affectionate and understanding family is the best milieu for the developing child. The facts that parents vary in their capacity for love and tolerance and that some are unable to create a warm home environment does not invalidate the generalization. A form of family organization exists in every society, whether it be the nuclear family of father, mother, brothers and sisters, an extended family comprising several generations or some form of collective. In many developed countries today, the nuclear family is tending to become smaller and to change its structure and function: thus when both father and mother work outside the home, their roles become interchangeable and the father's status as an authority figure diminishes. The single-parent family, with a woman as its head, is becoming commoner and more acceptable. Whatever its form, it is in the family that needs are met, socialization starts, and behaviour is moulded to an acceptable pattern. Approved behaviour varies in different communities, just as it does in different sections of the same community and in different families. The child-rearing practices of parents in poor housing in the centre of a city have been shown to differ from those of parents living in suburban areas of the same city (Newson & Newson, 1968), and these variations will be reflected later in divergent attitudes and standards of behaviour (see Ch. 2).

The real worth of family life becomes apparent when the consequences of its disruption are revealed. A single catastrophe, such as the death of the mother, may cause the immediate break-up of the family, but more frequently it disintegrates slowly under the strain of many repeated blows, especially where there is underlying inadequacy. Parental illness or incapacity, marital disharmony, unemployment, a family too large for a low income, and lack of a suitable home are basic difficulties which reinforce one another and give rise on the one hand to poverty, debt, and lack of adequate food and clothing, and on the other to neglect, desertion and occasionally cruelty. While poor material standards and inadequate parental care can and do frequently co-exist, it is important to realize that a dirty, poverty-stricken family may provide a warm accepting environment for a young child, while children may be unhappy and badly treated in the most affluent home.

Both in disease and in disability, the quality of family life and maternal care is of critical importance, for it helps to determine the physical and emotional resistance of the child as well as affecting the course and outcome. Most families are well able to withstand the strain of severe illness or chronic handicap affecting one of their members. Every member of the family responds so that the affected individual does not have to cope with the difficulty alone and the whole family acts as a buffer. Nevertheless the work of Kaplan and his associates (1973) makes clear that excessive or long-lasting stress impairs or destroys the buffering capacity of even the strongest family, though breakdown may be preventable by help and support from outside agencies.

Child abuse
The increasing number of young children who are maltreated by their parents is a matter of concern in many countries. Cruel and neglectful parents have existed in all societies in all ages, but there is a rising incidence of child abuse in urban industrial communities which is only partially due to greater public sensitivity and more intensive ascertainment of cases (see Ch. 7). Such maltreatment of children occurs in all racial, religious and educational groups and the strain of unsatisfied parental need is the principal precipitating factor. In the presence of predisposing personality characteristics and the stresses imposed by anxieties about marital relations, financial difficulty, unsatisfactory housing arrangements and a generally unsupporting social environment, the occurrence of some family crisis is likely to result in aggression directed at the child. While the resulting non-accidental injury may be damaging or fatal, it must not be forgotten that mental cruelty and passive neglect are also forms of abuse which may have deep and lasting consequences. The effective prevention and management of child abuse demand great understanding by paediatricians of the psychosocial background of parents who lack the capacity to care for their children.

Close co-operation with social and legal agencies is essential: in Britain, the Select Committee on Violence in the Family (1977) has made detailed recommendations aimed at ensuring that co-operation between all professions and agencies concerned is at a uniformly high level throughout the country.

Single-parent and substitute families
While difficulties can arise when both parents are present, they are compounded in the one-parent family. Whether the mother is single because she is unmarried, deserted or bereaved by death, the burden of trying to care for children while earning a living, and the inevitable loneliness and boredom, combine to create tensions which often prove intolerable. Support by providing financial aid, adequate accommodation and day care for the children or arranging for some form of group living in a residential complex, may help to keep the single-parent family together. If these measures fail the children sometimes have to be taken into care by government or voluntary agencies, as is more often the case when both parents are missing. Substitute homes for children in need of care and protection are essential, and their quantity and quality are a further index of the status of children in the eyes of the community (see Ch. 14).

Children who are deprived of a normal family life may be adversely affected even when a good and caring agency makes the best possible provision, by arranging adoption, foster care or residence in a children's home. Prompt action by the social service organizations to maintain the family therefore makes sound sense, on both humanitarian and economic grounds. On the other hand, the advantages must be carefully weighed, since a good adoptive home may afford a more favourable environment for the illegitimate child than any his natural mother can provide (Seglow et al, 1972).

Children of families rendered vulnerable by a combination of adverse circumstances are those most prone to mental and physical disability, intercurrent infection and cultural deprivation leading to educational difficulties. The handicap imposed by these problems is increased by the lack of a supportive family and so a vicious circle of disadvantage is created. The tensions and frustrations generated by such an unhappy and restricting childhood may culminate in delinquency and other forms of antisocial behaviour in adolescence, while the personality deficit frequently associated with these ensures parental inadequacy should the child later have children. Thus the unhappy pattern of distorted family life repeats itself yet again.

The handicapped child
The belief that there are two types of child, the handicapped and the non-handicapped, is deeply engrained in our society, yet the complexities of individual need are far greater than this simple distinction implies. In Britain, the Warnock Committee (1978) recommended that such categorization should be abandoned in favour of the concept of children having a range of special needs, varying with different children and at different ages in the same child.

Patterns of child care and the amount of early social experience afforded to children vary considerably between different cultures and individual parents within them. The young child with severe mental or physical disability is at risk of serious deprivation of social contact and stimulation whatever his social background and the resulting retardation of development must add further to his total handicap. Attention should therefore be devoted to ensuring that the child receives special training in social skills and has every opportunity to develop socially to the limit of his capacity, irrespective of the degree of his disability.

The difficulties of the handicapped child affect not only his own life but the lives of other members of his family and indeed of all who come in contact with him. Hewett et al (1970) have shown that most families meet the problems created by handicap with patterns of behaviour that differ little from the behaviour norms of families without a handicapped child. Young parents can usually make allowances for and expect less of their child but as he grows older the strain of such adaptation begins to tell. Adolescence is a particularly trying time, especially when the siblings begin to resent the restrictions which having a handicapped member places on the whole family, and on them.

Families, of course, vary greatly in their capacity for adaptation: a closely knit resourceful family may prove well able to cope with one or more severely handicapped children, whereas even mild disability in one child of weak incompetent parents may be sufficient to cause family disruption (Mitchell, 1973). The traumatic experience of being taken into care in such circumstances is likely to increase the child's handicap still further, so that every effort should be directed towards supporting the family of the handicapped child before it is stressed to the point of breakdown. The measures to be taken will vary according to need but intimate knowledge of the family's strengths, weaknesses and resources will make support more effective and may suggest ways in which assistance of a material kind can be given. The guiding principle must be to strengthen the parents' ability to care for their child at home and the temptation for professional workers to usurp their role should be resisted.

Adolescence

Some aspects of the transition from childhood to adult life are clearly of paediatric importance—the acceleration of physical growth, the process of maturation, the unwanted effects of puberty such as acne or gynaecomastia. However, paediatrics is also concerned with problems of adolescence which have their origins in environmental deficiencies (Rutter, 1979). Effective management in the early years, when disturbed behaviour is still only a protest by an essentially normal child, may help to prevent adolescent difficulties. The paediatrician has a part to play in the later years as well, when resentment and aggression have become established personality characteristics. Caution must be exercised when complaint is made about antisocial activities at adolescence, for the doctor himself may not fully realize how his outlook has been conditioned by his own development in a particular social stratum. Behaviour which appears deviant to him may be perfectly rational from the perspective of the separate youth culture. The adolescent who has really failed to adjust, perhaps because he comes from a broken home or is rejected by his family, is usually readily recognizable. He has a history of being difficult to control, hostile and inconsiderate of others in earlier childhood, and his aberrant behaviour gradually hardens into overt delinquency or manifests as physical symptoms which may be misinterpreted as due to disease. While adverse social conditions in early life are undoubtedly important in the genesis of such failure of adaptation, the work of Stott (1966) indicates that there is often a congenital predisposition to deviant behaviour which becomes manifest when the child is exposed to sufficient postnatal stress.

The abuse of narcotic drugs is a relatively new and sinister feature of adolescent life in some countries. It is a growing problem in Britain, although it has not yet assumed such large proportions as in the United States (Wiener, 1970) nor is it nearly so prevalent as the abuse of alcohol, especially in Scotland (Ritson & Plant, 1977). In no sphere of paediatrics is the need for close medical and social co-operation so cogent as in the management of the teenage drug addict.

Adaptation to adult life is difficult for any child from a deprived background, but is much harder for the handicapped adolescent. He feels isolated and frustrated by his disability, reacts with resentment and bitterness, and is likely to become increasingly unmanageable. Delinquency here may have social as well as medical roots—in family malfunctioning, the conflicts arising from rapidly changing social values and the pressures of gang expectations, all added to mental or physical handicap. The elucidation of these and other problems of adolescence demands not only medical knowledge but also familiarity with the pattern of teenage life in the paediatrician's own community and a readiness to act in concert with social workers, psychologists and other colleagues.

Health care according to need
In developed countries, the popular belief is that the health care of children is largely the province of health professionals. Clinical practice is traditionally based on answering calls for help, on the assumption that if help is not sought, there is no health problem. The reality is that mothers are by far the most important providers of care for their children (Haggerty, 1979) and the best mothers will only occasionally have to consult the nurse or doctor. However, less competent parents have more need of help and advice, although they may not always recognize this. There is increasing realization that high standards of health care depend on seeking out undetected illness as well as responding to demand and that children 'have a right to basic health care which comprehends not only treatment at times of illness or injury but also continuing surveillance to promote health and detect disability or handicap' (Court, 1976).

It is clear that even in countries where health services are highly organized, they are not equitably distributed and there are large areas of unmet need. This is especially true of child health, despite the fact that paediatricians generally are more aware of the importance of preventive medicine than are most other clinicians. In many parts of the world children are in poor health because medical care is not available but even where there are sufficient doctors and other medical services, some children do not benefit because parents are either unaware of their existence or fail to ask for help and advice. These are largely the same parents who are missed by social measures aimed at helping the underprivileged, conserving their resources and improving the quality of their lives. Thus they often do not claim welfare foods, grants for education, rent rebates and the like. This may be because they are ashamed of their state and unwilling to accept what they regard as charity, because they are put off by the complexity of application or the condescending manner of officials, or simply because they are apathetic, inarticulate and unequal to the struggle for existence in an industrial society. Such families tend to congregate in the least favoured areas, where rents are low, houses are old and ill-maintained, and there is a lack of space to play and other amenities. As time passes, overcrowding increases, the more competent families move away and those who can find nowhere else to live gravitate to the area—immigrants, large or single-parent families, the unskilled, the inadequate and the destitute.

Clearly we cannot take the detached view that it is the parents' responsibility and not the doctor's to see that children receive the attention they need. A pattern of care which is heavily used by children who enjoy good health and a privileged way of life and fails to reach those whose health is undermined by social disadvantage should not be accepted. Apart from the inequity of such a system, it ensures that the children of the poor, already at a serious disadvantage from malnutrition and a hostile early environment, will be further penalized by ill health which predisposes to educational failure. As a result, their competence in adult life will be less than it might have been and the cycle of social inadequacy and low status is repeated. The greatest challenge which faces those responsible for the health of all the children in their community is to provide services where they are needed and to ensure that they are used. The latter aim is more likely to be achieved by educating and stimulating parents to help themselves and claim their rights than by pressing care on unresponsive families with low expectations and passive acceptance of their powerlessness to alter their condition.

Relationships of the paediatrician to other professionals

Ill health in childhood, and particularly chronic disability, is a problem of paediatric medicine but not one for the paediatrician alone. We have seen that the mother bears the brunt of caring for her children, while the primary health care team of general practitioner, health visitor and community nurse, provide the main professional backing (see Ch. 11). The paediatrician must work in cooperation with all of these, with specialist colleagues and with members of other professions. He must be prepared to devote much time, not only to study of the child himself, but also to interchange of ideas with his associates.

The paediatrician has special knowledge of health and disease in the young, and skills in applying that knowledge. He cannot do so to best effect if he ignores or is ill-informed about other aspects of the child's life. He must understand the immense influence a child's experiences at home and in school have on his intellectual, emotional, physical and social development. He should know enough about educational failure, adverse environmental influences, and emotional disturbance to make him an effective physician. This does not mean that he must function as a social worker, a psychologist or a teacher, but that he should appreciate the basis of their professional work, their outlooks and methods, and the intricacies of the interfaces between their disciplines and his own. The unique contribution of the paediatrician to the child care team is his specialized medical competence. He can speak from knowledge and experience about the contribution made by social adversity to a child's ill health and the extent to which ill health affects a child's social behaviour. His first responsibility is to define and implement his own role but he must also consider how his actions relate to those of his professional associates. In some instances he may assume a co-ordinating or a leading function, but this should never become a dominating one, and his primary consideration must always be what is best for the child and his family.

Conclusion

The principles of social paediatrics are the same throughout the world, even if their application varies from country to country. The details of the difficulties encountered in a particular country are less important than a general concern for the quality of child life and effective action to enhance it. In Britain the health of children continues to improve but whereas we have progressed some way in the conquest of disease, we have been less successful in controlling ill health which originates in social disadvantage. In the words of the Court Report (1976) 'economic prosperity, a sufficient family income, adequate food, satisfactory housing, a widening education and a safe environment are still the foundation of good health in childhood and of services designed to maintain it'.

Familiarity with the community in which a child lives—the extent to which it is urbanized and the pattern of industrial employment, its people and their organization in neighbourhood, kinship and family, their social habits and beliefs—makes for better understanding of the external influences which determine the pattern of his health. The doctor who concentrates on the biomedical aspects of a child's illness and ignores his cultural environment, or who fails to advise on ways of improving the socio-economic background to ill health in childhood, is only fulfilling a part of his function as a paediatrician.

REFERENCES

American Academy of Pediatrics 1973 Committee statement: the ten-state nutrition survey. Pediatrics 51: 1095–1099
Arneil G C, McKilligin, H R, Lobo E 1965 Malnutrition in Glasgow children. Scottish Medical Journal 10: 480–484
Badgley R F, Bloom S W 1973 Behavioural sciences and medical education: the case of sociology. Social Science and Medicine 7: 927–941
Baird D 1975 The interplay of changes in society, reproductive habits and obstetric practice in Scotland between 1922 and 1972. British Journal of Preventive and Social Medicine 29: 135–146
Court S D M (chairman) 1976 Fit for the Future: report of the committee on child health services. HMSO, London
Cravioto J 1979 Effects of early malnutrition and stimuli deprivation on mental development. In: The child in the world of tomorrow. Doxiadis S (ed) Pergamon Press, Oxford
Field C E, Baber F M 1974 Growing Up in Hong Kong. University Press, Hong Kong
Finberg L 1969 Hypernatremic dehydration. Advances in Pediatrics 16: 325–344
Froggatt P, Lynas M A, MacKenzie G 1971 Epidemiology of sudden unexpected death in infants (cot death) in Northern Ireland. British Journal of Preventive and Social Medicine 25: 119–134
Goel K M 1979 A nutrition survey of immigrant children in Glasgow. Scottish Health Service Studies No. 40. Scottish Home and Health Department, Edinburgh

Haggerty R J 1979 Who provides health care for children? In: Doxiadis S (ed) The child in the world of tomorrow. Pergamon Press, Oxford
Haggerty R J 1980 Common happenings: the George Frederic Still Memorial Lecture. Developmental Medicine and Child Neurology 22: 391–400
Heisel J S, Ream, S, Raitz R, Rappaport M, Coddington R D 1973 The significance of life events as contributing factors in the diseases of children. Journal of Pediatrics 83: 119–123
Hendrickse R G 1972 Problems and future of paediatrics in pre-industrial countries: Africa. Helvetica Paediatrica Acta Suppl. 28: 23–31
Hewett S, Newson J, Newson E 1970 The family and the handicapped child. Allen & Unwin, London
Illsey R 1966 Early prediction of perinatal risk. Proceedings of the Royal Society of Medicine 59: 181–184
Kaplan D M, Smith A, Grobstein R, Fischman S E 1973 Family mediation of stress. Social Work 18: 60–69
McWeeny P M, Emery J L 1975 Unexpected postneonatal deaths (cot deaths) due to recognizable disease. Archives of Disease in Childhood, 50: 191–196.
Martin H P 1973 Nutrition: its relationship to children's physical, mental and emotional development. American Journal of Clinical Nutrition 26: 766–775
Mitchell R G 1973 Chronic handicap in childhood: its implications for family and community. Practitioner 211: 763–768
Mitchell R G, Dawson B 1973 Educational and social characteristics of children with asthma. Archives of Disease in Childhood 48: 467–471
Newson J, Newson E 1968 Four years old in an urban community. Allen & Unwin, London
Richards I D G, McIntosh H T 1972 Confidential inquiry into 226 consecutive infant deaths. Archives of Disease in Childhood 47: 697–706
Richardson S A 1970 Patterns of medical and social research in pediatrics. Acta Paediatrica Scandinavica 59: 265–272
Richardson S A, Birch H G, Hertzig M E 1973 School performance of children who were severely malnourished in infancy. American Journal of Mental Deficiency 77: 623–632
Ritson A B, Plant M A 1977 Drugs and Young People in Scotland. Scottish Health Education Unit, Edinburgh
Rutter M 1979 Changing youth in a changing society. Nuffield Provincial Hospitals Trust, London
Rutter M, Tizard J, Whitmore K 1970 Education, health and behaviour. Longman, London
Seglow J, Kellmer Pringle M, Wedge P 1972 Growing up adopted. National Children's Bureau, London
Select Committee on Violence in the Family 1977 First report: violence to children. vol I. HMSO, London
Singleton N, Tucker S M 1978 Vitamin D status of Asian infants. British Medical Journal 1: 607–610
Stacey M 1979 New perspectives in clinical medicine: the sociologist. Journal of the Royal College of Physicians of London 13: 123–129
Stott D H 1966 Studies of troublesome children. Tavistock Publications, London
Stunkard A, d'Aquili E, Fox S, Ross D L F 1972 Influence of social class on obesity and thinness in children. Journal of the American Medical Association 221: 579–584
Tizard J 1975 Three dysfunctional environmental influences in development: malnutrition, non-accidental injury and child-minding. In: Barltrop D (ed) Paediatrics and the environment. Fellowship of Postgraduate Medicine, London
Warnock H M (chairman) 1978 Special educational needs: report of the committee of enquiry into the education of handicapped children and young people. HMSO, London
Wiener R S P 1970 Drugs and schoolchildren. Longman, London
Working Party for Early Childhood Deaths in Newcastle (1977) Newcastle survey of deaths in early childhood 1974/6, with special reference to sudden unexpected deaths. Archives of Disease in Childhood 52: 828–835

Part Two: The Social Background

1   *David May and Philip Strong*

Childhood as an estate

The way we think about children, what we notice about them, our estimation of their capacities, what we value in them, what we dislike about them—all these things are shaped by the times in which we live. On one level the point is obvious; different cultures and different eras treat children differently. What is harder to grasp, however, is the way in which our own version of childhood is culturally determined. All societies tend to suffer from the delusion that the way they think about things is natural and right, a tendency reinforced in our own culture by the human sciences. It is tempting to think of these as unique devices for uncovering objective, impersonal and certain knowledge about the social world. Yet as Skolnick (1974) demonstrates, much developmental psychology can be treated as simply one more codification of current western concepts of childhood, as something which tells us as much about the experimenters as about their subjects. The same is undoubtedly true of sociology and also—or so we would strongly suspect—of both paediatrics and child psychiatry.

The aim of this chapter is to spell out some of the main features of the current western view of childhood, to indicate their historical origins, to argue that various organizations, groups and professions all have vested interests in the maintenance and development of particular features, and, finally, to note some of the important issues which may be obscured by conventional ways of looking at children.

The study of our attitudes to children is still in its infancy. A small amount of work, perhaps the better part, has been done by historians, but sociologists have barely started. We ourselves have studied some aspects of paediatrics and juvenile justice (and we shall be drawing on this work later in the chapter), but as yet our knowledge is fragmentary. We propose therefore to review some published research work, to speculate where we know of no research, and to suggest which areas need further study.

In essence, we shall argue that many of the properties which we ascribe to children are derived not from their innate qualities, but from adult interests. As these change, so do our image and treatment of childhood. Moreover, since our interests are varied and contradictory, so too are our expectations and judgements of children.

Some background assumptions

Let us begin by spelling out some of the assumptions surrounding the conventional modern view of childhood.

1. Childhood is first and foremost regarded as a 'natural' category, biologically determined and constituting a distinct period of life that spans the years from birth to the late teens. As such, it is imputed with its own psychology and special needs, and requires in its turn its own special institutions (Armstrong, 1979).

2. Children are characterized by dependence, subordination and exclusion. The distinguishing feature of all childhood, writes Skolnick, is incompetence. This in turn gives rise to a whole series of social and legal institutions (chief among which are the school and the juvenile court), which separate and suborn the child and the adolescent.

3. There is a further tendency, most marked in a great deal of sociological and psychological research, to treat children as curiously passive creatures, lacking in individual qualities or demands and only to be properly observed through the eyes of adults. Thus Dubin & Dubin (1963), in a review of work on the socialization of infants, noted that only a small minority of the studies examined reported on direct observation of actual child–parent interaction. Instead, children's behaviour was reconstructed from the responses of parents (usually mothers) to questions put to them by researchers. Here, as elsewhere, it was simply assumed that parents are able to speak for their children. In consequence a sociology of childhood—that is a sociology that treats the experience of childhood and the world of children as a topic in its own right, free from the preconceptions and concerns of adults—hardly exists outside the novel and the autobiography. There has instead been an overriding concern with the problems that particular kinds of children's behaviour—whether it be the toilet habits of infants or the delinquencies of adolescents—create for adults. Only through such pioneering work as that of the Opies (1959, 1969) have we begun to treat the child's world as an object of enquiry in its own right.

4. This proclivity is made possible because by and large the adult world looks on childhood as essentially a preparation for and a prelude to adult life. A principal moral, political and scientific concern is to discover how children acquire the skills and attributes that will transform them into fully competent adults, so that this process may be the more efficiently accomplished.

5. At the same time this does not prevent us from imbuing childhood with its own form of spirituality. Children may be at times irritating, messy and troublesome, but yet they are highly valued. 'Everybody loves a baby', and a childless marriage is, particularly in some sections of society, subject to a peculiar social stigma (see Klein (1965) for a discussion of adult ambivalence towards children). So childhood is sentimentalized and children are seen as inhabiting a special world of innocence, beauty, laughter and play—a happy childhood Eden from which adults have, alas, fallen, but which they may yet re-enter in a child's company—a version of childhood that perhaps reached its apogee in the work of Barrie and Lewis Carroll, but which still exercises its influence. Thus children viewed from this perspective are wonderful creatures at whom we can but marvel—indeed, at whom we have a duty to marvel if called upon to do so by others (Davis & Strong, 1976).

6. Above all, children are a problem. Public and private concern is manifest at all levels. It can be discovered in the perennial anxiety about juvenile delinquency and in the more recent debate over supposedly declining educational standards, as well as in the rise of such child-oriented occupations as paediatrics. Indeed, this present volume itself both reflects and reinforces that all-pervasive concern. And of course it exists, perhaps in its most agonizing form, at the level of the individual parent, as is nicely captured in the following quotation from one of the Newsons' mothers:

> People nowadays think more about what's good for the child from the child's point of view. Everything I do with him I try to do the best for him. I'm thinking about him all the time. I'm careful about his food, and I hold him on my lap after his bottle so he won't have tummy-ache; he's inoculated so he won't catch diseases; later on I take them to the dentist so they won't get toothache: I'm thinking in advance for his comfort all the time.... Nowadays, if they don't turn out right you wonder where you went wrong don't you? (Newson & Newson, 1963.)

Now while the natural impulse on being confronted with a 'problem' is to rush out and try to solve it, recent work, especially in the sociology of deviance, has suggested that an essential prior question is to ask 'for whom is this a problem and why?'. By and large, however, sociological work on children and childhood has not addressed itself to this question. Instead, whether in the areas of the family, socialization, mass media, education or deviance, it has simply taken for granted the problematic nature of children, and has approached the study of childhood essentially from the point of view of an idealized adult society as the abiding reality into which children of necessity must fit (Collins, 1975).

Age-grading

Linton (1942) has argued that all societies recognize seven basic age–sex statuses: infant, boy, girl, adult man, adult woman, old man, and old woman. But this is somewhat misleading, for the meaning of these terms varies significantly by time and place. At one extreme is the highly complex East African age–class system described by Prins (1953), while at the other stands Taleland where the 'social sphere of adult and child is unitary and undivided' (Fortes, 1938), the only differentiation being in terms of relative capacity; nothing in the adult world is hidden from the children who are actively and responsibly part of the social structure, of the economic system, and of the ritual and ideological systems.

Similarly Castle (1961), in discussing education in the classical world, notes the absence of any notion of childhood as constituting a period in itself, with its own character. The Spartans, who were outnumbered 10 to one by the helots, needed all adult male citizens for service in the army: childhood and youth were merely long training grounds for this end. The Athenians, with a very different state and system of education, had no firm views on the socialization of infants because they did not think it mattered. Children were regarded with amused tolerance until they were seven years old; they were allowed plenty of freedom so long as they did not make nuisances of themselves. Childhood was a period of waiting before the serious business of life commenced.

In the above examples, however different in detail, we can see some connection between the notions of childhood and biological age. But even this is not necessary, as Arensburg & Kimball's (1940) study of pre-war rural Ireland showed. Here was a society where 'you can be a boy for ever as long as your old fellow is alive'. It would be a mistake to think that this was even an approximation to a childhood concept. The dividing line was not between children and adults but rather between the 'married' and the 'unmarried', the 'men' and the 'boys'. At this extreme, status is determined by economic considerations; only the eldest son can inherit the farm and he cannot marry until he has inherited. Until then he is a 'boy' and excluded from the adult world.

Thus age-grades are essentially social constructs, based not so much on biological as on social time. The kinds of behaviour and motivation appropriate at different times of life depend more on cultural than on biological factors: 'Age–sex classificatory systems are sufficiently divorced from physiological considerations to make possible almost any amplification of formal categories, and almost any choice of transition points' (Linton, 1942). Not even birth and death can be assigned a universal and unambiguous meaning. (See, for example, Edmund Gosse's account (1976) of a mid-Victorian childhood and the influences thereon of strong religious convictions.)

No category stands alone. Each is part of a series, so that 'the character of an age-grade cannot be understood except in relation to those of other stages' (Eisenstadt, 1956). This does not mean that all categories flow into or prepare one for the next; grades may equally be defined by sharp opposition. Thus Musgrove (1966) distinguishes between those societies which integrate the youth grade with the adult world and those which segregate it. But, whatever the relationship, one can only be understood via the other: 'The boy is seen to bear within himself the seeds of the adult man; or else he must, as an adult, acquire new patterns of behaviour, sharply and intentionally opposed to those of his boyhood' (Eisenstadt, 1956).

The discovery of childhood
If the concept of childhood as we presently understand it is absent from many societies—ancient and modern—we should bear in mind that our own is a peculiarly modern discovery. As Aries (1962) particularly has shown, mediaeval Europe had no real conception of a child's personal individuality, and was little inclined to impute a distinct character to childhood. Few considered children as other than small adults. The unity of the social space of the adult and the child was apparent in all spheres. Until the tenth century, artists were unable to depict children except as small men; individual child portraits did not appear until the fifteenth century. Little distinction was made in terms of dress; what differences there were in fashion were class- rather than age-related, and not until the seventeenth century did clothing distinctively for children first appear. From the age of three or four years, children shared with adults many of the same leisure pursuits and enjoyed similar pleasures: children indulged in gambling while adults engaged in what we would now regard as children's games (e.g. blind man's bluff). Ballads, riddles and fairy stories were intended as much for an adult audience as for children. In matters of sex, little was hidden from

children. Aries quotes from the diary of Henry IV's physician a Rabelaisian account of the upbringing of the infant Louis XIII.

In the field of education, the schools that did exist catered for a wide age range, with few of the worries that the mixing of different ages would cause us today. Even the terms used to delineate different age-grades were extremely vague and fluid; they did not merely cover highly disparate stages of growth but, extending the notion of dependency, were applied also to servants of all ages. The French, for example, had no specific word for 'baby' until they borrowed it from the English in the nineteenth century; previously 'enfant' had been applied indiscriminately to both babies and adolescents.

The 'modern' concept of childhood as a separate and definable category of human existence, to be valued for its own sake, with its own particular pleasures and pace, was crystallized in the nineteenth century, and delineated through a whole series of institutional arrangements that marked off the world of the child from that of the adult—the imposition of compulsory schooling; the emergence of the juvenile court; the exclusion of children from economic activity; and the encroachment of the state into the lives of working-class families, all in the name of welfare (Platt, 1969).

It is customary to attribute this radical change in society's approach to children to changing patterns of economic and social activity consequent upon industrialization. One can distinguish two specific forces at work here.

First, there is the interaction between a declining birth-rate and a declining rate of infant mortality, brought about partly by expanding medical knowledge and technology, but chiefly through improved environmental and nutritional conditions (McKeown, 1965). Fewer children, who yet could be expected with some confidence to survive into adult life, made more resources available for each child and rendered individual children more valuable (Boli-Bennett & Meyer, 1978). This in turn made more rewarding a social and personal investment in specific children. It is difficult for us today to appreciate the matter-of-fact manner in which the mortality of infants was once regarded, but the historian Gibbon provides us with some insight:

> So feeble was my constitution, so precarious my life, that, in the baptism of each of my brothers, my father's prudence successively repeated my Christian name Edward, that, in case of the departure of the eldest son, this patronymic appellation might be still perpetuated in the family. (Quoted by Lorence, 1974.)

Caulfield (1931) estimates that in mid-eighteenth-century London two out of three children failed to survive to the age of five years. Under such circumstances a degree of psychological distancing between parents and their children was not only inevitable but indeed desirable. What is perhaps ironic is that the indifference to children that resulted from the high mortality rates seems to have produced child-rearing practices that reduced still further the chances of survival (Lorence, 1974).

The second change in pattern was the emergence of the home-oriented, bourgeois, nuclear family. Parsons (1963), Musgrove (1966) and Shorter (1976) have argued that the increasing separation of a whole series of functions from the family, the onset of contraception, and the decline in infant mortality have enabled the 'modern' family to specialize in affection. It does this because it need do little else. When there are difficult tasks to perform, intra-family relationships tend to be characterized by formality and restraint; the family becomes organized along authoritarian lines with a clear division of labour and chain of command. The modern, western family can provide friendship and an environment in which the romantic ideology of the child may flourish because there are comparatively few demanding jobs to be done.

Again, this concept of the family is a relatively recent phenomenon. Until the sixteenth century, the sociability and intimacy of social life rendered privacy—an essential ingredient for the development of the concept of family—difficult, and the idea of the family was much more diffuse than at present, not being particularly related to blood-ties. By the eighteenth century this was changing, as the family, more precisely defined along blood-lines, began to hold society at a distance, aided by important changes in the interior design of houses. These developments were completed with the emergence of an industrial economy that destroyed the working family as the unit of production and led to the separation of the work-place from the home. Boys no longer naturally took up their father's trade from an early age. The advent and prolongation of compulsory education removed children from the labour market and from the home, opening up a gap between the experience of parents and children, transforming the teenage years into a time of occupational choice, and creating the possibility of a separate youth culture (Aries, 1962).

It would be a mistake to see changes in the concept of childhood as wholly attributable to economic and demographic forces. As Aries and others have shown, intellectual theorizing about the nature of childhood goes back at least to the sixteenth century and pre-dates many of those changes discussed above. Moreover, once the category was established it became a subject both for investigation and for 'exploitation' in the sense that it was made available as a resource for use in theorizing about life in general. The nature of childhood was therefore rapidly established as a key area for ideological debate. Thus puritans and jansenists alike could preach a doctrine of infant depravity, while political theorists, like Rousseau, saw in children a natural goodness which society merely deformed. Despite the development of a gamut of academic and practising disciplines which probe, protect and control children, the issue is not resolved. Indeed, as we shall argue, it is irresolvable for the debate is itself a product of our separate categorization of childhood. (For a more extensive treatment of these issues the reader is referred to Skolnick's (1974) survey of theories of the child in psychology; to Coveney's (1967) analysis of the image of the child in nineteenth- and twentieth-century classic literature; and to Kessen's (1965) history of child study.)

Despite this centuries-old tradition of speculation and investigation, many researchers still make the fundamental mistake of ignoring the social context in which work is done. It is more than likely that many of the research findings about children's capacities and proclivities are the product, not of some universal childish nature, but of our particular cultural arrangements. For example, schools can perhaps better be understood as the cause of 'adolescence' than as simply a response to the needs of adolescents.

The professions, the State, and the child

At the same time as children were being excluded from the labour force, there occurred a complementary, although much less discussed, phenomenon: the rise of the child-oriented professions. From being workers themselves, children have been increasingly transformed into an object of formal, paid work for others. The servicing of children has, of course, deep historical roots; wet-nursing, for example, provided much-needed employment for many working-class women in the eighteenth century and earlier (Lorence, 1974). However, the nineteenth and twentieth centuries have witnessed a quite extraordinary expansion in occupations wholly or mainly concerned with children: from paediatricians and child psychiatrists to nursery nurses and health visitors; from schoolteachers and educational psychologists to youth leaders and social workers; and academics—sociologists such as ourselves, psychologists, and historians—who, though fewer in number, still make a living from children and their problems. (See Strong (1979) for a discussion of some of these issues particularly as they relate to medicine.)

All of these occupations have a vested interest in producing some distinct angle on childhood, in developing some unique skill or analysis, in finding some special problem which they alone can solve. Sometimes, they form a united front, for they share a common interest in the general formulation of childhood as an area of concern. At other times they engage in internecine struggle, seeking to expand their own small patches and diminish those of others. All this, of course, is done in the name of the child—and quite genuinely so. We do not mean to imply by any of this that the child-oriented professions are cynically motivated. Indeed, important advances may stem from professional interest. It has been argued, for example, that the current work on child abuse derives from the professional concern of radiologists (Pfohl, 1977). Nor is such a process unique to childhood, for it can be found in every aspect of our society. Nevertheless, whatever other purposes it may serve, it still works to reinforce and extend our conception of childhood as a separate and problematic estate. (See Platt (1969) for a discussion of these issues in relation to the rise of social work in the late nineteenth century.)

The professions are not the only sector of the economy with a vested interest in children; the commercial 'exploitation' of childhood is extensive and well developed, covering a range of important industries, among which food, toys, clothing, records, and publishing are perhaps the most prominent. As with the professions, it would be naive to see these industries as merely responding to an existing demand, ignoring all the while the many subtle ways they create and shape the market that they purportedly serve. The sale of proprietary baby foods to the Third World well illustrates this process, and the controversy to which it has given rise has brought into sharp focus many of the issues involved.

Whatever may be the particular and well-founded concerns of dietitians, dentists, and educationalists with some aspects of the commercial exploitation of the children's market, there can be no doubt that it has rendered the task of parenting much easier and pleasanter in many respects. For example, nappies can be more readily washed or thrown away, the range of 'bribes' we are now in a position to offer our children has been greatly extended, and television, games, books and comics provide not simply a distraction but a source of interest and education as well. At the same time, however, adults are caught in a series of classic consumer traps of which 'keeping up with the Joneses' is the most obvious. This takes the form of competitive parenting—who can provide the biggest and most expensive toys, the cleanest child on the street, the best-read boy in the class, the most well-balanced children in the neighbourhood? Different groups compete in different ways, but all call on the resources of industry to help them, and are, in turn, reinforced in their activities by those same industries. Thus bringing up children—in spite of all our new aids—now involves more work, a greater commitment, and a more professional orientation than ever before.

Children too are now trained as consumers from a very early age and they regularly watch themselves starring in the consumerist mini-dramas of television advertising. As with their parents, however, the effects of their consumption are far from straightforward. The development of a specifically child-oriented market was greatly stimulated by the advent of mass schooling which, by placing children together and yet apart from their parents, gave rise to a distinctive youth culture. With a growing economic surplus, the members of this newly strengthened culture found themselves with independent financial means and were therefore able, with the glad assistance of industry, to elaborate that life-style in ways that matched their own rather than adult interests. Thus capitalism has played a major role in strengthening the independence of the childhood estate, a process particularly marked in recent years.

Within this world one may note exactly the same process of competitive consumption as exists in the adult world, though here it takes on a slightly more febrile form; the 'crazes' of children, though the counterpart of adult 'fashions', seem even more encompassing in their sway and to have an even swifter rise and decline. The explanation for this lies, one imagines, in the 'hot-house' atmosphere of wholly separate age-graded institutions in which peer-group dynamics can operate at maximum intensity. But this is speculation, for we still await the application of Veblen's (1970) *Theory of the Leisure Class* to the world of children.

The creation and development of a concept of childhood have had major repercussions for the role of women in society. It is conventional in most feminist writings to see women as relegated to a form of domestic servitude by their child-rearing responsibilities. While there is much truth in this argument, the position is surely somewhat more complex. In their search for an identity outside the home, women have been able to extend their housewifely roles into public service and use their putative competence in child-rearing to secure a foothold in the professional world. Many of the nineteenth-century pioneers of education and social work were women and, as both these professions expanded, it was women who came forward to fill the posts available (Platt, 1969). That professional women are largely, and unfairly, restricted to such jobs is undeniable. It is equally true, however, that their creation offered opportunities not previously available to women and which women have not been slow to exploit. Even the rise of popular medical and child-care manuals for the home—that professional co-option of women so deplored by feminists—can be seen as an attempt to upgrade traditional women's work and render it less demeaning in a newly professional and scientific age.

Finally some mention must be made of the State in all of this, for the role it has played in the further development of our conception of childhood has been a crucial one. Children are no longer the sole property of their parents; they are now, at least in part, wards of the State. So much has their value increased that not only do their parents tend for them in distinctively new ways but the State also intervenes in, and watches over, their lives from the moment of their conception. Antenatal clinics, health visitors, social workers, schools, juvenile courts, truancy officers, and all the other assorted agents of the State regulate the life of the child and, on occasion, the lives of the parents too.

Contemporary studies in the making of childhood

So far in this chapter we have drawn on historical and comparative material to argue for the social and cultural relativity of the concept of childhood, and in doing so to hold up for consideration some of our taken-for-granted assumptions about children. In what remains of this chapter, we examine in a little more detail, using data from our own researches, the image of childhood that adults hold to and how that image is drawn upon, recreated, and further developed in our daily encounters with children.

We noted earlier that adults are essentially ambivalent towards children; on the one hand children are highly valued possessions, yet on the other they are a problem, a nuisance, trouble. In one sense these assessments of children are merely a popular expression of a long western tradition of theorizing about the properties of 'natural man' (Macintyre, 1967). In this, children join primitive tribes, gypsies, peasants, the working class, all of whom have been seen at various times and by various authors either as embodiments of all that was primitive and savage or, alternatively, as a repository of all that was virtuous and most natural.

This dualistic view of children's essential nature, which is what concerns us here, may be seen as a direct product of the creation of a separate childhood estate. For once childhood is firmly established as apart from adult life, it becomes possible to contrast it with adulthood and to judge it according to one's opinion of adult life. Moreover, although adults often talk about children as if their qualities were quite distinct from those of adult life—separate states inherent within childhood—these properties are in fact a direct product of the adulthood relationship and derive from that juxtaposition of adult knowledge and childish ignorance.

We proceed to explore these alternative characterizations of children in two rather contrasting settings—the paediatric clinic and the juvenile court—in which the different sides of children's nature are given different emphasis, reflecting in part the different tasks involved. Our principal thesis is that the characterizations that we make of children are shaped, firstly, by the high valuation we now place on them, and, secondly, by the imbalance of competence and power that exists in the adult–child relationship. That is, children are both less competent and held subordinate and excluded from much of the adult world. Our studies were restricted to particular—and in some respects, artificial—locales, so that our remarks should be treated as suggestions only.

The paediatric clinic—children as wonderful
Our first example comes from observational research carried out in paediatric clinics in Britain and the United States (Strong, 1980). While the ambivalence in which children are held was not absent from clinic encounters, the side of their nature which received the greatest attention was their rewarding, wonderful qualities. To the adults, children were objects of great amusement as well as admiration (Davis & Strong, 1976).

Clinic and therapy sessions were often punctuated by adult fun. Doctors, parents, nurses, students and researchers chuckled, giggled, and were occasionally overcome by mirth. There was a broad consensus that children were funny, that certain things in particular were very funny, and that it was perfectly reasonable to laugh at them, at least where younger children were concerned.

By the age of six or seven, a few children made jokes which were jokes in adult terms; in other words, one laughed at the joke. However with young children amusement centred around the child himself; one laughed at the child, and such laughter derived from the key features of the adult-child relationship; that is, around the child's ignorance of, and subordination to, adult life.

Fun could result when children behaved in a completely incompetent way as, for example, when young babies belched. On the other hand, given the general assumption of ignorance, an unexpected competence was also found amusing. Everyone laughed when a one-year-old child during a developmental examination refused to pick up a mug as instructed, having previously tested it with his finger and found there was nothing inside it.

Similarly, adults could find both children's subordination and their insubordination to have amusing aspects. On the one hand, the exercise of adult power seemed on occasion to be funny in itself. The sudden pacification of an angry young child with a sweet, or the prospect and immediate result of immunizing a baby were often occasions for joking and laughter. Fooling and teasing children could be most amusing but, just as their failure to be fooled could also evoke mirth, so too could their rebellion, as long as it was of short duration. A few older children were sometimes deliberately rude to adults, particularly to medical staff, and within limits this too could be found hilarious. More serious revolt was a different matter, and adults were ruthless in quashing this. Children who disrupted consultations seriously might be taken from the room by a nurse, and some rebellions were subdued by physical force. In all this, adults' attitude towards children bore some resemblance to that commonly displayed towards pet cats and dogs, for here too the themes of ignorance and competence, subordination and rebellion may elicit considerable amusement and occasional demonstration of power.

Though children were amusing, their most positive feature was their marvellousness. Every adult present could be called upon to marvel at a young child, and on such occasions adults would turn with smiles upon their faces and call forth similar smiles in others. Simply to have a child was deemed a wonderful thing for which mothers were to be congratulated. No one was heard to say that adults were marvellous, but all children were wonderful, even the most grossly handicapped.

This too follows from the assumption of incompetence, for, although children were ignorant of the adult world, knowledge of it was not felt to be an unmixed blessing: adults were not complacent about their own qualities. Thus, whereas adults were sometimes prickly and status-conscious, children were held to be far more open, far more ready to give and to receive affection and interest. The ignorance of social conventions that was revealed in their words and deeds could also be seen as bluntness and honesty. Their inability to manage an appropriate level of involvement could be portrayed as spontaneity. Their lack of future and past meant that only the present need be attended to in order to make them happy. Children's innocence meant that, for instance, female therapists did not have to worry about the sexual aspects of their relationship with male patients.

Although children were ignorant of the world, since they acted within it their actions could also be read as mocking that world. Subordinate adults were particularly pleased by certain childish acts. For a baby to urinate on the doctor was most amusing, if a little embarrassing for parents. Therapists enjoyed young children's inability to differentiate staff according to the medical hierarchy. Children, it was held by some, were a living reproof to the artificial conventions of the adult world; they simply took you for what you were. Children were also held to throw light on the adult world in quite another way. Since they were ignorant, the way in which they acquired knowledge revealed features about the world that adults simply took for granted. For example, their eternal questioning—asking 'why?' and 'what?'—displayed the fragility of all kinds of adult assumptions.

Since they owned their children, parents took a pride in their accomplishments even when these created problems for them. Throwing things out of a pram might be a nuisance but it could also be an occasion for pleasure at their clever child. Just as their subordination could be amusing, so too could it be wonderful. Dependency can be pleasing in itself. Further, since children knew no other world besides the one produced for them, they offered the opportunity to create a human being. One of the attractions of continuing therapy was the opportunity to mould the child in one's own way. Children were marvellous not just because they were apart from the adult world, but also because they themselves were potential adults. Here as elsewhere, however, there was ambiguity. They were wonderful both because you could train them up in the way that you wanted them to grow, and because in growing up they became themselves.

The juvenile court—children as a problem
The reality of how children grow up is not always so wonderful. For our second example of the making of childhood we turn to a study (May, 1978) of juvenile justice, as exemplified by the Children's Hearing system developed in Scotland.

Along with the schoolroom, the juvenile court stands as one of the major nineteenth-century instruments with which the modern concept of childhood was fashioned and enforced, its influence extending far beyond those children who are its direct concern. Its significance for us here lies not simply in its boundary-maintaining functions (Erikson, 1962)—that is, in its quite explicit concern with the limits to acceptable children's behaviour—but equally in its methodology. The juvenile court is a microcosm of a larger inter-generation struggle, and through its inspection we can learn something of the more fundamental aspects of that struggle. In its professed commitment to treatment and rehabilitation rather than punishment, the court is essentially future-oriented, concerned not so much with 'what has this child done?', as with 'what kind of child do we have here?'. In short, it is engaged in a search for 'moral character' and, by extension, in the construction of 'normal' childhood (Emerson, 1969).

The concern with 'moral character' springs in the first instance from a non-absolutist position on children's misbehaviour, and a general conviction that all children, whether unwittingly because that is their nature or from an absence of adult controls, stand permanently at risk of offending against adult norms and values, a belief nicely expressed in the following, slightly desperate plea from one member of a Children's Hearing to the young offender facing her: '*Try* and be good, nobody expects you to be good *all* the time. *No* children are good *all* the time.'

There is in fact a considerable degree of tolerance among adults for much juvenile misbehaviour, a willingness to recognize that children can at times become involved in quite unacceptable behaviour without deserving total denunciation or the epithet 'delinquent'. Except for cases of really serious offences (and not always then), the behaviour itself affords an unreliable and frequently misleading guide to diagnosis and prognosis.

The corollary to this quite laudable tolerance is, firstly, the transfer of attention from objective behavioural indices to the more elusive, not to say slippery concept of 'moral character'; and, secondly and perhaps rather perversely, the investment of apparently trivial behaviour with a significance far beyond its immediate potential for harm. One of the more striking features revealed by our research was the reluctance of those Children's Panel members interviewed to discount any misdemeanour, no matter how trivial in character or innocuous its consequences, as constituting inadequate grounds for intervention. In this they are sustained by one of the central assumptions of modern juvenile justice practice: 'What may outwardly appear to be minor offences may on occasion prove to be in fact the symptoms of more serious underlying emotional disturbance' (Kilbrandon, 1964).

It is no part of our argument that this belief is necessarily wrong or misplaced, although we do contend that it carries with it unanticipated consequences that have yet to be fully considered (May, 1971). Our concern here is for the situation of childhood. While it may be the case that the great mass of youthful misdemeanour excites little concern and is rarely in practice subject to more than mild rebuke, the child cannot know this for certain and in advance. His situation is therefore one of uncertainty and unpredictability, for he stands permanently at risk of inviting adult intervention and control—sometimes in most puzzling and perverse circumstances.

Adult concern with children's behaviour is, in the final analysis, subordinate to a more fundamental consideration—the eventual adoption by children of adult values and an adult world view. In her review of child-rearing practices,

Klein (1965) suggests that parental discipline, even in early infancy, is directed as much at 'the development of an approved adult character' as at the control or elimination of undesirable behaviour.

This commitment to the adult world of responsibilities is finally sealed with the acquisition of job and family, for in the absence of both lies the essence of childhood. The authorities' preoccupation with job and family is perfectly understandable, given that these provide youth with an escape route from the streets and from a life of delinquency (Werthman, 1967). Certainly their significance is not lost on gang-boys themselves, who reserve their especial anger and contempt for those of their fellows who announce their desertion to the 'enemy' by 'going steady' (Patrick, 1973). To acquire the attributes of adulthood, however reluctantly, is to promise a transformation of 'moral character'.

L.... was a teenage girl placed under supervision by a Children's Hearing for theft. Her conduct during that period of supervision was so deplorable that a subsequent Hearing recommended that she be sent to a List D (approved) school. That recommendation was about to be put into effect when L.... announced that she was pregnant, a piece of news which prompted the following declaration from the chairman: 'If she is pregnant, *and the boy is prepared to marry her*, then we might decide not to have her sent away. We want to make it quite plain that *we don't intend doing anything that would prevent her from marrying and settling down*. I'm sure that I speak for my colleagues when I say that we would be quite happy with this.' (Our emphasis.)

On the other hand, to flout or otherwise show indifference towards the *declared* values of the adult world—sobriety, respectability, reliability, deferred gratification, and a commitment to hard work—is to risk the 'moral indignation' of the guardians of those values. Young (1971) has argued in relation to drug-taking that the wrath of conventional (adult) society is aroused, not so much by the actual harmful consequences of the activity, but rather because the stereotypical offender is seen as someone who 'lives without work, pursues leisure without deferring gratification, enters sexual relationships without undergoing the obligations of marriage, and dresses freely in a world where uniformity in clothing is seen as a mark of respectability and reliability'.

Something of this attitude was manifest in the case of J...., another teenage girl placed under supervision for theft. Following a series of briefly held, low status and frankly exploitative jobs, J.... had 'retired' from the unpleasant world of work, apparently intent on 'living off Social Security'. Her stubborn refusal to consider seriously looking for new employment led to the following angry outburst from one Panel member: 'You see J.... we can't just leave jobs because we don't like them. Sometimes, especially at your age, we have to make sacrifices if we are to settle down. But no, you prefer not to work. You just want to sit down on your backside all day long, doing nothing. *This is what worries me. I just don't like it.*' (Our emphasis.)

What was particularly significant about this case was that J.... from her social security payments continued to make the same contribution to the family budget as her elder sister who was in work.

In pressing for a commitment to the world of adults a profound irony is involved for, as we have been at pains to emphasize, a central feature of childhood is precisely its exclusion from that world. Given this, how then is a commitment to the adult order inferred?

In the first instance it may be established by means of a simple declaration of intent. The child may in fact be excluded from the world of work but that in itself does not preclude the possibility of affecting a proper orientation to that world. This involves not merely a readiness to enter the adult world in due course (although that too is important as the case of J.... above shows), but an ability to demonstrate that one takes that world seriously, that one accepts the centrality of work to adult life, that one seeks not simply a job but, more importantly, a career. In short it demands that one professes ambition.

> 1st Panel member: 'What do you intend to do when you leave school?'
> 13-year-old child: 'I want to be a nurse.'
> 1st Panel member: 'Well, that's a good thing.'
> 2nd Panel member: 'Yes, a very good thing.'

A commitment to the world of work can be demonstrated at one remove, as it were, in the child's leisure activities. An invariable line of enquiry at Children's Hearings was the child's use of spare time. To what organizations did he belong? What interests did he have? What hobbies did he pursue? The emphasis at all times was on the constructive, purposeful use of time. For many Panel members this offered an infallible test of 'moral character', as is evidenced from the bewilderment shown by one Panel member when faced with an obvious incongruity.

> Here we have K...., the notable citizen, member of the Boys' Brigade, a keen footballer ..., a prospect for the Royal Air Force. On the other hand we have K...., the boy who has already committed three separate offences. Something obviously has gone wrong. Can anyone offer an explanation for this contradiction?

His own solution to the dilemma was in effect to deny one set of facts.

> I saw a split personality here. To me anybody who has been years in the Boys' Brigade, or is so interested in sport that he gets selected to go on a European tour, just isn't the same person as goes out and commits crime. I just don't see this.

What is really at issue in all juvenile court encounters is the legitimacy of adult authority. A commitment to adult values is most immediately and obviously revealed by the willingness of children to recognize adult authority over them. By the same token to reject that authority, even on minor issues, is to threaten the order of things and invites an instant display of adult power.

> B...., a vivacious young teenager who was being dealt with by a Children's Hearing for persistent non-attendance at school and who objected to attempts to set some limits to her weekend activities, was left under no doubt as to the consequences of her continued obduracy: 'We will do our best to help in any way possible, but I should say that if B.... consistently refuses to accept our help and advice then I'm afraid that eventually she will leave us with no option: we will have to send her away.'

The subordination of children to adult authority is at once so universal and so total, a general rule that covers all aspects of life and admits of few exceptions (the position of child kings, especially in the Middle Ages, is interesting but their authority was largely symbolic, real power residing with a regency), that it is regarded as part of the 'natural' order of social life. Even children themselves seldom question, let alone openly challenge, adult authority. Deference is so taken for granted by all concerned that when it is not forthcoming it tends to be seen, especially by the officially designated representatives of adult authority, as evidence of defective 'moral character' (Piliavin & Briar, 1964). Indeed Werthman (1967) goes so far as to suggest that those children, who in their attitudes and activities cease to accord adults general authority over them, should perhaps no longer be thought of as children.

> One could argue that the pre-adolescent who does not conceive of himself as dependent on his parents also does not really conceive of himself as 'a child', particularly when he loses his virginity at 8, and supports himself on lunch money taken from classmates.... Politically the child is not an adult, but sociologically it is hard to argue that he is still a child.

Conclusion

In this chapter we have sought to draw attention to the social meanings of childhood. As sociologists we reject a concept of childhood that holds it to be no more than (or even largely) a biological category. Of course, we do not deny the peculiar natural properties of children. All cultures recognize—indeed have to recognize—that children *are* different from adults in particular biophysical ways. Human children, like the young of all primates, are born relatively helpless and require a period of dependency, extending (for humans) at least into the seventh or eighth year, although thereafter its duration is more problematic (Skolnick, 1974; Gough, 1971). These truths constrained mediaeval practice towards children just as much as they do ours today. But acceptance of the special character of children does not alter our basic contention: that the concept of childhood—that is, the boundaries which at any time and place enclose it, the properties with which it is endowed, and, by extension, the experiences to which it gives rise—is essentially a social construction, a product of particular social, economic, cultural, and ideological forces—certainly in part shaped by biological constraints but not reducible to a biological formula.

To emphasize the social character of childhood is fascinating no doubt but scarcely of more than academic interest to those who must daily deal with children and their problems. We believe, however, that our argument has wider implications than that. What we demand from children and for children; what we consider to be their needs as well as their responsibilities; in short, those practical policies we develop to deal with children, either individually or in the mass, derive in the first instance from our taken-for-granted notions concerning the nature of children and childhood. Analysis of the work of the Victorian 'child-savers' (Platt, 1969; May, 1973) has convincingly shown how the reforms that were then proposed, and the institutions that were developed (chiefly the juvenile court, the industrial school, and the reformatory), reflected an idealized and highly sentimental middle-class version of childhood that was not, despite scientific pretensions, greatly informed by or dependent on any objective assessment of the physical or social possibilities of those children at whom the reforms were aimed. In seeking to rescue working-class children from the brutalizing anarchy that for the most part characterized their lives, the 'child-savers' advanced a version of childhood that in its own way was equally repressive and, whatever else it achieved, further increased the dependent status of children. Work on modern juvenile justice systems (Matza, 1964; Emerson, 1969; May, 1971) suggests that, despite a fund of good will and noble intentions, the problems of repression and class bias remain.

We do not wish to be misunderstood here; we are not impugning motive. We would not deny that public and private concern for children proceeds in good measure from a wholly laudable desire to improve the quality of their lives and to preserve them from the errors and miseries of earlier generations. These concerns inform the activities of those public agencies who have a statutory responsibility for children's welfare, just as much as they do our own dealings with our own children. But the concern is double-edged, for it leads also to intervention, regulation, and, in some degree, to confrontation. We showed above (in the case of the girl B....) how an expressed concern for behaviour is quickly transformed into an issue of authority.

In saying that cultures elaborate particular concepts of childhood and that these have no necessary relationship to physiology, we are *not* claiming that our culture has got it all wrong or that drastic reform is needed to bring our institutions into line with the 'true nature' of children. Children's nature, like that of adults, is as yet unclear, while the sorts of institutions that are appropriate in one kind of society may not work so well in another. These are matters for further investigation. Nor are we arguing, as some might do, that our culture has wrongly confined and controlled children, and that they are 'freer' elsewhere. Our point is rather that the particular type of control we exert has particular consequences. Other types of control such as integrating children at an early age into the adult work force—and we may see the beginnings of such a trend already in Sweden and Cuba—would have different consequences. Whether one is any better than the other is a matter of judgement. Exclusion, as Musgrove (1966) has shown, has potentially radical consequences and this may on some counts be a good thing. Incorporation, on the other hand, while it may solve many of the problems of juvenile delinquency, may also stifle other aspects of youthful peer-group innovation—whether cultural or political.

We have been at pains to show that, even within our own Western European culture, the meaning of childhood and attitudes towards children have altered radically over the centuries.

> The child's future at birth has changed from one of almost certain death to one of almost unlimited possibility. In the eyes of parents, the growth and development of the child has shifted from being the object of mild concern or indifference to the major emotional focus of the family. (Skolnick, 1974.)

Given what has happened in the past there is no reason, save for an indefensible 'chronocentrism', to believe that the present concept of childhood and the limits we impose on it are immutable. Already one can discern signs of change. Within childhood, as conventionally defined, age-grades are losing some of their force and distinctive character. The 'teenage' culture, itself a very recent phenomenon, has expanded to embrace younger and younger children, as any casual survey of the 'pop scene' will confirm. Current fashions, as Skolnick notes, are not only unisex, they are increasingly uniage, and 'where fairy tales once were shared by all age-groups, now television is'.

More significantly, perhaps, those institutional arrangements that once sharply defined the world of the child and which in a sense 'invented' childhood, are becoming looser. In particular, the schoolroom no longer occupies an exclusive position as the source of the child's knowledge about the world beyond his own immediate locality. Whatever its many other faults, television now provides a range of knowledge and experience unavailable to the child of just a generation ago. Under these and other pressures, education is being transformed from a once and for all preparation for (adult) life into an ongoing accompaniment to life. The expansion of higher education and its consequent availability to a far wider public offers the possibility to some of extending the years of childhood (in the sense of postponing the taking-up of adult tasks and responsibilities) almost into middle-age. In the opposite direction, work-experience courses, which are becoming an increasing feature of secondary education, promise to break down the once rigid barriers between the world of the school (the child's world) and the world of work (the adult world) and it is likely that the modern phenomenon of widespread youth unemployment will give further impetus to all these changes.

On another more general level, although we may yet be too close to appreciate fully their significance, we should not discount as forces for change the 'counter-culture' of the late 1960s that was associated with the 'hippies' and sundry other groups, or the present-day feminist movement. Both may yet exercise a profound and long-lasting impact on the role of women, the structure of the family, attitudes towards work and leisure and, by extension, the world of the child and practices of child-rearing.

REFERENCES

Arensburg C M, Kimball S T 1940 Family and community in Ireland. Peter Smith, London
Aries P 1962 Centuries of childhood. Jonathan Cape, London
Armstrong D 1979 Child development and medical ontology. Social Science and Medicine 13a: 9–12
Boli-Bennett J, Meyer J W 1978 The ideology of childhood and the State: rules distinguishing children in national constitutions 1870–1970. American Sociological Review 43: 797–812
Castle E B 1961 Ancient education and today. Penguin, Harmondsworth
Caulfield E 1931 The infant welfare movement in the 18th century. Paul Hoeber, New York
Collins R 1975 Conflict sociology: towards an explanatory science. Academic Press, New York
Coveney P 1967 The image of childhood. Penguin, Harmondsworth
Davis A G, Strong P M 1976 Aren't Children Wonderful?: a study of the allocation of identity in development assessment. In: Stacey, M (ed) The sociology of the National Health Service. Sociological Review Monograph No. 22, p 156–175
Dubin E R, Dubin R 1963 The authority inception period in socialization. Child Development 34: 885–898
Eisenstadt S N 1956 From generation to generation. Glencoe Free Press, New York
Emerson R M 1969 Judging delinquents: context and process in juvenile court. Aldine, Chicago
Erikson K T 1962 Notes on the sociology of deviance. Social Problems 9: 307–314
Fortes M 1938 Social and psychological aspects of education in Taleland. University Press, Oxford
Gosse E 1976 Father and son. Penguin, Harmondsworth
Gough K 1971 The origin of the family. Journal of Marriage and the Family 33: 760–771
Kessen W 1965 The child. Wiley, New York
Kilbrandon, Lord (chairman) 1964 Report of the Committee on Children and Young Persons, Scotland. Cmnd 2306. HMSO, Edinburgh
Klein J 1965 Samples from English cultures. Routledge & Kegan Paul, London

Linton R 1942 Age and sex categories. American Sociological Review 7: 589–603
Lorence B 1974 Parents and children in 18th century Europe. History of Childhood Quarterly 2(i): 1–30
Macintyre A 1967 A short history of ethics. Routledge & Kegan Paul, London
McKeown T 1965 Medicine in modern society. Allen & Unwin, London
Matza D 1964 Delinquency and drift. John Wiley, New York
May D 1971 Delinquency control and the treatment model: some implications of recent legislation. British Journal of Criminology 11: 359–370
May D 1978 The children's hearing system. Part 1. The limits to legislative action. The Journal of Social Welfare Law 1: 14–23
May M 1973 Innocence and experience: the evolution of the concept of juvenile delinquency in the mid-19th century. Victorian Studies 17: 7–29
Musgrove F 1966 Youth and the social order. Routledge & Kegan Paul, London
Newson J, Newson E 1963 Infant care in an urban community. Allen & Unwin, London
Opie I, Opie P 1959 The lore and language of schoolchildren. University Press, Oxford
Opie I, Opie P 1969 Children's games in street and playground. University Press, Oxford
Parsons T 1963 Youth in the context of American society. In: Erikson E (ed) Basic Books, New York
Patrick J 1973 A Glasgow gang observed. Eyre Methuen, London
Pfohl S 1977 The discovery of child abuse. Social Problems 24: 310–323
Piliavin I, Briar S 1964 Police encounters with juveniles. American Journal of Sociology 70: 206–214
Platt A 1969 The child-savers: the invention of delinquency. University Press, Chicago
Prins A H J 1953 East African age–class systems: an inquiry into the social order of the Galla, Kipsigis and Kikuyu. Wolters, The Hague
Shorter E 1976 The making of the modern family. Collins, London
Skolnick A 1974 The limits of childhood: conceptions of child development and social context. Law and Contemporary Problems 39: 38–77
Strong P M 1979 Sociological imperialism and the profession of medicine: a critical examination of the thesis of medical imperialism. Social Science and Medicine 13A: 199–215
Strong P M 1980 The ceremonial order of the clinic. Routledge & Kegan Paul, London
Veblen T 1970 The theory of the leisure class. Allen & Unwin, London
Werthman C 1967 The function of social definitions in the development of delinquent careers. President's Commission on Law Enforcement and the Administration of Justice. Task force report on juvenile delinquency and youth crime, p. 155–170. Department of Justice, Washington DC
Young J 1971 The role of the police as amplifiers of deviancy, negotiators of reality and translators of fantasy: some consequences of our present system of drug control as seen in Notting Hill. In: Cohen S (ed) Images of deviance. Penguin, Harmondsworth

2

Ross G. Mitchell

The social and physical environment

Introduction
The epidemiological background to health and the close relationship between illness and the environment are well recognized. However, earlier optimism that improvement in physical surroundings alone would solve environmental problems of child health has not been justified and there is growing appreciation of the role of social influences. This is not to say that high standards in public health are unimportant, but rather that physical improvements must be accompanied by changes in behaviour. As our concept of the genesis of ill health thus widens, the impact of the environment is increasingly seen as the combined effect of many cultural, social and physical factors. The task of unravelling the complicated meshwork of causation is a difficult one, for although the epidemiological method establishes connections, it does not by itself establish cause (Freidson, 1963). Clearly it is desirable to distinguish local effects from large-scale influences: the former relate particularly to the neighbourhood and family, while the latter cover whole classes or groups in a society. Children are greatly influenced by behaviour and relationships in the immediate surroundings of their home, their street and the community in which they live. Nevertheless, these local pressures cannot be isolated from wider forces and in particular changes in society. The important issue is the way these different influences affect the socialization of children as well as their growth and development.

Socialization
Socialization within the family remains a crucial determinant of child development (Eisenberg, 1979). Its consequences for childhood and later for adolescence are long-term, affecting growth to mature adult life and in due course the adult's capacity for engaging in the socialization of his or her own children. In this process the family plays a major role and so the relationship between environment and family is as important as that between environment and child.

The first indications of distorted socialization may occur quite early during childhood, arising from the combined impact of many adverse factors, biological as well as emotional and social. So far as the last are concerned, there are very wide variations in effect between different kinds of environment. Thus, for example, Spinley's (1953) study of children growing up in a London slum as compared with their counterparts at a well-known girls' public school provides an interesting contrast. Among people living in the slums, there is frequency of early marriage, absence of stigma over illegitimacy, ignorance of family planning and lack of care over feeding and toilet-training. Children move suddenly from the warmth of the home to the life of the street, where their care is largely the responsibility of older sisters, and the new baby becomes the centre of the mother's attention. The street group becomes a major influence in their socialization. At school the expectations of middle-class teachers provide a contrast to their own working-class homes. The standards set about ill manners, aggression and fighting are different from those of the street. Figures in authority are to be rebelled against rather than respected and public property is regarded as a legitimate objective of pilfering.

Other studies of deprived areas (Paneth, 1944; Kerr, 1958) also show the interrelationship between the physical environment, patterns of social behaviour and the problems of children and adolescents growing up in them. Paneth's work in a 'residual' and 'transitional' area of North London emphasizes the high rate of sickness and social pathology within its boundaries, a fact supported by more statistical studies such as that of Edinburgh by Philip & McCulloch (1966). Children live in the dangerous world of the streets, largely bereft of adult protection and with the rough companionship of their own age group. The environment is hostile and life unpredictable. Though close to their mothers as babies they are abruptly ignored as another baby arrives. The consequences of this change in child rearing for subsequent development of personality have been interestingly discussed by Robb (1954) in a study of anti-semitism.

It seems reasonable to suggest that the seeds of the aggressive behaviour shown by some adolescents and young men, for example at football matches, should be sought for in earlier failures in socialization. Their environment is frequently stigmatized by society but this stigma and the derogatory labels attached to many of the areas in which they live derive only in part from the facts. They are also rooted in the exaggerated stereotypes created by the mass media. As Cohen (1971) argues in his comment on the study by Armstrong and Wilson of the Easterhouse estate in Glasgow 'behaviour and reaction emerge as complementary processes. The image becomes the reality.' A vicious circle operates in which public attitudes themselves provoke a response from the adolescents who are stigmatized. The practical consequences of this process are well illustrated by the experience of youths seeking work with an employer or the employment services. They quickly recognize the need to disguise their home address if they are to stand a reasonable chance of getting employment.

The effects of environmental and social deprivation must also be seen in a much longer perspective than that of childhood and adolescence. These children themselves will become parents and the earlier experiences of their families during childhood are likely to be recreated later on for their own children.

Social class differences

Inevitably these variations in physical environment and social behaviour raise the very complex question of social class (see p. 143).

The Newsons (1963) discuss the influence of social class on the rearing of infants, at the same time drawing attention also to environmental factors, such as the equipment available in the home, and to the impact of the father's work, such as shift work or long absences from home. The study group on *The Origin of Human Social Relations* (Schaffer, 1971) supports similar conclusions about class differences in child rearing during infancy. The particular relevance of stimulation through talk, reward and encouragement is brought out in considering the mothers' treatment of girls as compared with boys. Douglas (1968) in his national survey points out that, in spite of the improvements in secondary education, middle-class children at secondary schools retain the advantage which they have earlier gained over the children of manual workers. The differences are comparable with those between the social classes in infant mortality, which have persisted despite the general decline in rates during this century.

The low attainment at age eight years of social class V children, or of children from large families where there are several brothers or sisters near to them in age, or of those with many symptoms of disturbed behaviour, has changed very little by the age of 15, compared with the higher achievement of elder boys in two-child families and of both boys and girls with median birth intervals of two to four years.

Concentration of social disadvantage

Many studies have drawn attention to the concentration of disadvantaged families within areas of deprivation. Some have made use of social indicators, especially those available from the Census such as housing, employment, education, assets, financial resources, housing tenure and residential mobility. In addition to these indicators, certain demographic variables such as the number of children under 14 have also been included. One such paper (Department of the Environment, 1975) shows that Scotland as a whole and Strathclyde in particular have very much more than their 'fair' share of deprivation in Britain on virtually all indices. For example on severe overcrowding, 24.7 per cent of Scotland's census enumeration districts and 43.9 per cent of Strathclyde's are in the worst 5 per cent of districts in Britain. Only London's inner districts and the West Midlands can bear comparison with this overcrowding in Strathclyde, which is repeated for nearly all of the housing indicators. However the most outstanding point about this study is the co-existence of several different indicators of deprivation in the same district, for example overcrowding, a severe lack of basic housing amenities and a high rate of male unemployment.

Moving away from area research, both cultural and statistical, to longitudinal studies of individuals and families, the same contrasts emerge. In the National Child Development Study (Wedge & Prosser, 1973), information on some 10 000 children born in March 1958 was collected in 1969 when they had reached the age of 11. One particular analysis of this mass of data was concerned with the facts about 'social disadvantage' in these children and the inequalities not only of health, but also of family circumstances, of educational progress and of housing, income and family size and composition. Social indicators similar to those employed in the DOE study were used, and the label of 'socially disadvantaged' was applied to children from families characterized by the three factors of adverse family composition (i.e. large numbers of children or one parent), low income and poor housing.

The number of children categorized in this way amounted to 6 per cent or one child in every 16. Once again, there is substantial variation between regions—one child in 16 for Britain but only one child in 47 in southern England, compared with one in 12 in northern England and Wales. The most disturbing evidence relates to Scotland where one in every 10 children was found to be socially disadvantaged. Although only 11 per cent of the 11-year-old British children lived in Scotland at the time, as many as 19 per cent of them were found in the disadvantaged group. This study shows again the interrelationship between physical development and ill health, the use of child health services, absence from school, accidents, impairment of speech, sight and hearing, performance at school and parental interest.

Changing needs of the family
A home environment suitable for a family at one stage may be quite unsuitable at another. When the home is first established by the married couple, it is thought of primarily as meeting the needs of the husband and wife rather than as a place where there will be children (Chapman, 1955). Later when children are born there is a marked difference between the arrangements made for them in the first year of life and those made in later years. Whereas the baby has special equipment such as a cot, bath, carriage and playpen, children who have grown out of these must use adult furniture and only in rare cases have a special desk for homework.

In a study of children's homework in a selected group of Merseyside secondary schools, Chapman (1955) showed the close relationship between domestic heating and the location of the child's work. The majority of children in winter faced the choice of either working in the family living-room or working alone in an unheated room and it was the temperature which determined the number of children working alone. There was a noticeable difference between the summer and winter samples: the better the conditions the better able the children were to concentrate on their work. It is evident from these and other studies that there is a striking contrast between the careful provision for the baby and the neglect of the play and educational needs of older children in furnishing and equipping the home.

There is general agreement about the value for child rearing of separate and self-contained housing. The relative ease of supervising children at play is a good illustration, for there is clearly a great contrast between arrangements for play under close observation from a kitchen window and the difficulties of control from a high-rise flat. The case for separate units is strengthened by children's enjoyment of activities which create noise of various kinds (Willis, 1955). Hence the problems created by shared buildings and poor sound-proofing, a point well made by Raven (1967): 'While it is true that people who live in flats suffer more from noise disturbance than people who live in houses, this is not the main complaint. More important is the restriction people feel on making noise themselves. This affects their whole pattern of leisure and makes for more sedentary hobbies such as television viewing.'

Several studies (e.g. Jephcott, 1971) have shown the unsuitability of high-rise flats for children and the difficulty for mothers of looking after children when living on higher floors: for example, lifts cause endless trouble because of their attractions for play and vandalism and the likelihood of their breaking down. Nevertheless high-rise flats, though inconvenient for families with young children, may be acceptable for some groups such as the single or couples whose income allows only the alternative choice of poorer housing.

The age of children must also be considered. Up to about the age of seven, children in high-rise flats keep closer to parents than children living in single-family houses, but after that age the opposite is the case. Older children in high-rise flats spend more time outwith the home and consequently beyond the control of parents. Nor should factors of economics be neglected. High-rise apartments for the well-off New Yorker, for example, may provide a range of facilities for play and recreation which are unknown in deprived areas.

When assessing the suitability of housing, the criterion of advantage for child rearing must be balanced against other criteria such as privacy, the convenience with which preferred activities can take place, and the ease of contact with neighbours. It seems clear from the evidence of family preference for flats or houses and for central areas or suburbs, that style of life is of equal importance to child rearing in influencing choice.

Yet again there is the question of the adolescent. Criteria appropriate for children and especially for the very young are not applicable to adolescents who want to get away from home and mix with their friends. As Michelson (1970) points out: 'There is nothing exciting in a neighbourhood designed for toddlers. The very same environment which is congruent for a style of life emphasizing the nuclear family becomes incongruent when, by virtue of a change in stage in the life cycle, a teenager *may* desire a life style different from that of his parents—at least temporarily. It is no wonder that cars and motorcycles play such a part in the lives and problems of teenage suburbanites.'

This observation on adolescents is that of an American living in Toronto, but it applies equally to British experience with the inevitable qualification arising from differences in culture and wealth. These and many other studies emphasize not only the crucial link between the physical environment and patterns of social behaviour but also the differences in children's needs as they grow from infancy to maturity.

Environmental change

In traditional societies, there is little impetus to change. Family life pursues its accustomed path, children adopt the values of their parents and patterns of living continue intact. If new forces precipitate social change, the 'normal' relationships undergo progressive erosion, old beliefs are challenged by children growing up in a more stimulating environment and the family structure is weakened. Society tends to become stratified into an older generation maintaining the standards of the past and a younger generation seeking new ways of life (Blood, 1972). The pace of such change has intensified in most societies during this century, with drift from village into town in agrarian communities and increased movement between cities in industrial countries. New patterns of behaviour are emerging and families are becoming smaller and less cohesive.

Stability and mobility

Change in an urban society stimulates economic growth and affords opportunity for industrial enterprise: these in turn create a demand for a mobile labour force responsive to new developments. There is a whole range of occupations in the modern affluent society which take the father out of the home for long periods or necessitate his moving to another area. The pattern of women's employment also changes and with it the attitude of women to work outside the home. The consequent increased social mobility has serious implications for children. When a family moves, its accustomed way of living and the supporting network of the extended family, which have provided stability for the growing child, are often lost. The child is further unsettled by the disappearance of familiar landmarks, the absence of trusted friends and the demands of new institutions such as school or health centre.

Two examples will illustrate this point. One concerns a group of children who are constantly on the move—those whose fathers are in the armed forces. Studies of army children show how much they suffer from continual changes of school and neighbourhood. The consequences of this movement from one garrison to another are also exacerbated by the absence of the father on military service and the problems which this creates for the family group. These children must continually form relationships with new schoolmates and neighbours and their success in doing so may be at the cost of a superficiality in those relationships and a need to over-assert themselves in the new group.

The second example comes from the experience of London children evacuated to Oxford during the Second World War (Barnett House Study Group, 1947). Children were asked how they compared the new world with the old. 'Parents and relatives' took first place in their lists of what they missed most but 'traffic and noises' came second. Once again there is the combination of personal relationships and environmental factors. The children missed not only their families but also the familiar shops and markets and the well-known figures in the streets such as the rag-and-bone man. Oxford by contrast seemed to them to be full of 'old ladies who were inclined to forbid everything'. Perhaps most important was the greater ability to adapt shown by children from stable and secure families when compared with unwanted and neglected children.

Effects of rehousing

Movement within cities is a feature of life in Britain today. Early housing reformers saw the destruction of the slum and the creation of housing estates in peripheral areas as a policy which would lead to improvements in health and also in social behaviour closely related to health. Their expectations were based on the assumption that the degrading conditions of slum life were such that healthy family living was prevented by overcrowding, lack of play space for children and rundown housing: that their optimism was only partly justified became evident on completion of the rehousing programmes carried out under successive Housing Acts. These included both the rehabilitation of old central areas, with accompanying changes in housing density and the design of houses (high-rise flats for example often took the place of small back-to-back dwellings), and the building of vast new housing estates on the outskirts of cities.

Doctors and social scientists among others have drawn attention both by reports of clinical experience and through research to the problems of living in these housing estates. Clearly, implementing the policy of rehousing has proved much more difficult than expected and the reasons are by no means only those of cost or of the shortage of land in the most convenient places. Some of the most significant in fact derive from the effect of change on patterns of social behaviour and social relationships. Families who live in crowded inner-city areas tend to rely on a wide range of relatives and friends for help, advice and companionship. After moving to suburbs or housing estates, they are no longer in physical circumstances which are congruent with the intense family interaction to which they are accustomed and on which they depend. In this connection, Michelson's (1970) distinction between what he calls mental and experiential congruence is interesting. Mental congruence is largely based on hearsay and opinion—often irrational, since people do not always analyse their feelings about the environment in an objective way. Experiential congruence on the other hand is based on the practicalities of daily living rather than on subjective preferences.

Many studies of life in housing estates and rehabilitated central areas have emphasized the loneliness and isolation of the families living in them and in particular the effects of loneliness on mothers left at home with young children. Some have recorded the prevalence of high rates of neurosis and mental illness among mothers and of delinquency among children. 'New town blues' was a label popularly applied to tenants of new towns in their early years of growth.

One of the earliest and most challenging studies came from the Institute of Community Relations in Bethnal Green (Young & Willmott, 1957). It showed the distinctive role of 'mum' in families of London's East End, an impoverished area which had retained a very stable way of life over many years. As in other areas of similar character, the life of the family centred on the mother—a pattern that clearly could not survive the splitting up and moving away of families consequent on slum clearance and rehousing. The process of environmental change thus produces a variety of problems for those faced with the task of adaptation to new surroundings. In emphasizing the social aspects, there is no intention to underrate the potentially serious effects of slum living on the physical health of children. Nonetheless, there is evidence that the adequacy of the housing and its amenities are less important for child development than the quality of maternal care (Pollak, 1979). The point here is simply to draw attention to the close relationship between changes in the environment and patterns of behaviour in the family. It is interesting to see how, over the last 25 years, ideas on rehousing and town planning have come to include consideration of social planning and the effects on people of altering their physical surroundings. The new towns built in recent years provide many examples of skill in meeting the needs of transplanted communities and present a vivid contrast with the drabness and the anonymity of the vast housing estates on the periphery of large cities such as Glasgow.

Community work

The current trend towards community care (see Ch. 14) should be seen both as a growing acceptance of the importance of supportive relationships in a neighbourhood and as the deliberate objective of health and welfare policy. This recognition of the role of the community in fostering social well-being is perhaps no more than a rediscovery of an old truth. In simpler forms of society the responsibility for the care of sick and deviant members rested very substantially on members of the extended family and on friends and neighbours. In spite of some popular beliefs to the contrary, the evidence suggests that in many areas it still does. A recent study of old people in the Border counties of Scotland provides yet further evidence of this (Gruer, 1975).

The conditions under which this care is given are very different in an industrial and urban environment. In the first place, there is no longer an extended network of relatives available to share the burden of, for example, a handicapped child. The task is more likely to fall on parents and the nuclear family itself. Second, there is the problem of mobility on which the foregoing discussion has placed such emphasis. Social relationships require time in which to grow and frequent movement is a disrupting influence. Third, the whole scale of the environment in which people live is much larger and this makes it more difficult for individuals and families with differing values and traditions based on class, age and wealth to create an active community life. These adverse features of modern living operate even when the family unit is a stable and happy one. All too often, however, there is in addition parental disharmony or family breakdown, which compounds the difficulty of providing effective community care. The report of the Finer Committee (DHSS, 1974) considered the position of children growing up in single-parent families and gave rise not only to renewed discussion on policy but also to specific proposals for environmental change aimed at strengthening support for the mother and her child, such as better housing and facilities for day care.

Concern over children and their families is a central feature of community work because of the importance of promoting healthy child development and also for the interest which it stimulates within the community. Thus children provide a focus for local activity and initiative on the part of parents, and constitute an integrating force in districts where common interests, such as the occupations of fathers, no longer exist to any substantial extent.

The pre-school playgroup movement is one excellent illustration. It serves the double purpose of providing young children with opportunities for playing in a group before school age and of giving mothers the experience of working for the group and sharing in learning about the children. Although the supervision of play may be less professional than in the nursery school, this experience of participation by mothers is of great value. Another example from the field of play is the adventure playground. This movement, originally adopted from Denmark, is much more than merely a reaction against the drabness of municipal playgrounds. It provides scope for initiative and creativity as well as adventure in play, in which children may build their own dens and create a world of their own with adult encouragement (Spencer, 1964).

In recent years there has been a rapid growth of play schemes for schoolchildren during the summer holidays. Like the pre-school playgroup movement, these schemes also are an effective stimulus to community self-help. Yet in spite of such encouraging developments, the scope for further work of this kind is enormous, for play and recreation offer opportunities for redressing some of the stresses imposed by an antagonistic and overcrowded environment.

In adolescence, personal mobility is of increasing importance, for as children grow up their interest is in gaining independence from parents and home and in movement further afield. Hillman et al (1973) emphasize the dependence of adolescents on public transport, especially in areas of heavy traffic, where the dangers of cycling are a serious limiting factor to the use of the bicycle. They conclude that the transport planners appear to have paid little attention to facilitating the mobility of the young.

Conclusions: the environment and the doctor
In the course of their medical practice doctors, as well as other staff in the health service, become acutely aware of the impact of the environment, social as well as physical, on their patients. Above all they see these influences on the lives of children and their parents and the consequences for children's health. In poor communities and in more affluent ones at times of economic crisis, the question of scarcity of resources becomes dominant and priorities in spending are essential. In this short chapter it has not been possible to consider the many serious consequences of poverty and the cycle which leads to ill health, poor educational attainment, unemployment and back to poverty. The effects on the lives of children are abundantly illustrated by a number of studies, especially those carried out over a period of years (e.g. Douglas, 1968; Wedge & Prosser, 1973). Recent surveys of poverty in the United Kingdom and of child labour throughout the world underline the magnitude of these problems (Townsend, 1979; Challis & Elliman, 1979).

For the doctor, as well as for the policy maker, the purpose of social analysis must surely be to search for better methods of dealing with those environmental factors which contribute to illness, to social breakdown and to unhappiness, and to implement these if it is in his power to do so. The family doctor in particular is well placed to effect improvement, as may the clinic or school doctor be in certain circumstances. In this context, it may be important to know not only about the relationships between husband and wife and between parents and children but also about the family's relationship with their relatives and the community. Such enquiries will be particularly relevant when the family is isolated from both kin and neighbours. For example, a study of battered children and their parents (Smith & Noble, 1973) pointed out the frequency of social isolation and loneliness in these families, as well as the cramped accommodation and lack of amenities. In recent years the development of work with groups has gradually emerged as a great source of help for the isolated and the lonely. Although there are great variations between different areas both in the skill and in the availability of such resources, the encouragement of group membership, both for parents and children, may be particularly helpful.

The doctor may be in a position to promote environmental and social improvement in other ways as well. In many communities in Britain, doctors play a leading part in community organizations, such as voluntary and statutory associations concerned with the conduct of local affairs. Although the community association movement initially grew from a voluntary foundation, the recent reorganization of local government has brought community councils within a statutory framework and in some respects parallel with local health councils. In work of this kind doctors, by virtue of their education, experience and position in the community, have much to contribute. Of great importance also is the more recent role of the community medicine specialist, whose new social responsibilities extend substantially beyond those of the former medical officer of health.

Changing the child's physical and social circumstances is a deliberate process which cannot be left to the interplay of market forces. Although in times of economic stringency there are restrictions on new developments as well as on refurbishing the old, opportunities for renewal and improvement of the social environment will continue to arise with the help of doctors, and through collaboration between local authority social work departments and the health service. If the deprived children of today are the delinquents, alcoholics and neurotics of tomorrow (Ashton, 1979), improving the quality of child life must surely rank amongst our highest priorities (Stacey, 1980).

REFERENCES

Ashton J R 1979 Poverty and health in Britain today. Public Health, London 93: 89–94
Barnett House Study Group 1947 London children in war-time Oxford. Oxford University Press, London
Blood R O 1972 The family. Free Press, New York
Challis J, Elliman D 1979 Child workers today. Quartermaine House, London
Chapman D 1955 The home and social status. Routledge & Kegan Paul, London
Cohen S (ed) 1971 Images of deviance. Penguin, Harmondsworth
Department of the Environment 1975 Census indicators of urban deprivation. EcUR Division: Working Note No. 6. Department of the Environment, London
Department of Health and Social Security 1974 Report of the committee on one-parent families (Finer Committee), vol I. Cmnd 5629. HMSO, London
Douglas J W B 1968 All our future. Peter Davies, London
Eisenberg L 1979 The human family in a changing world. In: Doxiadis S (ed) The child in the world of tomorrow. Pergamon Press, Oxford
Freidson E 1963 The sociology of medicine: a trend report and bibliography. Current Sociology X/XI. Blackwell, Oxford
Gruer R 1975 Needs of the elderly in the Scottish Borders. Scottish Health Studies No. 33. Scottish Home and Health Department, Edinburgh
Hillman M, Henderson I, Whalley A 1973 Unfreedom road. New Society 24: 234–236
Jephcott A P 1971 Homes in high flats. Glasgow University Social and Economic Studies: Occasional Papers No. 13
Kerr M 1958 The people of Ship Street. Routledge & Kegan Paul, London
Michelson W H 1970 Man and his urban environment: a sociological approach. Addison-Wesley, London
Newson J, Newson E 1963 Infant care in an urban community. Allen & Unwin, London
Paneth M 1944 Branch Street. Allen & Unwin, London
Philip A E, McCulloch J W 1966 Use of social indices in psychiatric epidemiology. British Journal of Preventive and Social Medicine 20: 122–126
Pollak M 1979 Housing and mothering. Archives of Disease in Childhood 54: 54–58
Raven J 1967 Sociological evidence on housing: the home environment. The Architectural Review 142: 236–240
Robb J H 1954 Working class anti-semite: a psychological study in a London borough. Tavistock Publications, London
Schaffer H R (ed) 1971 The origin of human social relations. Academic Press, London
Smith S, Noble S 1973 Battered children and their parents. New Society 26: 393–395

Spencer J C 1964 Stress and release on an urban estate. Part IV. Tavistock Press, London
Spinley B M 1953 The deprived and the privileged: personality development in English society. Routledge & Kegan Paul, London
Stacey M 1980 Realities for change in child health care. British Medical Journal 280: 1512-1515
Townsend P 1979 Poverty in the United Kingdom. Allen Lane, London
Wedge P, Prosser H 1973 Born to fail. Arrow Books and National Children's Bureau, London
Willis M 1955 Living in high flats. London County Council, Architects Dept
Young M, Willmott P 1957 Family and kinship in East London. Routledge & Kegan Paul, London

The child in his family

Introduction
Family relationships are so subtle and complex that to delineate them precisely has always posed a major challenge. The optimum perhaps, as between parents and child, is an enduring interaction of love and approval, without qualifying 'strings' to the parental role. This means that parents, however much they disapprove of certain aspects of their child's behaviour, should never imply rejection of the child himself—a distinction by no means always easy to achieve.

The character of this relationship keeps changing all the time. Initially, it is all-embracing, embodying overall control; but as the child grows older, so he gains in independence and autonomy. Without sacrifice of affection, the parental sphere of influence is gradually reduced, until finally in adolescence there is ultimate assumption of full personal responsibility. That at least is the optimum.

In everyday life however, parent/child relationships do not always evolve so smoothly. When things go wrong, and symptoms erupt, emotional pathology takes one of two main forms. Either the relationship is deficient in *quantity*, i.e. lack of love through 'opting out', or even physical absence of parents (death, desertion, divorce): or there are defects in the *quality* of interaction. These range from overprotection to overt rejection, and from overindulgence to domineering suppression. Quantitative defects yield emotional deprivation; qualitative defects yield a greater variety of reactions, for example from overanxiety to excessive aggression; from undue compliance to undue defiance; and from dependence to delinquency. These responses are differently expressed in different children, according to age and individual make-up. The channel of expression may be disordered behaviour, disordered body function, or a combination of both.

Diagnostic guidelines
Prodromal signs of physical disorder in childhood are not too difficult to identify—the 'runny' nose, lack-lustre eyes, fretfulness or lack of energy—each has a story to tell, as often as not of similar significance the world over. By and large, the same applies to principles of medical treatment. Not so however with emotional problems. There are several reasons for this discrepancy.

1. No child can be assessed in isolation from his family; yet family interaction is far more difficult to interpret than standard physical signs.

2. Even when emotional pathology is suspected, no two children react alike. To a far greater extent than in physical illness, presentation varies with individual make-up (Thomas et al, 1968).

3. Presentation also varies with the age of the child or, more correctly, his level of emotional development. As a general rule, the younger he is, the more vulnerable to noxious stimuli, be they physical or mental. Similarly, at the senior end of the development spectrum, teenage flux leads to recrudescence of instability.

4. Even within the same age group however, identical symptoms may have widely differing significance. For example, soiling in one child could represent a regressive reaction to anxiety; in another child an aggressive response to pressure; while in yet a third, the soiling might be overflow from a basically constipated bowel. In this instance, retention of faeces would then be the primary problem.

5. Moreover, circumstances alter cases, i.e. the circumstances which have evoked the particular problem. For example, social adversity such as overcrowding, new housing estate isolation, or parental fecklessness can all generate reactive symptoms in the child, quite different to those arising from more personal disturbance.

With so complex a matrix of contributory factors, how best to formulate a practical framework for classifying the presenting problem? A useful starting point is to consider *where* the problem mainly presents, i.e. its *locational* setting. Does it arise chiefly in school (including playgroup, kindergarten, day nursery and nursery school), on the housing estate or community complex as a neighbourhood hazard, or largely within the home? Despite inevitable overlap between these three, this approach does help to narrow down the area of presentation.

Next we might consider *when* the problem erupts, i.e. at what stage in the child's development. Are we dealing with a pre-school issue (say) of separation anxiety, or a teenage state of rebellious revolt; with negativism in the toddler or failure to adjust to senior school pressures?

Thirdly, in this diagnostic exercise, it is helpful to ask *how* the problem presents. Is it predominantly 'acting out' in calibre, i.e. conduct disorder disturbing to others, yet indicative of underlying subjective disturbance; or is it more in the nature of an inwardly directed presentation such as anxiety state, phobic disorder, depressive state or sleep disruption?

Defining its character may materially help to identify the source of the problem, which brings into focus the fourth facet of the diagnostic process: determining *why* the problem has arisen.

Irrespective of where it comes to light, what is it a reaction to? Does the stress really emanate from school, from threats within the community, from conflict within the home or from a mixture of all three? If the trouble lies predominantly within the domestic setting, does it stem mainly from parental overinvolvement or its converse, parental non-involvement? Only by establishing diagnostic guidelines for the individual case can any rational therapeutic programme be worked out.

The school setting (Table 3.1)

Introduction to any new group, however small or informal, poses fresh challenge to the average child. Hence those already under strain for any reason tend to develop reactive symptoms that much more rapidly; but reactive to what? Essentially the demand is two-fold: to conform in behaviour to an accepted standard pattern, and to concentrate in absorbing what is being taught: in other words, the social and academic aspects of schooling. Should there be problems in adapting to either, what are the early warning signals? What should the teacher, nursery nurse, play supervisor, or educational psychologist be alerted to look for?

Broadly speaking, *how* the child reacts depends on whether he 'takes it out' on his environment, or 'takes it out' on himself (Pinkerton, 1974), i.e. whether he directs the reaction outwards or turns it inwards against himself (Table 3.1).

Table 3.1 *Where? The school setting.* A schematic representation of school-based symptoms

When? Maturational level	How? Character of symptoms		Presenting problem	Why? Parental attitude
Junior age range	Directed	inwards	Undue sensitivity Social isolation Reluctance to attend school	Overinvolved
		either way	Wetting, soiling Feeding difficulty	Varies
		outwards	Aggressive, disruptive Acting-out behaviour	Opting-out Neglectful Rejective
Senior age range	Directed	inwards	School phobia Daydreaming, moodiness Cosmetic sensitivity Fainting at assembly	Overinvolved
		either way	Learning block	Pressurizing
		outwards	Truancy, delinquency Drug experimentation	Opting out Neglectful Rejective

The first leads to 'conduct problems' (aggressive acting out); the second to 'personality problems' (regressive withdrawal) (Peterson, 1961).

To try to codify patterns of disturbance in primary schoolchildren, a large-scale research project was mounted in 1973 by Kolvin and his co-workers in Newcastle upon Tyne. The study is still going on but has already yielded significant findings. For example, to tabulate behaviour, information was collected on a major random sample of infant pupils, reported upon by their mothers. These data were then formally itemized and submitted to statistical processing (Kolvin et al, 1975).

What emerged confirms the bi-polar character of presenting complaints. Under the heading of conduct disorder on the one hand, the listed problems included wayward behaviour disruptive of class discipline (overactive, destructive or gratuitously aggressive children); temper tantrums; and such descriptions as reckless, inattentive, heedless of danger or actually given to wandering off. In the older child, comparable problems would encompass stealing, lying, vandalism, truancy or flagrant menaces, all the more disquieting in the absence of guilt feeling.

By contrast, certain symptoms elicited by Kolvin would fall within the category 'inwardly directed'. These would include undue sensitivity, excessive anxiety, specific phobias, social isolation or actual resistance to attending school at all—what Achenbach (1966) designates 'internalizing' symptoms. This same label incorporates tension habits such as tics, clothes chewing, nail biting and stammer.

More difficult to evaluate as they present in school, are disturbances of body function such as diurnal wetting, soiling, abdominal pain, vomiting and headache; together with symptoms like finicky appetite or greedy eating in the child taking meals at school. The difficulty lies in diagnosing correctly just what these symptoms mean in any given pupil. Thus wetting and soiling may both be either aggressive in character (what Kolvin calls 'externalizing vegetative') or regressive in significance in response to anxiety. Similarly, disordered appetite may be regressive or perversely defiant in character. The implication of the symptom is thus dictated by the factors which evoke it—in other words, the *why* of symptom formation.

One of those determining factors is the child's temperament, a notoriously difficult dimension to classify. Nevertheless, Kolvin and his colleagues have directed their research towards clarifying this aspect as well, i.e. temperamental organization. A principal component analysis of their data, within the infant school sample under review, highlighted four significant dimensions of temperament. These were: poor adaptation, withdrawal, dependence; high level of activity or distractability; moodiness or sulkiness; and irregular pattern of basic functions such as bedtimes, sleep rhythm, mealtimes and bowel action (Garside et al, 1975).

To help identify these dimensions of temperament within the standard classroom situation, the Newcastle team developed a questionnaire for routine use in schools. While still experimental, this could have obvious potential as a future diagnostic probe. More recently, the group has applied its research resources towards trying to identify, within their overall sample, those pupils considered at risk of either social maladjustment, learning difficulties or more overt nervous disorder. From a battery of tests with which they experimented, three proved helpful as diagnostic pointers. These were behavioural deviance on the Rutter Scale, as rated by teachers; reading retardation below the level of a reading quotient of 75; and a sociometric instrument involving choice of companions from among the child's immediate classmates. This yielded a measure of peer rejection (Kolvin et al, 1977).

The whole issue of how far children with special needs can first be identified and thereafter helped within the ordinary school setting, has recently been the subject of official enquiry (Warnock, 1978). One of the most revealing findings of that committee is the percentage of children—as high as one in five—who qualify for special treatment (of one kind or another) at some stage in their school career. With a prevalence of this order and the need to husband scarce resources, projects such as Kolvin's are of prime importance in helping to refine our screening programme for children at risk of educational disorder.

However, symptoms also vary in significance with the maturational level of the child. In other words, *when* or at what stage the problem erupts is as important as *where* or in what context it shows up.

The younger the child, the more vulnerable he will tend to be to stresses like separation anxiety; conversely, the older he gets, the more effective his emotional defences should become. Thus initial reluctance to separate from home at five years of age to attend school for the first time is neither very unusual nor particularly worrying as a temporary phase. However, its presentation as a neurotic response *de novo* at the age of 11-plus is always more significant and usually indicates pathology of long standing in relationships within the family. It is no accident that this represents the peak age incidence for school phobia or school refusal.

The same holds true for feeding, soiling and wetting problems (the oral–anal–bladder complex). The older the child in whom these symptoms present, the more serious their potential significance.

By the same token, fantasy in the younger child is acceptable as part of his developing ideational world; so that richly embroidered 'tall tales' may signify nothing more sinister than a vivid imagination. In the older child however retreat into fantasy, especially of recent origin, may well indicate serious underlying disturbance. These are examples of normality shading into pathology with advancing age in childhood.

However, the converse is equally true. While conformity is the general rule during the junior school years, there is an increasing trend towards defiance of authority as childhood merges into adolescence. What might be regarded as distinctly precocious in the seven- or eight-year-old therefore, by way of rebellious intolerance, becomes much more typical of the teenager, and should be interpreted as such. Making too much of an issue of it at this time could thus create a crisis of confrontation which it would be far better to avoid by diplomatic management if at all possible.

Drug experimentation
One aspect of the teenage school years merits particular emphasis because of its increasing incidence and potentially sinister significance. This is experimentation with drugs. In certain districts of large city conurbations, the problem is now alarmingly widespread, a reflection perhaps of increased permissiveness in society generally. Teachers should be wary therefore of any sudden change in the pattern of behaviour of a particular teenage pupil, especially if this is out of keeping with his or her acknowledged life-style. Inexplicable variations in mood or application, bizarre or odd reactions in the classroom, or an insidious falling off in concentration or animation—all are potential danger signals.

Nevertheless, unaccountable changes in teenage personal behaviour do not invariably signify the toxic effects of drugs. For one thing, the teenage 'drug scene' has latterly been overtaken, in the same age group, by increasing indulgence in alcohol. In some cities and suburban estates, this now represents the more immediate focus of concern by police, community workers and education welfare departments alike. Again it reflects the current laxity in control, the increasing tendency by parents to shelve responsibility, and the shift of spending power towards younger and younger age groups. Alcoholic excess is not perhaps a major problem as yet, numerically, but prodromal signs are already in evidence which should not be lightly dismissed.

To maintain a sense of balance, however, it is as well to keep in mind that this is a notoriously fluid phase of maturation, both physiologically and psychosocially, so the implications of behaviour change are not necessarily all that sinister. What then are possible alternative reasons for conduct aberrations in this age group? *Why* do symptoms erupt when and where they do?

Pubertal instability

In early adolescence, the aetiology is as likely to be intrinsic or endogenously determined as to be engendered by environmental factors. Puberty with its attendant flux plays temporary havoc with emotional and social stability, so that in youngsters already sensitive or prickly by nature, overreaction is commonplace and capricious mood swings are perhaps the rule more than the exception. As transition proceeds however through teenage to adolescence, with secondary sex characteristics developing and crystallizing, so stability is regained and clinical symptoms gradually subside. Features such as fainting at school assembly, cosmetic sensitivity and locomotor gaucheness are all characteristic of this phase and are largely endogenous (Table 3.1). Bear in mind however that the teenager *is* hypersensitive and self-critical, so that slights are exaggerated and authority all too readily resented, whether stemming from home or school. There is increased danger at this time that affinity will be sought with neighbourhood gangs who are not always wholesome in their influence: thus calling for mature understanding and monumental patience by parents and teachers alike, more than ever before.

Incipient schizophrenia

Occasionally, but important enough always to bear in mind, oddities in behaviour out of keeping for the particular youngster may herald the onset of an insidious psychotic change. Especially is this so if the pupil has been under particular strain—academic, religious, personal or domestic—and especially if there is a family history of schizophrenia. The peak incidence of this illness after all is in late adolescence, hence its original title of dementia praecox (premature dementia).

At the lower end of the school-age spectrum, failure to conform in the infant or nursery class is almost always diagnostic of prior mishandling on the domestic front, so that the newly enrolled pupil is poorly equipped to make the additional group adjustment. An alternative possibility, however, is that a child of limited endowment, hitherto unsuspected as such, will fail to match up to academic expectations, however elementary these may be to start with. Add to this, unwitting pressure by ambitious parents, and the scene is set for reactive symptoms of one or other kind; acting out, 'show-off', defiant behaviour, or 'opting out', anxious withdrawal. Although they present in the setting of school, the evocative stimulus is really the home, or at least certain facets of parental management within that home. As in organic disease, symptomatic presentation does not always reflect the true origins of the problem. This is why the Warnock recommendation (Warnock, 1978) to promote fuller participation by parents in educational programmes for their pre-school children, is so apposite a suggestion. What is envisaged is a partnership between parents and school; and since this need not be a costly innovation, it ought to be adopted expeditiously.

The neighbourhood setting (Table 3.2)

Overlapping with school as a focus of symptom presentation, neighbourhood stresses commonly bring to the surface problems which might otherwise remain submerged. In the larger city conurbations, for example, the policy of rehousing families in peripheral estates, or in high-rise blocks of flats, has brought with it two new hazards, the 'horizontal' isolation which follows banishment to a

Table 3.2. *Where? The neighbourhood setting.* A schematic representation of community-based symptoms

When? Maturational level	How? Character of symptoms		Presenting problem	Why? Parental attitude
Junior age range	Directed	inwards	Sleep disturbance Nightmares Excessive clinging Regressive soiling and wetting	Overinvolved Tension-ridden
		either way outwards	Pre-school hyperactivity Destructiveness Accident prone-ness Disobedience Wandering	Varies Opting out Neglectful
Senior age range	Directed	inwards	Social isolation Multiple phobias Gang victimization	Overinvolved Tension-ridden
		outwards	School refusal Gang violence Vandalism, lawlessness Sexual promiscuity	Opting out Neglectful Rejective

distant estate, and its 'vertical' counterpart of feeling trapped on the top floor of a multi-storey flat complex (Pinkerton, 1974).

Usually, it is the young mother who first shows signs of breakdown. Cut off from supportive contact with her own family, denied the communal facilities of inner-city living, and faced with higher rental and transport charges, she often reacts with marked anxiety or depressive features. These inevitably affect the younger members of her family and, as they in turn develop symptoms, their mother becomes increasingly harassed and progressively less able to cope. If her husband is working at all, his move out to the new estate has usually meant increased travelling time, curtailed leisure hours at home and therefore less opportunity to cushion the tensions experienced by his family. Indeed, he may add to those tensions himself.

Nevertheless, for the health visitor, school welfare officer or family doctor, consulted in the early stages of the rehousing process, it is more than likely that one of the children will be paraded as the ostensible problem.

Predictably, against this background, anxiety features will tend to predominate. Thus sleep disturbance is a common complaint among the younger age groups, i.e. initial insomnia, restless sleep, nightmares, night terrors, head banging and teeth grinding. Often there is associated nocturnal enuresis.

Complementary to these, feeding problems, soiling, excessive clinging and fearfulness are characteristic of the child's waking hours. All are symptomatic of personal insecurity which simply reflects the young mother's own anxiety state. Each represents a withdrawal or regressive response (Table 3.2).

Among more robust personalities, however, the presentation may be very different. Here the response could well be, as in school, wilful disobedience, destructiveness, temper tantrums or generalized motor overactivity—the last being the hallmark, in the active pre-school child, of incarceration in a high-rise flat.

Range of reaction notwithstanding, what this illustrates once again is dichotomy of direction concerning *how* each child responds to underlying domestic tension.

As for the timing of reactive disturbance, i.e. *when* it occurs, or how it ties up with developmental level, the older and more independent the child, the greater his disenchantment over absence of social facilities in his immediate neighbourhood. This is still too often a discouraging feature of stark new housing developments, so that to fill the vacuum, bored youngsters drift into vandalism, gang violence, defiance of school authority and general lawlessness, which gets increasingly out of hand.

Disturbed and disturbing behaviour alike are by no means the exclusive hallmark of rehousing. They can and do present in certain urban, as well as suburban, settings. For example, by comparing the life styles of senior school-age children on the Isle of Wight (a stable, settled and cohesive community) with a comparable age group of children in an inner London borough, Rutter (1973) has convincingly demonstrated how the various unsettling influences of metropolitan city life are reflected in the greater incidence of delinquency among the London schoolchildren. These disruptive influences include more frequent changes in school staff (compared to the Isle of Wight sample), less closely knit families and greater scope for law breaking. The very real impact of community factors is thereby only too convincingly substantiated.

In recent years, Brown and his sociological colleagues at Bedford College, London, have undertaken complementary research into the mental state of women in a large-scale psychosocial study in the Borough of Camberwell. Though concerned primarily with maternal depression, this work has very real relevance to paediatric practice through a number of its findings. As with the Rutter research, Brown has shown that mothers residing in metropolitan city areas are particularly prone to psychiatric disorder (especially depression), given a combination of four distinct vulnerability factors. These are: early loss of their own mother (not father) before the age of 11; three or more children under the age of 14 living at home; unavailability of outside employment, even part-time, beyond the home; and denial of a supportive relationship with a confiding adult consort—husband, steady boyfriend, or stable cohabitee (Brown & Harris, 1978). These factors have summative impact in that in their presence any intercurrent crisis or stressful provocation is much more likely to precipitate maternal breakdown than in their absence.

The implications for community paediatrics in underprivileged urban areas are obvious. Where mothers are burdened by young families without the support of a stable male consort, with no opportunity for even temporary 'escape' into part-time outside employment, and especially where their mothering competence has been potentially undermined by losing their own mother in early childhood, they and their children are equally at risk—the mothers, of frank psychiatric breakdown; and the children, of reactive disturbance arising from that breakdown. Community workers must therefore be alert to the potential repercussions for children in their locality of pathological factors affecting such mothers, whether the stress be psychosocial, socioeconomic, inter-generational or a combination of all three, with the ultimate danger of frank maternal breakdown.

Even when the mother's mental stability is not called into question, her children, especially her pre-school children, are still at risk of retarded development if her level of maternal care is inadequate. But while 'poor', unstimulating, or neglectful home environments have long been associated with impaired scholastic achievement, behaviour disorder and even frank psychiatric disturbance, exactly what it is about these homes had never been very clearly defined. Now, however, a recent research study has confirmed (Pollak, 1979), in a sample of 200 pre-school children from an inner London borough, that however inadequate the housing standards, including overcrowding, spatial restrictions and lack of basic amenities, no convincingly adverse link emerges affecting overall level of development. In sharp contrast, the adequacy or inadequacy of maternal care within the families studied does show a highly significant relationship to child developmental levels assessed by modified Gesell parameters. In other words, between housing (a neighbourhood factor) and mothering (a home factor) quality of care clearly transcends physical and material provisions in overall importance for child health.

The home setting (Table 3.3)

To recapitulate, both school-based and community-based problems undoubtedly contribute to emotional disorder in childhood. Nevertheless, their impact can be cushioned by the right kind of protective home environment. Adequate mothering is clearly one vital aspect of the 'protective home'; but in more general terms, it is family solidarity which buffers outside stress. In other words, neither neighbourhood pressures nor stresses at school are likely in themselves to exert significantly adverse effects, so long as family cohesion remains intact; for that is the ultimate determining factor. But family ties can be too close as well as too loose, overinvolvement can be as inhibiting as non-involvement, parental cosseting as counter-productive as constant carping. To achieve a balance in bringing up children calls for commonsense, emotional maturity, a sense of humour and a willingness to shoulder the responsibilities of parenthood without expecting too much in return—a tall order. Yet the majority of parents do prove equal to the challenge. Is it therefore possible to predict those less likely to, and by so doing, anticipate problems and *why* they

Table 3.3. *Where? The home setting.* A schematic representation of home-based symptoms

When? Maturational level	How? Character of symptoms		Presenting problem	Why? Parental attitude
Junior age range	Directed	inwards	Socially inept Immature Anxiety-prone Overdependent Phobic, obsessional Emotional stunting	Overinvolved
		outwards	Battering Negativistic defiance Sleep refusal Food refusal Faecal retention	Rejective Abusive Pressurizing Overcontrolling
Senior age range	Directed	inwards	Socially inept Immature Anxiety-prone Overdependent Phobic, obsessional	Overinvolved
		outwards	Defiant, rebellious Stealing, lying Absconding Socially deviant	Overcontrolling Opting out Neglectful

are liable to emerge? In this context, experience has shown that certain life circumstances are especially likely to influence parental management (Pinkerton, 1974).

Predictive signs of overvaluation
Should this be an only child, or one born after a prolonged interval, maternal overinvolvement is all the more likely. The same holds true if fetal viability has been endangered by threatened abortion, toxaemia or antenatal bleeding: or for obstetric hazards such as birth before term or a difficult delivery.

Similarly, the nearer to the menopause the baby is born, the greater his emotional value, the more so if previous pregnancies have been abortive and future prospects are receding all the time.

After birth, a stormy neonatal period or serious illness in infancy are factors which may equally promote undue concern; as may the death of any older sibling. Most pernicious of all perhaps is the guilt that builds up from original rejection of an unplanned, unwanted pregnancy when realization leads to compensatory overprotection.

All such children are potentially at risk, not of deprivation, but its converse—emotional smothering. The signs are plain enough to identify, if only the right questions are asked.

Given this kind of background, virtually any childhood handicap, physical or mental, is bound to generate overprotection by parents, the more so if they are anxious by nature. Hence the importance of keeping in mind when counselling that circumstances can affect the most level-headed of parents to make them overanxious.

If anything is 'to blame', it is the particular life situation, not the parents themselves. This is of tremendous import in counteracting feelings of guilt and the natural sense of failure universally experienced at some time by virtually all parents of handicapped children.

Invalid response. But natural or not, overvaluation *is* a hazard, bringing with it the prospect of resulting overdependence. Is this so potentially serious? In one research study after another, almost irrespective of the lesion, the same conclusion has been reached—undue dependence encourages 'caving in', with exaggeration of symptoms, leading to negative outlook, and invalid life-style— the opposite of optimal coping.

This is as true (say) for congenital heart disease (Linde et al, 1966) as for haemophilia (Mattsson & Gross, 1966) and for juvenile diabetes (Travis, 1975) as for childhood asthma (Pinkerton, 1971a).

But is such a reaction inevitable? By no means. The more robust the patient's make-up, the more likely he is to resist parental cosseting, a further example of variation in *how* the child reacts. The optimum is for him to accept, in realistic terms, what the disability still allows him to achieve and what it prevents him from doing: rough and tumble sports in haemophilia, sustained running in asthma, unsupervised swimming in epilepsy, etc. That is the commonsense attitude.

Denial of handicap. At the opposite extreme, however, there is danger of an equally pathological response, denial of handicap in the effort to flout its limitations. This if it occurs is more typical of the older child, which emphasizes that *when*, or at what age, therapeutic strategy comes to be mounted, can materially affect its prospects of success.

Mattsson & Gross (1966), for example, refer to rebellious defiance by certain haemophilic teenagers revolting against irksome restrictions on their activity; Mattsson (1972) also mentions resentment of epileptic adolescents against continuing adult surveillance, while similar problems present in teenage diabetes and cystic fibrosis (Pinkerton, 1969; Pless & Pinkerton, 1975). Their management, in other words, differs materially at this stage from management of the same disorder in younger and more compliant age groups (as a rule).

There are younger children, however, already so stoical in outlook and so determined to play down the problem, as to create a false impression of coping, at variance with how handicapped they really are. By nature, they tend to be super-stable or counter-neurotic (Pinkerton, 1973), and if encouraged by equally unrealistic parents to deny the gravity of their condition, the outcome can be potentially serious and even fatal (Pinkerton, 1971b). It is important, therefore, always to look behind the superficial presentation at the underlying substrate of pathology.

What holds true for organic disease applies equally to disorders which are emotionally determined—parental attitude and self-attitude significantly influence the clinical reaction. Are there therefore recognizable syndromes to be looked for in response to parental overinvolvement? Undoubtedly there are, and indeed they appear throughout the whole range of childhood development (Table 3.3).

Spectrum of response to overinvolvement. For example, in infancy, focus on feeding with excess concern over food intake and eating schedules can lead to problems in establishing a regimen, and even greater problems in maintaining it. The same holds true for toilet function and sleep rhythm. The toddler in particular is especially prone to perverse contrariness. Therefore, show him an area of parental overconcern and he will be tempted to exploit it with all the artfulness at his command.

Weary young mothers driven frantic through lack of sleep, or distracted with anxiety over failure by the child to gain weight, or refusal to 'perform' in normal bowel action, bear ample testimony to the dangers of overemphasis in early training schedules.

Too close a relationship in the pre-school years spells problems for the child in squaring up to later demands for social self-reliance. It is in this area that the seeds are sown for overt separation anxiety, should some outside challenge eventually occur, be it urgent admission to hospital for acute intercurrent illness, or the 'disappearance' of mother through her own admission to hospital, or simply the standard enrolment of the child at school.

Continuing overinvolvement during the middle years of childhood further stifles freedom of expression with varying results. The immature youngster continues to feel dependent and lacking in self-confidence in asserting himself. Thus when faced with any crisis, in home or school affairs, he still tends to react with undue symptoms of anxiety. These can range from phobic states, through obsessional preoccupation or hysterical behaviour, to actual disorder of body function: wetting, soiling, vomiting, frequency, recurrent abdominal pain or equivalent systemic disturbance. Because the repertoire of response is relatively limited however, broadly similar symptoms may well be indicative of widely differing stresses. All that can be said is that they signify erosion of personal security and thereby draw attention to environmental challenge.

Response to pressurizing. Emotional stifling is usually associated with positive feeling for the child; if anything, overattachment. On occasion, however, 'smothering' assumes a negative connotation aimed at pressurizing or dominating. The response then is correspondingly different. Now there is more tendency for the child to look cowed, and if critical overtones persist, the level of disturbance becomes heightened in proportion. This is the kind of aura which fosters multiple habit spasm, 'emotional block' in school work, or in children of histrionic make-up, florid hysterical symptoms such as functional 'paresis', 'deafness', or 'blindness'.

How the child responds is to some extent easier to define than *why* that particular reaction should have taken place at all. For example, not all children withdraw in face of stress, nor for that matter do they elaborate their withdrawal into obsessional defence or hysterical dissociation. Some, the more robust in make-up, may well react with defiance, reflected in aggressive behaviour, flouting of authority, destructiveness or even physical violence.

As a general rule, the older the child, the greater the likelihood of rebellious challenge to parental authority, be it overprotective and cossetting, or overcontrolling and carping. Indeed ultimately the most reasonable of parents are likely to encounter teenage resistance, however liberal the code of discipline they try to maintain. Such is the progression of response from childhood into adolescence.

Nevertheless, there are exceptions to the rule. In place of self-reliance, there is sometimes continuing subservience; in place of maturation, persisting dependence, in which case chronological advances fail to be reflected in comparable growth emotionally. When that happens, the clinical outcome is discouraging. This is, for example, the kind of morbid symbiosis commonly at the root of school phobia persisting into the senior school years. Nor does the problem automatically resolve at school leaving. There is evidence, on the contrary, that school-shy pupils become work-shy adolescents (Warren, 1965; Berg, 1970). In other words, parent/child relationships far transcend the period of formal schooling in their overall significance.

Teenage depression. Nor is this by any means the only hazard of persisting immaturity. For while emotional unfolding lags behind, physical and endocrine development continue, with resulting conflict and confusion in the mind of the unfortunate youngster. Small wonder therefore that this is the age group reflecting paramount flux in emotional stability; and in these more vulnerable children, depressive mood swings are especially commonplace, in the struggle to identify with their new self-image. Yet at the same time they are afraid to shoulder individual responsibility. In the circumstances, it is easy to understand how suicidal gestures come to be made as one way out of an intolerable dilemma. Indeed in the United States, suicide now ranks as the fourth most frequent cause of death in adolescence (Bakwin & Bakwin, 1972).

But depression and preoccupation with suicide are not exclusive to immature teenagers unable to break away from parental domination. They occur just as frequently at the opposite end of the relationship spectrum, in response to deprivation through parental opting out.

Alternatively, the depression may be endogenous, i.e. not determined by mismanagement at all, but 'coming from within', though this is much less commonly encountered. In other words, affective responses being just as limited in range as their somatic counterparts, it is never wise to assume that a specific situation has sparked off a specific response. The clinical state must always be evaluated as a whole.

Nevertheless, diagnostic pointers can be useful and just as overinvolvement was seen to produce a characteristic spectrum of reaction in the child, so may parental non-involvement evoke equally typical repercussions. Naturally, they too will vary with age and temperament, but still provide some basis for further exploration.

With what object? the object of identifying, as early as possible, children at serious risk of deprivation. How may these hazards be recognized, what are their early warning signs, and what are the clinical consequences of ignoring them?

Predictive signs of non-acceptance
Once again, maternal attitude to the pregnancy is as reliable a point as any from which to start. This applies particularly to the younger mother. Older women as a rule enjoy the more settled circumstances of a stable married home; in which case, if they do become pregnant and feel initially rejective because it was unplanned, they are more likely to develop compensatory guilt feeling later on.

By contrast, the less experienced mother, in less settled circumstances, and perhaps with more problems to cope with, may well find the unwanted pregnancy a much greater burden. If so, she will feel less charitably disposed to the baby despite the popular idea of its helpless appealing state at birth.

The situational setting of the pregnancy may thus be of critical importance in determining the prevailing attitude. As such, it always repays careful assessment. A particularly significant clue, if it can be established at the time, is the mother's very first reaction to the knowledge of being pregnant.

Especially do these considerations apply to the young *unmarried* mother, the more so if her consort is equally immature, unready for parental responsibility, work-shy or at least uncertain in his work prospects, and similarly uncommitted to long-term cohabitation. All these are potential danger signals militating against the baby's prospects of untrammelled thriving after birth.

Discussing disadvantaged children and their backgrounds, Kellmer Pringle (1974) has listed five groups with a higher than average chance of developmental damage or stunting because of personal, family or social factors. They are:

1. Children from poorly housed large families on low incomes—an obvious socio-economic 'target' group.

2. Children being brought up by one parent.

3. Children obliged to live apart from their parents (e.g. in local authority care).

Situations 2 and 3, i.e. single-parent families as well as children in care, both tend to create adjustment problems almost inherently, but these are usually all too apparent even at first encounter.

4. Not so apparent as a disadvantaged group are children with physical or mental handicap. Traditionally, parents are thought of as being overprotective towards their handicapped children but, in practice, a significant minority are found to express rejective feelings, either overtly or covertly. This is particularly true of some fathers who in a curious way seem to resent the implication of their own impaired virility. They cannot accept that biological 'damage' could possibly be attributed to their defective germ plasm, even when no such implication is being made (Pinkerton, 1970).

Undoubtedly, chronic handicap of any kind in one child is likely to throw additional strains on other members of the family. Ann Gath's in-depth study of mongol children and their siblings convincingly demonstrates this (Gath, 1972, 1973), especially in respect of the older sisters in the family (Gath, 1974); for it is upon them, predictably, that most of the burden falls. Even for parents, chronic disability by no means invariably leads to cossetting. Parents may experience negative feelings, especially if the condition is physically burdensome, socially embarrassing or disappointing because of their fond ambitions for the child.

In her most recent research, Gath has focused upon just this facet of the problem, i.e. the impact on parents of having to bring up an abnormal child (Gath, 1977). In a prospective, matched follow-up of 30 families with a newborn mongol baby, she looked at parental relationships in detail for each of the couples in the study, i.e. the control group as well as the 'mongol' group. Compared with the 'normal' parents, all her negative ratings for marital disharmony were higher in the mongol group, for example severe discord or breakdown in nine couples versus none in the controls. Conversely, some of her positive ratings were also higher among the 'handicapped' families. In other words, for some couples, family adversity increases the risk of marital breakdown, whereas in others, the additional challenge seems to cement the relationship, no doubt through the experience of sharing the burden. Similar findings have been reported for parents of children with cystic fibrosis (Burton, 1975), although these were based upon a less rigorous research design.

The implication for management of handicapped children is that assessment must include family function, with particular focus upon parental relationship (Pinkerton, 1978). During crisis periods support can then be concentrated on 'suspect' or unstable marriages. The role of the Health Visitor expressly assigned to paediatric practice is tailor-made for crisis intervention of this kind, as so presciently envisaged by the Court Committee (1976). Failure to acknowledge the need for such support, in spina bifida for example, is highlighted by the increased incidence of marital breakdown among families with a spina bifida baby, compared with the position in unaffected families (Tew et al, 1977). All the more significant is the disparity between frequency of breakdown where the child fails to survive beyond the first 12 months and the three-fold increase in broken marriages among those who do survive. The implication is obvious. The more protracted and sustained the period of burdensome duress, the greater the risk of marital schism, so that chronic disability in childhood by no means invariably brings out the best in harassed parents.

5. It is Pringle's fifth category of children at risk, however, which is the most difficult to recognize with certainty. These are the cases in which the parents are 'mentally handicapped, socially deviant, or (themselves) emotionally damaged'. The subnormal or mentally ill parent is perhaps not too difficult to identify and deal with, by arranging for appropriate surveillance. But how to recognize the 'social deviant'?

A major error is to focus exclusively on parents in social classes IV and V. By the same token, absence of material squalor or financial hardship is no guarantee that more subtle factors may not be operating to undermine stability. In their study of social factors associated with child abuse, Smith et al (1974) clearly showed that temperamental instability is not confined to a particular social group or set of adverse home circumstances. The important point is not to be deceived by a father's or mother's well-groomed appearance, brittle brightness, or brash confidence in apparently coping with problems. Often this is more illusory than real, and breaks down rapidly under duress, to reveal the underlying character defect.

A knowledge of personal background, if it can be procured without risking offence, is always a helpful pointer. Clinical experience confirms the link between a 'rootless' childhood, in local authority care perhaps, and later difficulty in adjusting to parental responsibilities. Accommodation over long periods in large community homes can add to these difficulties, but even shorter periods of separation are not without pernicious repercussions on occasion.

Recent research by Wolkind (1977) confirms this clinical deduction. In a sample of primigravidae attending at antenatal screening, Wolkind found that

7 per cent had a history of residential care in childhood of at least one month under local authority provision. Compared with the sample as a whole, this 'in care' subgroup carried a disproportionate number of unmarried teenagers. Equally significantly, the subgroup reported poorer housing conditions and less stability in their basic domicile, and scored higher on the 'malaise' inventory of health level during their pregnancy. There seems no doubt therefore that erosion of personal security in early childhood can affect the subsequent quality of 'mothering' in girls exposed to this deprivational experience.

Defective mothering. The earlier study by Eva Frommer (1973) of British-born married primigravidae, also undertaken at antenatal screening, represents the prototype for this kind of research. As part of the assessment, each was asked to recall any period of separation from either parent, occurring before the age of 11, and long enough to have left an impression. One hundred and sixteen returned positive replies. Some referred to permanent separation (e.g. death or desertion of parent), others to more temporary breaks. All were matched for age and social class with controls in the same series unable to recall any such experience. Both groups were subsequently followed up for 12 months after confinement, without the reviewer knowing which was which. Important differences emerged.

The mothers with separation experience consistently reported greater problems in several areas of behaviour, their own and the baby's. For example, the baby cried more often and had more disturbed sleep; the mother herself was significantly more anxious, irritable, tired and depressed than her counterpart in the control group; and the marital relationship was more often threatened. Why should this be?

One explanation is that in their own childhood, these young 'separated' mothers have restricted opportunities to build sustained relationships within their own family circles. When in due course each is called upon to construct similar ties with husband and baby, she finds the task more challenging because of her own deprivational history.

This sequence is not of course inevitable, but quality of motherhood is so important a factor in successful child rearing that routine screening for suspect personal histories is surely worth promoting along these lines.

The original Frommer study which pointed out this conclusion has been amply confirmed by Wolkind and his colleagues, who have replicated but expanded her approach on a much larger sample of 534 obstetric cases (Wolkind et al, 1976). Nevertheless, such background information is not always readily forthcoming. There are many reasons for this. For example, families move around more freely than they used to do a generation ago, which means that histories may not be so easy to trace. In the absence of clues of this kind, could there still perhaps be certain warning signs, of more immediate import, to alert the schoolteacher, social worker, doctor or nurse, to whom a parent may turn for guidance in the first instance when tensions begin to mount intolerably on the home front?

Impending breaking point. In this context, Pringle (1974) refers to expressions of parental anxiety about the child which even if unjustified, need to be taken notice of. What does she mean? Commonly, under duress, one or other parent begins to sense loss of control in tolerating a particular child. It may be a sleep problem which tips the balance, or persistent soiling, or hyperactive behaviour especially if it brings constant complaints from neighbours. Each of these is almost certainly reactive to pre-existing marital strains, but which follows which is really immaterial. The point at issue is how exasperated the parent has become in trying to contend with the additional stress, on top of overcrowding or new estate isolation or financial pressures already crowding in. It is almost impossible to appreciate objectively the feeling of desperation subjectively engendered by psychosocial duress of this kind. Yet it is the subjective impression alone which brings that parent closer and closer to breaking point.

Repeatedly in these circumstances an appeal will be made to the doctor, health visitor or welfare worker for urgent intervention otherwise 'something will snap'. More often it is the mother who seeks help. She can no longer carry on because she is 'terribly afraid she will do something desperate' to the child. This is the immediate danger signal, the *cri du cœur*.

Admittedly, she could be exaggerating or even overdramatizing her ordeal, and the experienced family doctor who knows his patient is in a good position to judge. For workers less familiar with the family, however, it is never wise to dismiss the situation lightly. Better a misjudgment of commission than one of omission which fails to diagnose and thereafter 'defuse' a genuine crisis.

Bonding. Over and above environmental pressures which operate postnatally and the quality of mothering so often established long before pregnancy, a further area of potential pathology remains to be considered, associated with the birth itself. This is the phenomenon of bonding between the mother and her newborn baby. Traditionally, after labour, it was believed helpful to a mother to encourage her recuperation by separating her for a time from her baby to allow her to rest. When in addition there is biological risk due to frank perinatal pathology and intensive care is indicated for the baby, segregation becomes almost mandatory, because so few special care baby units include accommodation for mothers. Yet the evidence is mounting that separation in this way for more than very brief intervals in the period after birth can seriously undermine the bonding process—with potential impairment of long-term relationships between that mother and her child. This coupling is akin to the pattern of imprinting first described by Lorenz in newly hatched goslings. It does not, however, have the same primitive instinctual basis. On the contrary, in human mothers the sequence is more subtle but also more conscious, reinforced as it is by fondling, eye-to-eye contact and extended opportunity for physical handling of the baby. Klaus & Kennell (1976) are the paediatricians commonly credited with pioneering this concept, but acknowledgement of its significance is now extensive, with obvious implications for modified obstetric practice. Nevertheless, pockets of resistance among more conservative practitioners still persist, with genuine danger of permanent threat to the mother's acceptance of that particular child unless traditional practice can be brought into line. Otherwise, the prospect of later problems developing is very real indeed.

Syndromes of deprivation
So much for defects in the adequacy of parenthood—the *why* so to speak which

lies behind syndromes of deprivation. But what about the form in which problems present—the *how* of clinical practice? Are there comparable warning signs to indicate children at risk? Again a great deal hinges on *when* or at what age the exposure takes place (Table 3.3).

As a rule, the older the child, the stronger his emotional defences in standing up to adversity. Even so, how he reacts depends partly on temperament and partly on circumstances.

Somatic symptoms, for example diffuse recurrent abdominal pain, hysterical loss of motor function, relapse into bed wetting, are typically the response of sensitive or inarticulate children unable to give vent to their feeling of abandonment at being deserted or let down, bereaved or betrayed. More robust youngsters better able to express their anger openly, may respond with acting-out behaviour to a similar situation of broken faith. Conversely, the death of a parent, by its untimely withdrawal of stabilizing authority, can lead to indiscipline in the meekest of teenagers by way of filling the 'power vacuum'. As always, the significance of symptoms can only be interpreted in the light of prevailing circumstances.

By contrast, at the lower end of the age scale, vulnerability is greater, the risk of serious trauma higher, but correspondingly the pattern of response is so much more stereotyped that it is easier to recognize as an indication of abuse. What is there to look for?

Non-accidental injury. The campaign for recognition of non-accidental injury to children originally mounted by Kempe et al (1962) has now gained such momentum that doctors are increasingly alert to the atypical lesion, especially when contracted under dubious circumstances or if it keeps recurring. But these are retrospective clues in that injuries have to be reported before action can be taken. Prospective suspicions are obviously of much greater value. They include recognition in the child of '... a depressed or withdrawn attitude ... avoidance of eye contact, a refusal to speak to adults and/or children' (Pringle, 1974). Ounsted has a phrase for it—'frozen watchfulness' (Ounsted & Lynch, 1976).

Couple such observations with suspect quality of parenthood, and the picture emerges of a child at risk of damage, physically, emotionally or both. Wife battering, moreover, overlaps in incidence with child battering (Scott, 1974), so that suspect evidence of one points to increased likelihood of the other. Both result from violence based on episodic upsurge of paternal aggression, rather than a baseline of sustained rejection. Nevertheless, the threshold of tolerance to frustration is so relatively low in these fathers that it takes precious little to provoke them. Yet so long as they are not provoked, they may not be too unkindly disposed to their wives and children. It is this capricious variation in attitude and behaviour which makes positive recognition so difficult. Paradoxically however, although father, by his uncertain temper, more often aggravates domestic tension to crisis point, it is the mother who more often perpetrates the actual assault. Hers in a sense is a double burden of family responsibilities and personal duress, under which eventually the abused herself may become the abuser.

Emotional stunting. By contrast, children who are treated to *sustained* rejection, persisting over long periods, more commonly present with stunted development. This is not to preclude their ill treatment through physical assault, and indeed a more apposite concept would be child abuse, to indicate the breadth of spectrum involved. One third of the children studied by Martin et al (1974), for example, were below the third centile for growth at first recognition, and even at follow-up further progress was disappointing in half the cases studied. Alternatively, abuse may take the more sinister form of actual drug poisoning (Rogers et al, 1976). As a general rule, 'the battered child is more often the object of parental ambivalence, the stunted child more often the target for cold and constant rejection. He is in fact being emotionally disowned' (Pinkerton, 1975).

McCarthy has made a special study of these stunted children. He too concludes: 'Children who eventually show physical signs of this syndrome have suffered from rejection from an early age, probably right from birth or even before birth' (McCarthy, 1974). That emotional deprivation can lead to retardation of growth has been repeatedly confirmed: reversible failure of growth hormone has been demonstrated in disadvantaged children (Powell et al, 1967). There could be no more convincing evidence of the link between pre-existing psychopathology and resulting pathophysiology.

The dramatic progress made by stunted children when they are admitted to hospital for investigation is itself diagnostic. Like the battered child, they 'thaw out' rapidly in the ward even without special treatment, simply in response to humane management.

But what about the families to which these stunted children are ultimately obliged to return? In the eloquent words of Margaret Lynch (1978) 'While parents can respond positively to intervention... they do not thereby automatically gain knowledge of how to rear their children successfully' (and) 'yet for many families the only help given is emergency medical treatment for the child and social case work for the parents'.

No less discouraging is the outcome for the child who is removed by the local authority from his suspect home and placed outside his family for fostering or even adoption. All too often, sadly, there is breakdown here too, with disastrous undermining of the child's self-image (Loadman & McRae, 1977). To quote Lynch again, 'If the prognosis of child abuse is to improve, those working with these families must be prepared to look behind and beyond the overt abuse and ... to commit themselves to more than "crisis intervention".'

Battering and stunting do have in common the element of being visible and to that extent discernible to the alert clinician. There are, however, less tangible sequelae of deprivation no less significant in the long term, even though they may be less dramatic. They include delay in scholastic attainments (Neligan, 1974), more overt intellectual retardation (Lynch, 1978) and delinquency (Robins, 1966), all well documented. Aside from these, Pringle (1974) has drawn attention to more general impoverishment in the quality of living. Indeed, as demonstrated so conclusively in the Newcastle Survey of Child Development for 1960/62, as prospects for survival improve beyond the immediate postnatal period, obstetric hazards recede in significance in inverse ratio to socially determined factors (Neligan, 1974). In other words, at birth and immediately thereafter, biological faults take precedence over adversity in affecting developmental progress; but once viability has been established, psychosocial factors play a progressively greater role in any subsequent adaptational failure.

Cot deaths. There is one striking exception to this chronological sequence; the role of psychopathology in the sudden infant death syndrome (cot deaths). Although, as the name implies, cot deaths tragically occur at a stage in early infancy when biological factors are still in the ascendancy, inadequacy of mothering cannot be discounted as a contributory factor. The aetiology to be sure is multifactorial and organic pathology remains a major determinant even when it is cryptic. Undeniable, nevertheless, is the very real suspicion that if more of these young mothers could be alerted earlier to the subtle deterioration taking place in their babies' health, the ensuing tragic outcome could well be averted more often (Stanton et al, 1978). There can be no more poignant argument in favour of global assessment encompassing emotional as well as organic pathology.

Conclusion

A wide spectrum of problems has come under discussion. Despite their diverse character, they all exemplify two things—the inextricable linkage between intrinsic and extrinsic factors as regards causation and the all-pervasive import of family relationships irrespective of where or in what guise the problem presents.

In fact, parent/child interaction is central to every aspect of child health. Whatever the nature of the challenge—pressures at school, social stresses within the community, or the impact of disease or chronic handicap—a warm and mutually supportive cohesion acts as a buffer enabling the child to cope more effectively. Conversely, if the relationship is pathological and thereby unsupportive, any threat to personal security, whatever its source, becomes that much more difficult to contend with.

It follows that any programme of treatment to be effective must take cognizance of family function, however unrelated the setting in which difficulties seem to arise. This calls for greater parental involvement on the one hand and greater concentration of health care resources 'on the spot' to tackle problems at their source. This increasing focus on community paediatrics is reflected in the sponsorship of official Reports, first by the Court Committee (1976) governing general child health trends, and latterly by the Warnock Committee (1978). Both stress the importance of a firm community foundation, to keep the child so far as possible within his familiar fold by reducing segregation to a minimum. Warnock's emphasis for example is on special schooling rather than Special Schools (Anderson, 1976), to meet the special needs of different handicaps; and always in collaboration with the child's parents. Court lays equal emphasis on health care provision in the field, delivered primarily by designated family doctors and Health Visitors collaborating with school medical officers and community child health specialists.

Not all these recommendations can be implemented at once, but their intent is surely positive and their trend undeniably in the right direction.

REFERENCES

Achenbach T M 1966 The classification of children's psychiatric symptoms: a factor analytic study. Psychological Monographs 80: 1–37

Anderson E M 1976 Special schools or special schooling for the handicapped child? The debate in perspective. Journal of Child Psychology and Psychiatry 17: 151–155

Bakwin H, Bakwin R M 1972 Behaviour disorders in children, 4th edn. Saunders, Philadelphia and London

Berg I 1970 A follow-up study of school phobic adolescents admitted to an inpatient unit. Journal of Child Psychology and Psychiatry 11: 37–47

Brown G W, Harris T 1978 Social origins of depression. Tavistock Publications, London, p 181

Burton L 1975 The Family life of sick children. Routledge & Kegan Paul, London

Court S D M (chairman) 1972 Report of the Committee on Child Health Services. HMSO, London

Frommer E A, O'Shea G 1973 Antenatal identification of women liable to have problems in managing their infants. British Journal of Psychiatry 123: 149–156

Garside R F, Birch H, Scott D McI, Chambers S, Kolvin I, Tweddle E G, Barber L M 1975 Dimensions of temperament in infant school children. Journal of Child Psychology and Psychiatry 16 (3): 219–231

Gath A 1972 Mental health of siblings of congenitally abnormal children. Journal of Child Psychology and Psychiatry 13: 211–218

Gath A 1973 The school-age siblings of mongol children. British Journal of Psychiatry 123: 161–167

Gath A 1974 Sibling reactions to mental handicap: a comparison of the brothers and sisters of mongol children. Journal of Child Psychology and Psychiatry 15 (3): 187–198

Gath A 1977 The impact of an abnormal child upon the parents. British Journal of Psychiatry 130: 405–410

Kempe C H, Silverman F N, Steele B F, Droegemuller N, Silver H K 1962 The battered child syndrome. Journal of the American Medical Association 181: 17–24

Klaus M H, Kennell J H 1976 Parent-to-infant attachment. In: Hull D (ed) Recent advances in paediatrics, Churchill Livingstone, Edinburgh, ch 5

Kolvin I, Garside R F, Nicol A R, Leitch I, MacMillan A 1977 Screening schoolchildren for high risk of emotional and educational disorder. British Journal of Psychiatry 131: 192–206

Kolvin I, Wolff S, Barber L M, Tweddle E G, Garside R, Scott D McI, Chambers S 1975 Dimensions of behaviour in infant school children. British Journal of Psychiatry 126: 114–126

Linde L M, Rasof B, Dunn O J, Rabb E 1966 Attitudinal factors in congenital heart disease. Pediatrics 38: 91–101

Loadman A E, McRae K N 1977 The deprived child in adoption. Developmental Medicine and Child Neurology 19: 213–223

Lynch M A 1978 The prognosis of child abuse. Journal of Child Psychology and Psychiatry 19: 175–180

McCarthy D 1974 Physical effects and symptoms of the cycle of rejection. Proceedings of the Royal Society of Medicine 67: 1057–1061

Martin H P, Beezley P, Conway E S, Kempe C H 1974 The development of abused children. In: Advances in pediatrics. Year Book Medical Publishers, Chicago, p 21, 25–73

Mattsson A 1972 Long-term physical illness in children—a challenge to psychosocial adaptation. Pediatrics 50: 801–811

Mattsson A, Gross S 1966 Adaptational and defensive behaviour of young hemophiliacs and their parents. American Journal of Psychiatry 122: 1349–1356

Neligan G 1974 The paediatrician's role: a contribution towards a discussion of the cycle of deprivation. Proceedings of the Royal Society of Medicine 67: 1055–1056

Ounsted C, Lynch M A 1976 Family pathology as seen in England. In: Helfer R E, Kempe C H (eds) Child abuse and neglect: the family and the community. Ballanger, Cambridge, Mass.

Peterson D R 1961 Behaviour problems of middle childhood. Journal of Consulting Psychology 25: 205–209

Pinkerton P 1969 Managing the psychological aspects of cystic fibrosis. Arizona Medicine 26: 348–351

Pinkerton P 1970 Parental acceptance of the handicapped child. Developmental Medicine and Child Neurology 12: 207–212

Pinkerton P 1971a Childhood asthma. British Journal of Hospital Medicine 6: 331–338

Pinkerton P 1971b Depression v denial in childhood asthma: equipotent fatal hazards.

Proceedings of the 4th Union of European Paedopsychiatrists Congress, Stockholm, p. 187. Almqvist & Wiksell, Stockholm

Pinkerton P 1973 Paediatrics and child psychiatry. The case for collaboration. Archives of Disease in Childhood 48: 970–974

Pinkerton P 1974 Childhood disorder—a psychosomatic approach. Crosby Lockwood Staples, London

Pinkerton P 1975 Why not an 'at risk' register of deprivation? Update 10: 723–725

Pinkerton P 1978 Family function in fibrocystic disease. Update 16: 1449

Pless I B, Pinkerton P 1975 Chronic childhood disorder—promoting patterns of adjustment. Kimpton, London

Pollak M 1979 Housing and mothering. Archives of Disease in Childhood 54: 54–58

Powell G F, Brasel J. A, Raiti S, Blizzard R M 1967 Emotional deprivation and growth retardation simulating idiopathic hypopituitarism. New England Journal of Medicine 276: 1279–1283

Pringle M K 1974 Identifying deprived children. Proceedings of the Royal Society of Medicine 67: 1061–1062

Robins L N 1966 Deviant children grown up. Williams & Wilkins, New York

Rogers D, Tripp J, Bentovim A, Robinson A, Berry D, Goulding R 1976 Non-accidental poisoning: an extended syndrome of child abuse. British Medical Journal 1: 793–796

Rutter M 1973 Why are London children so disturbed? Proceedings of the Royal Society of Medicine 66: 1221–1225

Scott P D 1974 Battered wives. British Journal of Psychiatry 125: 433–441

Smith S M, Hanson R, Noble S 1974 Social aspects of the battered baby syndrome. British Journal of Psychiatry 125: 568–582

Stanton A N, Downham M A P S, Oakley J. R, Emery J. L, Knowelden J 1978 Terminal symptoms in children dying suddenly and unexpectedly at home. British Medical Journal 2: 1249–1251

Tew B J, Laurence K M, Payne H, Rawnsley K 1977 Marital stability following the birth of a child with spina bifida. British Journal of Psychiatry 131: 79–82

Thomas A, Chess S, Birch H G 1968 Temperament and behaviour disorders in children. University Press, London

Travis L B 1975 Care of children with diabetes. In: The care of children with chronic illnesses: report of the 67th Ross Conference of Pediatric Research. Ross Laboratories, Columbus, Ohio

Warnock H M (chairman) 1978 Special educational needs: Report of the Committee of Enquiry into the Education of Handicapped Children and Young People. HMSO, London

Warren W 1965 A study of adolescent psychiatric inpatients and the outcome six or more years later. Journal of Child Psychology and Psychiatry 6: 1–17, 141–160

Wolkind S N, Kruk S, Chaves L P 1976 Childhood separation experiences and psychosocial status in primiparous women: preliminary findings. British Journal of Psychiatry 128: 391–396

Wolkind S N 1977 Women who have been 'in care'—psychological and social status during pregnancy. Journal of Child Psychology and Psychiatry 18: 179–182

The adolescent years

The German word for adolescence, *Entwicklungsjahre*, means the unfolding years. Adolescence is a period of rapid change which can be confusing for the young people going through it and for the adults who have dealings with them. But because it is a period of change it provides opportunities for affecting personality development which may be lost if put off until adulthood.

A theoretical model

Because adolescence can be such a confusing period, it is important to have a theoretical model, or framework, within which to think about the problems of adolescents. There are a number of such models available and they have been succinctly reviewed by John Coleman (1974). The model that is presented here is based on the ideas of Erik Erikson.

As a child enters upon adolescence, he must begin to withdraw from his parents and to work towards achieving an adult identity. By the end of adolescence, he should be able, if he so wishes, to make his own way in the world and to choose a partner with whom to start up a new family.

The period between the beginning of withdrawal from parents and the achievement of an adult identity can be a very perplexing and lonely one. Some young people have to seek special ways of coping with their feelings of vulnerability. Adolescent gangs, for example, can act as a support to hold on to until they feel able to stand on their own feet. Often these gangs have colourful names which conjure up vivid pictures quite at variance with the impoverished emotional and intellectual lives of the individual gang members. It is as though the gang gives them a corporate identity which they lack individually.

Adolescents may also try to cope with their vulnerability by adopting what Erikson (1968) has called a 'negative identity': an adoption of attitudes and ways of behaving which seem to be the reverse of adult, particularly parental, ways of doing things. Such an identity is an extreme form of the negativistic behaviour which is characteristic of so many young people. Adolescents who have adopted a negative identity can be infuriating to adults, but it is helpful to remember that such an identity betokens an adolescent's underlying doubt about his ability to cope on his own.

The concept of identity is a difficult one. It is fully discussed by Erikson in the prologue to his book *Identity: Youth and Crisis* (1968). Erikson talks about a personal and a cultural identity. By a personal identity he means 'a subjective sense of an invigorating sameness and continuity'. By a cultural identity he means the affirmation of an individual's personal identity by those groups in society which are significant for him. For example, a doctor's professional identity is affirmed and reinforced because he belongs to a profession which has its own internal laws and even its own language.

In this chapter, the term 'adult identity' is simply defined in terms of the achievement of certain maturational tasks. If these tasks have been successfully negotiated then the individual is defined as having achieved an adult identity. There are five of these maturational tasks to be considered:

1. There is a work task. The adolescent has to begin to think about and prepare for the part that he will play in the world of work. Many adolescents find this difficult and drift from one job to another, or cease working altogether for a time (Evans & Moloney, 1974).

2. There is a peer group task. The adolescent must find a niche for himself in his peer group: a social role which, it is to be hoped, will be a satisfying one for him and his peers. Few young people get through adolescence without, at some time, feeling lonely and isolated. For a few of them this can be a major problem which they need help to overcome.

3. Adolescents have the task of mastering their newly acquired sex drive. This presents some young people with almost intolerably anxiety-provoking problems. A few of these will be discussed later. It is worth noting here, however, that contrary to the beliefs of some adults, most adolescents do not indulge in sexual activities with the degree of freedom and wholesale enjoyment that is commonly imagined.

4. Young people have to master the increase in aggressiveness that adolescence brings. Young people who have academic ability are able to channel some of this aggressiveness into passing examinations and getting on in the world. For them, there is the promise of a valued place in adult society. Many young people, however, can find no legitimate outlet for their aggressiveness and they find themselves clashing with the adult world. Unless they can be helped they can end up feeling embittered and hopeless.

5. Adolescents have the task of resolving the independence–dependence dilemma that they find themselves in. How do they begin to separate away from grown-ups when in many ways they are still dependent on them?

Alan, a 14-year-old, was referred to an adolescent unit for getting into trouble at school. His parents were separated, but not divorced, and they both came to the interview. Alan's mother complained that he never cleaned his teeth and never wore suitable clothes: he wouldn't do anything he was asked. In the interview Alan vigorously defended his right to use and abuse his body and to clothe it as he wished. When his parents started to talk about divorce, however, Alan became very upset. He was then able to talk about his need for his parents to stay together and about his desolation at the prospect of their splitting up for good.

Alan needed to assert his independence, but, at the same time, he felt dependent upon the combined support of his parents. It is this aspect of adolescence that many adults find most bewildering and disturbing. Young people want to have their cake and eat it.

With these five maturational tasks in mind, the question then follows what sorts of difficulties may commonly be encountered by those trying to help adolescents?

The neurotic adolescent

Younger adolescents tend to deal with feelings of anxiety and depression by taking some sort of action rather than complaining of anxiety and depression as such. This can be puzzling for adults who are trying to help them. Adolescents have a limited ability to talk about distress because of the immaturity of their cognitive faculties. The ability to think about thinking and so to handle concepts such as 'anxiety' and 'depression' is one that develops as adolescence progresses: it can baffle younger adolescents to be introduced to such concepts (Elkind, 1967).

Beryl, a very grown-up-seeming 14-year-old, kept getting into trouble at school and also had violent rows with her parents. She tended to stay out late and was in with a very bad set. She was sent to an approved school because of truancy and because she was outwith her parents' control. Her home seemed a good one and her bad behaviour was a mystery. Beryl herself was unable to talk about her difficulties and left adults feeling that they could not get through to her. Beryl's behaviour settled rapidly in the approved school, but as she became happier, her mother became more and more depressed. It soon became clear that this woman had been coping with feeling bad for years. Beryl had undoubtedly been affected by this, but had been unable to talk about her feelings—instead, she had behaved badly.

Older adolescents can present with symptoms of neurotic illness which conform more to adult patterns and they can express themselves in terms of feeling anxious or depressed. Their symptoms should always be viewed, however, against the background of their attempts to work out their adolescent maturational tasks and an effort should be made to relate their symptoms to such tasks, rather than trying to treat the symptoms in isolation.

Carol, aged 19, developed a choking sensation in the chest when she went on holiday with some girl-friends. On her return to her parents the sensation persisted and she also became agoraphobic. Anxiolytic and antidepressant drugs failed to help her and she had to be admitted to an adolescent unit. It became clear that Carol's choking symptoms during her holiday had started when one of her girl-friends went off with a young man. Carol seemed to be having difficulty in working out an adult sexual identity but, initially, the reasons for this were not clear. Eventually, when Carol and her parents had grown to trust the unit staff, Carol's father was able to talk about his adultery. Carol's father and her mother had, for some time, been using her as a confidante: each telling her about their own unhappiness. Carol had come to view sexuality as dangerous. It was some time before she felt able to free herself from her symptoms and to start having dealings with boys.

As happened in Carol's case, the effect of anxiolytic and antidepressant medication can be disappointing in adolescent patients. This is, in part, due to the fact that adolescents often resent taking prescribed medication and take it haphazardly or not at all. The use of drugs in children and adolescents has been discussed by Frommer (1967).

The self-injuring adolescent

The term 'attempted suicide' is an interpretation of behaviour rather than a diagnosis. It is doubtful whether most adolescents who cut or drug themselves are trying to kill themselves, and so the term 'attempted suicide' will not be used in this section. The term 'self-injury' will be used instead and it will include physical methods of injuring, such as cutting, and chemical methods, such as the taking of drug overdoses.

The incidence of self-injury rises sharply during adolescence, particularly at the age of 14. Many more girls than boys are referred to psychiatrists because of self-injury (Evans & Acton, 1972). Boys tend more to aggressive attacks on other people than to mutilating themselves.

The two most commonly encountered methods of self-injury in young people are the taking of drug overdoses and cutting. In the case of drug overdoses, these drugs have often been filched from the family medicine cabinet, and were originally prescribed for one or other parent. Cutting (often just superficial scratching) is generally of the wrists and arms, but not infrequently of the belly and face. The overdose or cutting is often carried out in a highly dramatic way and is exceedingly alarming for the other members of the family. The parents will often assume that an act of self-injury automatically indicates that their child is suffering from a serious mental illness and they will need to know that this is not necessarily the case. They will also need considerable support to contain their panic.

There are three typical situations involving self-injury which are likely to be encountered:

1. Very ill adolescents—for example those in a psychotic state—may attempt to injure themselves and will almost certainly need immediate admission to a psychiatric unit. Such young people, fortunately, crop up relatively infrequently.

2. The following is a much more common story.

Dinah, aged 16, had taken to staying out late at night. This upset her parents very much. She was an only child and had been adopted at the age of six weeks. Her parents doted on her. Dinah's mother was prone to depressions and had been particularly 'down' since having a hysterectomy. One night Dinah did not return home at all. When she turned up the next day, there was a tremendous row which culminated in Dinah's rushing upstairs and swallowing some of her mother's tablets. She immediately told her parents, was admitted to a medical ward overnight and then referred to a psychiatric unit. On examination, it was clear that Dinah needed help in achieving independence from her very loving parents. The sudden overdose was seen as an urgent attempt to draw attention to her difficulties: an act of independent defiance, as well as an expression of her need for help. In particular, Dinah needed support in separating from her mother whom she felt she was damaging by trying to achieve independence. Dinah's mood, and behaviour, improved when her father was helped to give more support to her mother.

3. From time to time, epidemics of self-injury will sweep through an institution, such as an approved school, which is looking after a large number of disturbed young people. Epidemics of this sort commonly take the form of arm scratching, or the infliction of friction burns, but almost anything can happen such as glass swallowing or ear poking. The outbreaks of crude self tattooing

that occur in ordinary secondary schools seem to be a milder form of the same phenomenon. Adolescents in general often seem to have a disregard, even a positive loathing, for their bodies: they are capable of abusing themselves in a way that can be very perplexing for adults.

School epidemics of self-injury usually run a natural course and, unless too much fuss is made about them, they cease as suddenly as they begin. In the course of them, however, school staff may need considerable support. On occasion, staff tensions will be found to have contributed to the epidemic.

In conclusion, all attempts at self-injury by young people should be taken seriously, but they do not in themselves necessarily indicate serious mental illness. Indeed young people are often alarmed by the reaction to their self-injury.

The school-refusing adolescent

The distinction between truanting and school phobia was first clearly made by Adelaide Johnson and her colleagues in the early 1940s (Johnson et al, 1941). The term 'school refusal' is now more commonly used than 'school phobia' because the latter term implies that a specific irrational fear of school is the central psychopathological feature. In practice, this is not necessarily the case.

Hersov (1960), distinguishing between truancy and school refusal, wrote: 'Persistent non-attendance (at school) may take the form of truancy—that is, unlawful absence from school without the parents' knowledge or permission—or it may manifest itself as a refusal to go to school in the face of persuasion, recrimination and punishment from parents, in addition to pressure from school authorities. Truancy is most often part of a rebellion against adverse home circumstances, associated with a lack of satisfaction at home and at school, whereas school refusal, without truancy, may be an outstanding symptom of psychoneurotic disorder.'

There is a high incidence of school refusal at about the time of starting secondary education. At least one of the causes of this must be the transition from the relatively undemanding primary school environment to the more formal world of the secondary school. Nevertheless, school refusal is usually just one aspect of an adolescent's difficulties in coping with maturational tasks. Traditionally, it has been seen as resulting from a child's over-close relationship with his mother. During adolescence such a child has more than usual difficulty in working out his independence–dependence task. His attempts to separate and grow up are perceived by him as damaging to his mother. He therefore withdraws from the task and opts for safety by remaining inappropriately dependent; by refusing to go to school he contrives to stay close to his mother or at any rate to home. This is a safe solution, but a frustrating one: school refusers are often very angry young people, although at first their anger may be cloaked by apparent complaisance.

Skynner (1974) has pointed out that the fathers of families with a school-refusing child may also play a key part in the development of the symptom. Because of their lack of authority, they do not claim the mother, sexually or socially, so that she is forced to remain in an over-close relationship with her child.

The choice of method of management of school refusal will depend upon the level of personality development that has been achieved by the individual adolescent; some are more firmly tied to their mothers than others. The management will also vary from therapist to therapist. Some therapists will invariably try to look at family difficulties and will regard the adolescent's school refusal as just one aspect of these difficulties. Other therapists will prefer to treat the problem symptomatically, using anxiolytic or antidepressant drugs (such as diazepam and trimipramine). Alternatively they may set up a system whereby the adolescent can be escorted to school: at first for a short period only, and gradually staying for more of the school day until they have fallen back into the habit of school attendance. If the problem proves intractable to such measures, admission to a psychiatric unit or to a boarding school for maladjusted adolescents may be necessary.

School refusers are capable of stubbornly resisting all attempts to help them and they have a knack of making people feel that they are being hard and insensitive when they try to help them to get back to school. It is, however, usually a mistake to give in to the school refuser's entreaties: if a course of management has been decided upon this must be adhered to (Bruggen & Pitt-Aikens, 1975).

Eating problems

Anorexia nervosa
There are few situations more frightening, both for parents and doctors, than being faced with a child who seems determined to starve to death. Perhaps it is the sense of urgency provoked by this symptom that has led to anorexia nervosa being studied so extensively.

This condition is characteristically found in girls in mid-adolescence: only about one in 20 anorexic patients are boys. The patient is very likely to have been overweight before the onset of her illness, which is typically ushered in by an attempt to lose weight through dieting. Once the girl has started to lose weight she seems to be unable to stop and may even resort to subterfuges such as vomiting and purging. Secondary amenorrhoea may occur quite early in the illness as a result of complex hormonal changes that occur as weight is lost (*British Medical Journal*, 1975).

Anorexic patients seem to be particularly anxious to avoid carbohydrate-rich foods. On occasion, however, they will go on eating binges in which they stuff themselves. After such binges they feel racked with guilt.

Once the illness has become established, hospital admission is usually necessary. The details of in-patient management differ from unit to unit, but a successful outcome depends upon the presence in that unit of nursing, medical and social work staff, who are able to work closely and efficiently together: such a team provides mutual support for its members when they are faced with the anxieties that the anorexic patient and her family can generate. The initial management of the patient must be based on a firm policy designed to make quite sure that the patient does eat. It is important for the staff to be absolutely in control so that the patient is not allowed room to manipulate her diet. Where there are lapses in control the patient will exploit them and be left feeling panicky and hopeless.

It is generally accepted that anorexic patients have what amounts to a phobia of weight gain. The individual and familial determinants of this phobia have provided a rich field for psychopathological speculation: a commonly held view is that by remaining underweight the patient can put off dealing with adolescent maturational tasks which are experienced by her as being overwhelming: in particular the task of achieving an adult sexual identity (Crisp & Kalucy, 1974).

Obesity
Adolescents are very preoccupied with their appearance and constantly compare their clothes and bodies with those of their peers. The obese adolescent can feel acutely unhappy and may come in for a great deal of teasing. Nevertheless, it is only a minority of fat adolescents who are disturbed enough to warrant medical help. There are many causes of overeating in adolescence and it is difficult to isolate any one psychopathological feature. However, Hilde Bruch (1971) writes: 'In the disturbed group (of obese young people), with their great individual differences, certain common features can be recognized. In all cases the development of obesity is related to the fact that food and eating are used to appease non-nutritional needs and tensions which are erroneously interpreted as "desire to eat". In some instances the ordinary demands of adolescence are experienced as threatening and dangerous.' She goes on to say that the parents of obese children are 'apt to superimpose their feelings and values on the developing child, expressing this in every detail of his physical and psychological care'. Thus, when faced with the maturational tasks of adolescence, these young people are ill-prepared to begin the withdrawal from their parents and gradual achievement of an adult identity. In severe cases, the obese adolescent may even feel that he has no right to his own body. Overeating seems to be an attempt to deal with this feeling—as though by feeding his body he may get it to come alive for him.

In trying to help these young people it is not enough to rely upon dieting: symptomatic treatment is usually only effective when combined with attempts to help with individual and family problems.

Sexual problems
With puberty, adolescents find themselves with the task of working out an adult sexual identity. In other words they must work towards feeling free to choose a partner of the opposite sex with whom they can have a mutually satisfying genital and intimate social relationship.

There can be few adolescents who manage to work out their sexual identity without some qualms, and many experience very considerable difficulties. It would be wrong to assume that because young people are having sexual intercourse, they are fully mature sexually. There is a distinction to be made between physiological maturity and an adolescent's capacity to commit himself fully to a relationship with another person. Those teenagers who do marry are often opting for an instant pseudo-maturity as an alternative to tolerating a period of uncertainty. Frequently there are young people to whom the prospect of uncertainty is particularly daunting because of bad and confusing experiences earlier in their lives.

Despite the fact that many adolescents harbour doubts and even fears about their sexuality, young people do not necessarily welcome well-meaning attempts by grown-ups to enlighten them. They can perceive such attempts as tantamount to seduction. Usually they are happiest with rather formal instructions about the 'facts of life'. They will tend to shy away from discussion of their personal sexual doubtings.

Paradoxically adolescents tend to expect high moral standards from grown-ups with whom they have dealings. They feel acutely let down when these are not lived up to. It is a grave mistake for adults to try to win over young people by talking with them in the same kind of florid sexual language that adolescents can use among themselves. Often, particularly in the course of group counselling and group psychotherapy sessions, they will appear to be inviting one to join in, but this pressure should be resisted.

Schofield (1968) has made a useful contribution to the writings on adolescent sexual behaviour. Certain sexual difficulties are commonly encountered in work with adolescents.

Homosexuality
Homosexual tendencies in adolescent boys and girls are so common that it is very nearly meaningless to attach the label 'homosexual' to a particular boy or girl. When young people (they are usually boys) are referred for help because of homosexual activities, it is best to think in terms of their having difficulties in working out an adult sexual identity; and to look for factors in them, and in their families, which may be leading to such difficulties.

Edward, aged 15, was a boarder at a public school. The school doctor had been asked to help with him because the headmaster felt that Edward's homosexual activities were getting beyond what could normally be coped with: he persisted in getting into bed with other boys in his dormitory in spite of punishment, and there had been complaints from other boys' parents.

When Edward was seen by a psychiatrist, it became clear that he was a very unhappy boy indeed. His parents had separated about six months before and Edward didn't know where he would be staying during his next holiday. He described his father as a frightening, cold, academic man, on whom he felt he could make few demands. There was very little that could be done about Edward's miserable home situation, but he was helped by having someone to confide in, and his blatant 'homosexuality' subsided.

Occasionally, a complaint of homosexuality can be the presenting symptom of a severe psychiatric disturbance.

Frank, aged 14, had told his school housemaster that other boys were calling him a 'queer'. Frank felt that they were referring to incidents which had occurred at his preparatory school about which he felt very guilty. On examination by a psychiatrist it soon became clear that Frank was so out of touch with reality that he bordered on the psychotic. He warranted in-patient treatment, not for his homosexuality, but for his psychotic illness.

A complaint of homosexuality by an adolescent or by adults responsible for him, should always lead to a full assessment of the difficulties of both the adolescent and his family. For both Edward and Frank the complaint of homosexuality was only one aspect of a much larger problem.

Sexually promiscuous girls
In our society, sexually promiscuous girls are always unhappy girls. This may not, at first, be apparent because their promiscuity is a way of dealing with their unhappiness. Such girls often appear tough and woman-of-the-worldish, but those who work with them know that they are often quite naive about sexual matters, and that they suffer great embarrassment when talking about sex.

The sexual promiscuity of these girls is often an aspect of their inability to trust in another person. They move from boyfriend to boyfriend because it is safer to leave than to risk being left. Their inability to bestow trust generally has its origins in their having been let down in various ways throughout their childhood. At the same time, their ability to attract members of the opposite sex reassures them about their desirability. They and their families may derive help from psychiatric in-patient treatment, or they may need the more restricted setting of some approved schools. As these girls shift away from their sexual promiscuity into new ways of coping with their difficulties, they often have to endure a period of depression through which they will need to be supported. Where a girl has become established in a life of prostitution, with the secondary gain that such a life can provide, she may be beyond radical help.

Adolescent girls who get themselves pregnant often start off by feeling very happy at the prospect of having a baby. They have a tendency, however, to change their minds, generally at about the third month of gestation, when the fantasy about having a baby finally, and undeniably, becomes a fact. The question of abortion is one to which there is no right answer. It is useful to bear in mind, however, that these girls (and their families) can change their minds frequently: the doctor will usually have to take the onus of decision upon himself, and carry his decision through with as much courage and conviction as he can muster. Doctors are frequently requested to consider putting sexually promiscuous girls on the contraceptive pill. Unfortunately, these girls are as impulsive about the taking of medication as they are about their sexual relationships: they cannot be relied upon to stick to the recommended pattern of dosage. The prescription of the 'pill' also leaves out of account the desire that many of these girls have to become pregnant.

Exhibitionism and inverted sexuality (transvestism and transsexuality)
Most adolescent boys harbour at least some doubts about their sexual capabilities. Many of them are also rather hazy about the details of where babies come from. They frequently, openly or surreptitiously, compare the size of their penises with those of other boys, and their indulgence in flamboyantly dirty jokes acts both as a reassurance and as a way of comparing their own sexual fantasies with those of other boys—in this way, they get to an approximate understanding of the realities of sex. All this is normal, and is in the nature of a way-station on the road to an adult male sexual identity.

However, a few boys get stuck and feel themselves forced to give expression to their sexual drive in outlandish ways which society finds unacceptable. Boys who exhibit themselves, and boys who dress in women's clothing, are encountered quite frequently by those who work with adolescents.

Exhibiting boys, and their families, often conform to a typical pattern. The father is distant, and is perceived by the mother as weak. He is perceived by the boy as an unattractive person with whom he feels reluctant to identify. The boy and his mother, however, are very close. This closeness leads to a difficulty in separating because of the security that the relationship provides. But since inevitably such a relationship smothers the boy's drive towards independence, it results in the boy's impotent fury with the mother and with women in general. This fury gains partial expression in the act of exhibiting (Rooth, 1971).

Dressing-up in women's clothing (transvestism) and the fixed idea that one is a girl, although biologically a boy (transsexualism), are syndromes which may blur into one another, although not all transvestite boys feel that they are transsexual. Boys who cross-dress, but who are not transsexual, often have a family constellation which is similar to that of boys who exhibit: they perceive their fathers as distant and their mothers as close.

It has been suggested that transsexual boys and men have a defect in their 'core gender identity' (Stoller, 1964) which dates from very early childhood.

Exhibiting and sexually inverted boys are often in need of in-patient treatment; they and their families can present very complex psychopathological problems.

Adolescents and drugs

It has been said that there are more people addicted to the drug problem than to the drugs themselves. Certainly adults can overreact to drug abuse by young people, but there can be no doubt that adolescents are experimenting with drugs far more now than they were some years ago. Boyd (1971), quoting United Kingdom Home Office figures, makes the point that between 1967 and 1968 there was a 93 per cent increase in opiate addiction in the under-20 age group.

A considerable variety of drugs are abused by young people. Those that are commonly encountered include cannabis, amphetamines, lysergide, barbiturates and Mandrax. It should not be forgotten, however, that young people abuse tobacco and alcohol far more than any other drugs and, indeed, there is growing alarm about the apparent increase in alcohol abuse by adolescents.

There has been much written about the chemical composition of drugs and about their physiological and psychological effects. Boyd (1971) has provided an excellent review of the field. For practical purposes, it is useful to divide adolescent drug abusers into three groups.

1. Those who try drugs on a few isolated occasions as part of a current fad or experiment. They want to find out what all the fuss is about and don't want to feel left out. The great majority of these young people feel pretty unimpressed by their drug experience and soon move on to something more interesting. However, these group fads can be very alarming for parents if they happen to find out about them. A psychiatrist was asked for some advice by a colleague whose daughter had been caught sniffing glue in the local youth centre. It turned out that this had been going on for a week or so and that a large number of young people were involved. It was clearly impracticable to try to help each individual family which had a child involved, and so the psychiatrist met with all the parents to talk about the whole issue of drug abuse. This meeting was successful

in allaying the anxiety of most of the parents, and a week or so later the whole affair had blown over. The young people's glue sniffing had to some extent been perpetuated by their parents' alarm—when the latter abated, the young people lost interest.

2. Those who, for various reasons, are having difficulties with their adolescent maturational tasks and use drugs to allay their anxieties. Their use of drugs also qualifies them to adopt a negative identity which helps them to cope with at least a few of their uncertainties. These young people find the prospect of uncertainty overwhelming and, whilst masquerading as radicals, they can present themselves and their views in a manner which is tinged with infuriatingly conservative dogmatism. Such young people (and their families) need help with the personal problems that their negative identity and drug abuse are cloaking.

Graham, aged 17, was referred to a psychiatrist because he had failed to get a job since leaving school and seemed to be drifting. He was associating with a like-minded set of young people and he admitted to the habitual use of cannabis and the not infrequent use of other drugs such as lysergide and amphetamines. He was a bright young man who had passed a large number of 'O' levels. His parents were in despair and whilst making endless demands on them, Graham treated them with contempt. Graham was seen individually by a psychiatrist for about nine months, whilst his parents met with a social worker. At the end of this time, Graham felt able to meet in the same room with his parents and the three of them were able to work out a number of issues with the psychiatrist and social worker. It became clear that many of Graham's difficulties had arisen because he had been born with deformed legs, and had needed extensive orthopaedic treatment. He had been in plaster for a long time as a small child, and his parents had had to carry him about until he was quite old; for them, he was a very special baby. When Graham came to his adolescent maturational tasks he, and his parents, faced difficulties in separating. Graham dealt with his closeness to his parents by careering in the opposite direction and trying to achieve independence through a negative identity which was reinforced by his gang of cronies. The psychiatrist and the social worker acted as a bridge between Graham and his parents whilst they worked out a new relationship; and Graham was able to find himself a job and cut down his drug consumption.

3. The young people who, for various reasons, have deeply flawed personalities and who seem able to get through life only by the severe abuse of drugs—in particular by the persistent use of intravenous opiates and especially heroin (diacetylmorphine). They often seem to be quite indiscriminate in their drug abuse, and will try anything that they feel might be psychoactive. They can present as charming, reasonable, even self-composed, but this veneer covers a deep disturbance and it is a good rule always to consult a specialist when considering the management of these young people. Many of them require admission to a special drug unit before they can really be helped: unfortunately, such units, and the staff qualified to work in them, are few and far between.

The psychotic adolescent
Adolescents are very frightened by madness and not a few harbour secret fears that they are themselves going mad. Certainly, the disorganized thinking and labile emotional state of some young people can lead a doctor to suspect a psychotic illness where none exists. 'Early schizophrenic illness' is a diagnosis which is quite frequently applied to disturbed young people, but in only a very few

of such cases does the diagnosis turn out to be correct. To some extent the fault here lies with psychiatry. A formal examination of mental status, looking for such phenomena as thought-blocking, thought-alienation and auditory hallucinations, can be a very frightening experience for an adolescent, and can actually precipitate disorganization in their thinking, as well as rendering them suspicious of and hostile towards the examiner.

An 18-year-old girl, Hannah, had just moved to a job in a large town from her home in the country. She felt depressed and 'strange' and was referred to a psychiatrist. He felt worried about her and admitted her to a psychiatric ward for observation. Her condition seemed to deteriorate: she maintained that she still felt strange and, in addition, now had the idea that she was the reincarnation of an Egyptian mummified cat. It was thought that she might be developing a schizophrenic illness, but the histrionic quality to her symptoms left room for doubt. She was discharged to the out-patient care of an adolescent psychiatrist who arranged to meet her with her parents. It soon became clear that there were very considerable family problems and that Hannah's move to the town was an attempt to escape from them. Her 'symptoms' subsided rapidly when her difficulties were viewed against the background of her attempt to separate from a disorganized family.

A diagnosis of schizophrenia in an adolescent can generally only be made with certainty after a prolonged period of careful observation. The treatment is largely that for adult schizophrenic patients. Phenothiazines and butyrophenone drugs are of immense value, and particularly valuable are depot phenothiazines, such as fluphenazine enanthate, because of the tendency of adolescents to shun medication prescribed by doctors. Adolescents may have to be chased up to make quite sure that they are getting their injections: it is no good relying on them to organize themselves. Also adolescents will often try to persuade the doctor that they no longer need their injections and he may have to be very firm with them. Some schizophrenic adolescents have great difficulty in coping at home and for them closely supervised hostel accommodation can prove a great support.

It should, of course, always be borne in mind that schizophrenic adolescents, like other young people, have maturational tasks to accomplish and that they need particular help and support with them.

From time to time, a practitioner working with adolescents will encounter a young person who seems to have developed an acute psychotic illness in response to a specific stressful situation.

A 14-year-old, Ian, was referred to a psychiatrist because he seemed to be very frightened, and had been keeping his family up at night following his discharge from hospital four days before. He had had a hernia repaired and all had gone well during the operation. Ian maintained, however, that the man in the bed next to him had made homosexual advances: there seemed to be some doubt about the truth of this. Ian had no previous history of psychiatric disorder. On examination, he appeared to be terrified and was almost incoherent; he seemed to want to bolt from the room. He was given large doses of oral chlorpromazine for a week or so, and his illness settled rapidly.

The prognosis for such 'reactive psychoses' (Warren & Cameron, 1950) seems to be favourable. Acute psychotic episodes may, of course, be triggered off by such drugs as amphetamine and lysergide and this possibility should always be borne in mind.

Assessment of adolescents in difficulties

In working with adolescents it is hard to think neatly in terms of assessment, diagnosis and treatment. Young people demand a directness of relationship which makes it difficult to retain any sort of objectivity in one's dealings with them. But for this very reason it is important to have some sort of assessment scheme in mind in order to avoid being swamped by their demands.

Because adolescents do not have their existence in isolation, an assessment of an individual adolescent's difficulties must consist of three parts:

of the adolescent;

of his family or the people who are standing in for them;

of those members of society who are involved with the adolescent and his family.

Let us consider each of these separately.

The adolescent

1. The assessor must try to decide which of the adolescent's difficulties lie primarily in the present and which have their roots in the past: that is, are the adolescent's difficulties in working through maturational tasks principally the result of present problems, or are his difficulties being exacerbated by earlier childhood problems? If childhood problems are being exacerbated, these will have to be taken into account even though they appear to be remote from the present difficulties.

Jane, aged 16, had, as an infant, suffered from bilateral congenital dislocation of the hips and from pyloric stenosis. She was in hospital on a number of occasions. Subsequently, she was also found to have slight brain damage. All in all, she was a difficult baby to mother, and her mother felt a failure. Jane was a quiet girl until the age of 14 when she started to take drugs and to indulge in sexual promiscuity: it was clear that her struggles to cope with adolescent maturational tasks were being made more difficult by the upsets in her earliest infant relationship with her mother. Both Jane and her family needed prolonged psychotherapeutic help before they were able to achieve even a semblance of normal relationships.

2. There must be an assessment of the ways in which the adolescent is trying to cope with his difficulties: for example, by adopting a negative identity or by trying to deny the need to become independent by remaining immature and clinging to parents.

3. To what extent are the ways of coping with difficulties in working out maturational tasks going to prejudice the adolescent's future prospects? For example, is his adoption of a negative identity wrecking his progress in school? Some ways of coping can be potentially useful, although they may also lead to difficulties: for example an excessive sublimation into academic studies and academic achievement may be paid for with impoverished relationships.

4. If the adolescent presents with psychiatric symptoms to which a definite diagnosis can be attached, this should of course be noted. The Group for the Advancement of Psychiatry (1966) classification of psychiatric disorders of adolescence is a helpful guide. It should, however, be accepted that diagnostic labels are of limited usefulness in adolescence: young people can seem to shift from one diagnostic category to another, perhaps from day to day, and even from

hour to hour. Also, a diagnostic label can be seized upon by an adolescent as a ready-made identity allowing him to retreat from his maturational tasks. 'I am suffering from a depressive illness so how can I possibly be expected to cope with life's problems?'

5. Which are the particular maturational tasks that the adolescent is having difficulty with? All of them—or just one or two?

The adolescent's family
An assessment should always be made of the adolescent's family or of those standing in for the family. One must ask whether they also need help and to what extent the parents' difficulties are the cause of, or the result of, the adolescent's difficulties. The latter is often a very difficult question to answer. Is the adolescent relatively healthy but being used as a ticket of entry to gain help for another member of the family?

> Keith, a bright 15-year-old, started to refuse to go to school. When seen by a psychiatrist, he seemed a pleasant, healthy boy. It soon became apparent however, that his mother was developing a schizophrenic illness of paranoid type. When help was arranged for her, Keith returned to school.

The adolescent and other members of society
The referral of an adolescent for help may be the culmination of a complex series of events which constitute a covert reason for referral. This possibility must always be borne in mind.

> Twin girls, Linda and Margaret, were referred to a psychiatric unit from a girls' hostel. One of the girls was described as being a truant, and the other as a fantastic liar. On examination it became clear that the girls' difficulties had started about two months previously, at the time, that the deputy matron of the hostel had left. This woman had kept the hostel together, and since her departure everybody, girls and staff, had been upset: almost any one of them could, reasonably, have been referred for help. When the psychiatrist arranged extra support for the hostel staff, everybody in the hostel, including the twins, settled down. It would have been a waste of time to have tried to treat the twins while disregarding their social situation.

An adequate assessment, taking account of the factors listed above, should give the basis for a provisional plan of management and treatment.

Management and treatment
In this section, the various methods of treatment and management will be dealt with in separate sections: but of course in any given case two or more of these methods may be used in combination.

Individual counselling and psychotherapy
The essential difference between counselling and psychotherapy lies in the fact that whereas counselling is confined to talking over with an adolescent his day-to-day difficulties, the aim of psychotherapy is usually to give the patient some insight into the part his unconscious is playing in his attempts to deal with his difficulties.

The form that individual psychotherapy takes will vary according to the age of the adolescent. For older adolescents, psychotherapeutic techniques suitable for adults can be used. These rely heavily upon the use of words and upon the therapist's use of himself as a blank screen: his aim being to introduce his own personality as little as possible. The therapist working with the middle range of adolescents (age 14½ to 17½) needs to be much more direct and confronting. He is required to act as an interpreter, helping the adolescent to find a language in which to express thoughts and feelings which have hitherto been expressed in actions. Younger adolescents (age 12 to 14½) are preoccupied with beginning to separate from grown-ups and they do not take easily to being closeted in a room with a stranger who asks them probing questions. Young adolescents can sometimes find it easier to talk if the discussion takes the form of a game. Winnicott's (1971) squiggle technique can be of particular use here: it can act both as an assessment tool and as a vehicle for treatment.

Group counselling and psychotherapy
Group psychotherapy, like work with individual patients, aims at giving insight to the group members, whilst group counselling provides a forum in which to discuss particular difficulties (MacLennan & Felsenfeld, 1968). An example of the latter would be the course of weekly meetings held in a girls' approved school, in which the aim was to talk about baby care, child health and sexual relationships. If it is planned to set up group counselling in a school, it goes without saying that it is very important to keep the head teacher informed about what is being discussed from week to week. If he is left in the dark, all sorts of obstacles will crop up which will inevitably wreck the counselling programme.

In adolescent psychotherapy groups, as opposed to adult groups, much of the therapist's time and energy is spent in setting limits, and in directly confronting the young people with the outcome of their behaviour. The effect of this is to make such groups immensely difficult to work with, and for those who run them it is essential to have someone available to talk to about the problems that have arisen, and to offset the strain of holding their own with the adolescents (Bruce, 1978).

Residential management and treatment
It is important to note that to cover the whole spectrum of adolescent disorder, it is essential to have available a range of residential facilities. Any residential unit which tries to cater for all types of adolescent problem is sure to find itself in grave difficulties.

In this section, the term residential unit includes psychiatric units, drug units, approved schools, boarding schools for maladjusted adolescents, and hostels, but the principles hold good for any residential unit dealing with adolescents.

Each unit has to develop its own philosophy. In this context, philosophy means both day-to-day policy and the theoretical assumptions that underlie such a policy. On the whole, residential units will admit those adolescents who they feel can be helped by their particular unit philosophy. They will only admit other adolescents if they are forced to do so by external circumstances, or if they feel that they can learn something by admitting an adolescent whom they would not normally feel able to help.

One important reason for the need in residential units for a consistent philosophy is the tendency for disturbed young people to play adults off against each other. In the absence of a philosophy, such manipulation can lead to staff anxiety and to tensions between staff members which ultimately prove intolerable—at worst, staff morale can break down completely.

There are five main types of residential unit philosophy.

1. *The medical philosophy* in which the aim is to diagnose psychiatric disease and to treat it with the most effective means available. Not all psychiatric units have this as their philosophy.

2. *The training and educational philosophy* in which the aim is to train young people to behave better, and to provide them with basic social, educational and work skills. Such a philosophy is found in many approved schools.

3. *The punishment and containment philosophy* in which the aim is to remove from society those young people whose behaviour is intolerable, and to teach them that such behaviour is unacceptable. Some approved schools still use this model, and it is certainly applied by many penal institutions dealing with young people.

4. *The child-care philosophy* in which the basic assumption is that young people in serious difficulties have suffered from a lack of love in childhood. Units with this philosophy aim to make good such lack of love. This will frequently involve them in handling very regressed, child-like, or even baby-like behaviour, and is very demanding of staff time and emotion. Redl & Wineman (1965) have provided a good account of such a unit.

5. *The therapeutic community philosophy:* this developed during the Second World War when psychiatrists were asked to try to help large numbers of servicemen who had dropped out of active service for emotional reasons. Therapeutic communities attempt to get away from the traditional medical model of psychiatry and to shift the focus away from individual patients to the functioning of the institution as a whole. This approach can be particularly useful with adolescents. It provides them with support, and at the same time it allows them to work out, through participation in the running of the unit, more adult ways of coping with their difficulties.

The therapeutic community approach also allows some modification of behaviour through peer group pressure—young people often find this more acceptable than being told what to do by adults.

In any particular unit, there may be elements from a number of these philosophies, but if a unit dealing with adolescents is to survive, it has to have one basic philosophy to fall back upon in times of crisis.

Family therapy
There is at present considerable interest in psychotherapeutic treatment involving the whole family. Although family therapists differ as to their particular

techniques, most base their work on the systems theory of Ludwig von Bertalanffy (1950). According to this theory, the symptoms presented by an adolescent are indicative of a malfunctioning family system rather than of psychopathology within the adolescent Some family therapists (Minuchin, 1974) pay no heed whatsoever to the past history of family members and work entirely with family interaction as it is observed in the here and now. Other family therapists (Dare, 1979; Cooklin, 1979) have tried to integrate psychoanalytical theories of personality development with systems theory.

Family therapy is particularly important in work with adolescents. The adolescent very readily feels under attack from adults and may believe that parents and therapists are ranged against him. The presence of siblings during therapy helps to offset this suspicion and in the course of therapy his own problems find their proper perspective in the context of the problems, as they emerge, of his parents and siblings.

A concise account of theories and techniques of family therapy has been given by Walrond-Skinner (1976).

Vocational guidance

It is common for young people to have difficulty in deciding what sort of work they want to do. In the United Kingdom they can seek help from a number of sources.

Most schools now have a careers master (or mistress) who is available to discuss job prospects with children leaving school. Too often, however, such teachers have had inadequate training in vocational guidance, and are given little support in their work by their colleagues.

Alternatively, young people can turn to the Careers Service of their local education authority. Careers officers can be a great help because they are in touch with the job market in their area and can also direct young people to training courses. Not infrequently, however, careers officers find themselves trying to place young people with very considerable cognitive and personality difficulties who need help of a specialized kind. Such specialized help is offered by a few psychologists who have a special interest in vocational guidance. The aim of such a psychologist is usually to assess, as far as possible, the adolescent's intelligence using a test such as the Wechsler Intelligence Scale for Children, and then to look for specific areas of difficulty: for example, perceptual defects, impulsiveness, and inability to tolerate stress. When this basic information has been obtained, a comparison can be made between the adolescent's expressed interests and job preferences, and those that he reveals in a more objective test situation, using, for example, the Kuder Preference Record. The aim is to help both the adolescent and his family to get a more realistic idea of his capabilities and potential. To this end, the information obtained in the course of testing must be fed back to the adolescent, and to his parents. This can be a difficult task requiring some understanding of psychodynamics. Indeed, if the adolescent has considerable personality difficulties, vocational guidance may need to go hand in hand with psychotherapy (Boreham, 1967).

Consultancy
Dealing day after day with emotionally disturbed adolescents is exhausting. Increasingly the staff of residential units and, indeed, of ordinary day schools, are asking for help from outside consultants. It is useful for such consultants to bear in mind three vital points. First, they will be on the receiving end of much of the staff's angry feelings. Second, they must keep their sights low and not expect to alter the institution in any radical way. Third, they must be able to achieve a working relationship with the head of the institution—if they cannot do so, they are wasting their time (Caplan, 1959).

Conclusion
There exists a school of thought which sees adolescence as being by its nature a time of turmoil and considers that the only course of action needed to help troubled adolescents is to wait until they 'grow out of it'. In fact, psychiatric pathology is only slightly commoner in adolescents than in younger children and adults (Rutter et al, 1976) and alienation of young people from their parents is not a common feature unless adolescents are already showing signs of psychiatric disorder. There is absolutely no evidence that psychiatric disorders arising during adolescence follow a more benign course than those arising at any other period of life. The development of psychiatric services is therefore quite as important for adolescents as for children and adults. The Royal College of Psychiatrists has recently produced a memorandum on the psychiatry of adolescence. It recommends a three-fold expansion of existing manpower in services to deal exclusively with adolescence: the aim being to make possible the existence of an adolescent psychiatric team for every 500 000 total population.

REFERENCES

Boreham J L 1967 The psychodynamic diagnosis and treatment of vocational problems. British Journal of Social and Clinical Psychology 6: 150–158
Boyd P R 1971 Drug abuse and addiction in adolescents. In: Howells J G (ed) Modern perspectives in adolescent psychiatry. Oliver & Boyd, Edinburgh, ch 13
British Medical Journal 1975 British Medical Journal i: 52–53
Bruce T J R 1978 Group work with adolescents. Journal of Adolescence 1: 47–54
Bruch H 1971 Obesity in adolescence. In: Howells J G (ed) Modern perspectives in adult education. Oliver & Boyd, Edinburgh, ch 11
Bruggen P, Pitt-Aikens T 1975 Authority as a key factor in adolescent disturbance. British Journal of Medical Psychology 48: 153–159
Caplan G 1959 Concepts of mental health and consultation: their application in public health social work. Children's Bureau Publication No. 373. US Department of Health, Education and Welfare Administration, Washington
Coleman J C 1974 Relationships in adolescence. Routledge & Kegan Paul, London and Boston
Cooklin A A 1979 A psycho-analytic framework for a systemic approach to family therapy. Journal of Family Therapy 1: 153–165
Crisp A H, Kalucy R S 1974 Aspects of the perceptual disorder in anorexia nervosa. British Journal of Medical Psychology 47: 349–361
Dare C 1979 Psycho-analysis and systems in family therapy. Journal of Family Therapy 1: 137–151
Elkind D 1967 Egocentrism in adolescence. Child Development 38: 1025–1034
Erikson E H 1968 Identity: youth and crisis. Faber & Faber, London
Evans J, Acton, W P 1972 A psychiatric service for the disturbed adolescent. British Journal of Psychiatry 120: 429–432

Evans J, Moloney, L 1974 Adolescents and work difficulties. British Journal of Psychiatry 124: 203–207

Frommer E A 1967 Treatment of childhood depression with anti-depressant drugs. British Medical Journal, i: 729–732

Graham P, Rutter M 1973 Psychiatric disorder in the young adolescent: a follow-up study. Proceedings of the Royal Society of Medicine 66: 1226–1229

Group for the Advancement of Psychiatry 1966 Report No. 62. Psychopathological disorders in childhood: theoretical considerations and proposed classification

Hersov L A 1960 Persistent non-attendance at school. Journal of Child Psychology and Psychiatry 1: 130–136

Johnson A M, Falstein E L, Szurek S, Svendsen M 1941 School phobia. American Journal of Orthopsychiatry 11: 702–711

MacLennan B, Felsenfeld N 1968 Group counselling and psychotherapy with adolescents. Columbia University Press, New York and London

Minuchin S 1974 Families and family therapy. Tavistock Publications, London

Redl F, Wineman D 1965 Children who hate. The Free Press, New York

Rooth F G 1971 Indecent exposure and exhibitionism. British Journal of Hospital Medicine 5: 521–533

Rutter M, Graham P, Chadwick O F D, Yule W 1976 Adolescent turmoil: fact or fiction? Journal of Child Psychology and Psychiatry 17: 35–56

Schofield M 1968 The sexual behaviour of young people. Penguin, Harmondsworth

Skynner A C R 1974 School phobia: a reappraisal. British Journal of Medical Psychology 47: 1–16

Stoller R 1964 Contribution to study of gender identity. International Journal of Psychoanalysis 45: 220–226

von Bertalanffy L 1950 The theory of open systems in physics and biology. Science 111: 23–29

Walrond-Skinner S 1976 Family therapy: the treatment of natural systems. Routledge & Kegan Paul, London

Warren W, Cameron K 1950 Reactive psychosis in adolescence. Journal of Mental Science 96: 448–457

Winnicott D W 1971 Therapeutic consultations in child psychiatry. Hogarth Press and Institute of Psychoanalysis, London

5

Phyllida Parsloe

Troubled and troublesome children

Behaviour and health, growth and disturbance, learning and security are interdependent. No clear dividing lines exist between these aspects of a child's being and no one discipline has a monopoly in any one area. Doctors who are in touch with their patients and who have shown a concern for suffering, backed by the authority of their medical knowledge, are likely to be consulted about a wide range of problem situations and problem behaviour amongst their child patients. This chapter is particularly concerned with troubled and troublesome behaviour in children and young people* which can eventually bring them within the jurisdiction of the juvenile justice system. The fact that the subject is here defined in relation to the juvenile justice system should not be taken to mean that there is any inevitable connection between certain types of behaviour and a court appearance. More and more the emphasis is upon prevention, to use the British term, or diversion from the juvenile justice system, to use the language of the United States. This means that when a doctor feels that his troubled child patients need help of a kind that he has neither the training nor the facilities to provide, there are likely to be resources available in the community. Doctors need to build up knowledge of the particular resources of their area: this chapter will attempt to give an over-view of the legal and social framework, as it relates to troubled and troublesome children in the United States, England and Scotland.

That children should receive special protection or treatment from the law is a twentieth-century innovation although it is based upon ideas and practices which developed earlier. Until the end of the nineteenth century children who committed criminal offences were dealt with by the same courts in which adults were tried. Many were sentenced to imprisonment and served their sentences alongside adult prisoners. The situation caused growing concern as it became recognized that prisons were schools of corruption and that children were not just miniature adults but particularly malleable personalities. This recognition led to concern not only about children who committed offences but also about children being brought up by criminal and pauper parents, being taught to beg

---

* English juvenile courts deal with 'children', who are those up to 14 years old and with 'young people' age 14 to 17. Young people are not a category in Scottish or American law. In Scotland a child for the purposes of compulsory care is someone up to 16 years old and in the United States the upper limit of juvenile court jurisdiction varies from state to state. In this chapter 'child' will mean a person of an age to be liable to compulsory measures of care, and to avoid repetition will include young people.

or to become prostitutes, or being subjected to harsh physical treatment from adults. Such ideas led to the establishment in 1899 in Chicago of the first juvenile court. Most of the other states rapidly followed Illinois and in 1908 the Children Act established juvenile courts for England and Scotland.

From the beginning, juvenile courts had jurisdiction over children who committed offences and those whose behaviour did not contravene the criminal law but who were considered to be in need of care. In other words they had both criminal and civil jurisdiction.

There are differences between the American and British courts, and Scotland has recently developed a completely new system of lay hearings for children in trouble: however the grounds providing jurisdiction for courts or hearings are very similar. Children who can become subject to this jurisdiction can be divided into four groups.

1. Those who commit acts which, if they were committed by an adult, would be a criminal offence. Most of such acts are offences against property, particularly stealing, but offences against the person, which seem to be a feature of city life, are on the increase amongst juveniles. In the past it was often suggested that juvenile crime was not a particularly serious matter. It is difficult to hold this view today, when Berlins & Wansell (1974) point out that in 1972, 22 per cent of all indictable offences in England and Wales were committed by under-17-year-olds. This figure included 40 per cent of all burglaries and 16 per cent of all crimes of violence against the person.

The reason why this group of children is described with such carefully chosen words is that in the Scottish system and in most American states a child cannot be charged with a criminal offence. The act, which would be a crime if he or she were an adult, can however be used in Scotland as the basis for a claim that the child needs compulsory measures of care or, in the United States, that the child should be adjudged a delinquent. In England, children and young people can still be charged with criminal offences, although it was the intention of the Labour government, which was responsible for drafting the 1969 Children and Young Persons Act, that the possibility of criminal charges should be greatly restricted. However the Labour party was in opposition when the Act, which was to be implemented in stages, became law and by the time it returned to power the juvenile justice system had come under so much criticism that the government had little impetus while in office to act on its original intentions.

2. The second group comprises children who behave in ways which are illegal because of their age. The most usual behaviour of this kind is truancy, but the group also includes certain sexual acts which are prohibited below specified ages.

There is considerable argument about this category of behaviour and a growing feeling, particularly in the United States, that courts should deal only with criminal acts. However a great many children both in the United States and in Britain are subject to compulsory measures of care because they truant from school. This may have more to do with society's apparent inability to change its often irrelevant school systems, than with any shortcomings in the individual child.

3. The third group comprises children who are said to be in a particular state

or condition rather than to have committed specific acts. They are children who are 'incorrigible', or 'in moral danger'. They include children who are said to be beyond the control of their parents. Such children may display all kinds of behaviour, but frequently they stay out late or all night and run away from their homes. The idea of parents having to tell a court that a child is beyond their control is distressing and seems to bode ill for future child–parent relationships. For this reason in England restrictions are placed upon the parents' right to bring their children before a court: they must consult the local authority social service department and can only initiate proceedings where the social workers cannot help and also refuse to take the case to court themselves. As with the non-criminal acts so with these so-called 'status offences' there is considerable disagreement as to whether such children should be subject to compulsory powers and particularly whether they should be dealt with alongside children who have committed criminal acts.

4. There is a fourth group over which the juvenile justice systems are given jurisdiction, comprising children who are neglected, or actively harmed by their parents either by battering or by sexual assaults. This group is of particular concern to family doctors but is outside the scope of this chapter.

Theories about the causes of troubled and troublesome behaviour

Juvenile delinquency
There is a considerable literature on the causes of juvenile delinquency. Delinquency is a term which has no legal meaning in Britain although it is usually used to refer to children who have committed criminal acts. In the United States it is a legal term since the court finds a child to be a delinquent if it is satisfied that the child falls into one of the groupings discussed above.

Until recently, research about the causes of delinquency has focused upon the child, and has been based on the underlying assumption that children who commit offences are in some way different, either personally or socially, from those who do not. Now sociologists interested in deviance have begun to study the part played by society, through its schools, police, social workers and courts, in creating juvenile delinquents. The various theories tend to exist in isolation from one another: nevertheless, the doctor faced by an individual child who is said to be truanting from school or stealing from the local shops needs some way of understanding how this particular child relates to his social world and how this world has contributed to making him what he is.

Nineteenth-century writers blamed poverty, drunken and criminal parents, theatregoing and lack of religion for juvenile crime. Their works were impressionistic and the first scientific study of criminals is usually attributed to Lombroso (1911), although he is remembered more for his theory that criminals were physically different from other men than for the methodology for which he was responsible. His ideas were discredited by Goring (1913) who found that English prisoners could not be distinguished physically from members of a non-penal control group.

The idea that there may be a physical basis, which if it does not cause crime may at least predispose people to impulsive acts, continues to intrigue researchers. Sheldon (1949) developed a scheme which linked body type with personality and claimed that the mesomorph, who is muscular and aggressive, is most likely to become a criminal. The Gluecks (1968) too have studied physical characteristics, this time of juvenile delinquents, in an attempt to develop a prediction tool. The latest interest in physical characteristics is in the possibility that men with an additional Y chromosome may have violent or criminal propensities. The evidence for this is at best sketchy (Fox, 1971) but it has renewed interest in the field of criminal biology. These researchers were hoping to find a single physical factor which might determine criminality. While we cannot rule out the possibility that future research may uncover some factor which determines some criminal behaviour, the present view is that physical abnormalities and defects are likely to play a part in making a child who is vulnerable in other ways yet more likely to be involved in delinquent behaviour.

Acknowledged juvenile delinquency is predominantly a feature of city life and of the poorer parts of cities. These observations led sociologists to explore the social background from which delinquents come and to develop theories to explain the apparent urban, male, working-class nature of juvenile delinquency. One set of theories built on the ideas of Durkheim (1951). Merton (1938) made use of Durkheim's theory of anomie or normlessness and applied this to delinquency. He suggested that when children are taught the goals at which they should aim and are then denied the means to achieve them because of their place in the social system, stress and frustration result and norm breakdown and deviant behaviour develop. In an age when most children watch television they are exposed to success symbols and life-styles which they are unlikely to be able to achieve if they live in a poor district with overcrowded schools and limited employment openings. Other sociologists (Cloward & Ohlin, 1960) built on Merton's idea, showing how gangs or groups of adolescents develop in such areas and how the gang provides the support and success opportunities which school and employment may be failing to do. The gangs and the neighbourhood also offer the opportunities to learn delinquent behaviour since, like any other behaviour, delinquency has to be learned. Some researchers, such as Miller (1958), have suggested that delinquent behaviour is very similar to working-class behaviour and that the features of toughness, smartness, excitement and a belief in the power of fate which characterize working-class culture find expression in delinquent behaviour.

The sociological theories have been characterized by Hirschi (1969) as falling into three groups. Those which he calls 'strain theories' rest on the assumption that legitimate desires which a person cannot satisfy create a strain which forces him into delinquency. Merton, Cloward and Ohlin are typical of strain theorists. Other theorists postulate that the reason why a person is free to commit delinquent acts is that his ties to the conventional order have been broken or failed to develop. It is not that delinquent children have legitimate but unattainable ambitions but that they never develop the ties to society which create such ambitions. Matza (1964) and Reckless (1967) are exponents of 'control theories'. The third group Hirschi calls 'theories of cultural deviance': these suggest that delinquents conform, not to the standards of the larger society, but to their own local culture. Miller is an exponent of such a theory. Hirschi claims that his own research shows that a social control theory provides the best explanation of the facts. He found that the child with little stake in the community is the most susceptible to the prodelinquent influences in his environment.

Sociological theories are concerned to explain tendencies in groups of people, not individual behaviour. However even in the most deprived ghetto area all children do not get into trouble and it is the factors which cause one individual to offend and another not to which have interested psychologists. There is a major division amongst them between those who see a delinquent act as having an unconscious, or at least a hidden, meaning and those who see it simply as a response which has occurred because of faulty learning.

The first group draw their ideas from the psychoanalytic schools and in particular from those which emphasize the importance of family relationships. Winnicott (1963) has suggested that delinquent behaviour in the form of stealing means a child has not given up hope that somehow the environment, in the shape of his parents, will meet his needs. In the past it was thought that early mother–child separation would lead to later stealing by children who developed an affectionless character (Bowlby, 1946). While there is no doubt that separation can have long-lasting effects, we know now that its evils can be minimized if the child's world is not too seriously disturbed and if a substitute for his mother is available. None of the psychoanalytic explanations of juvenile delinquency is either specific or direct. They link behaviour in the present to deprivation or trauma in the past and the exact way in which stealing comes symbolically to mean a demand for love is obscure. This is not to say these theories are unhelpful. They often seem to mean something to parents who will produce past events as explanations of present behaviour without any prompting.

Faulty family interaction
So far the focus of the research we have considered has been upon children who commit criminal acts. However, an area of work with families has developed in attempts to understand and to treat the many emotional problems of children, some of which may take forms such as school phobia or running away which may lead to appearance in court. One interesting set of ideas sees the child as the agent for the family. The most familiar role which a child agent plays is that of scapegoat. Doctors will be familiar with families where one child is represented as being everything that is bad and the family feel that if only this child could be placed in a Home all would be well. Unfortunately all too often all is not well and another child may be selected as scapegoat to cover the family badness. This theory of the child as agent, albeit a willing agent, seems to offer some help in understanding situations where, for example, a family complain about their thieving son and yet always leave their purses and wallets, stuffed with money, in readily accessible places for him. A similar example is of the adolescent girl whose mother seems to drive her into a pregnancy by endless talk of how she fears her daughter will become pregnant and no provision for sex education or contraception. Psychoanalytic theory suggests that the child in these situations acts out the parent's unconscious wishes.

The possibility that the child is agent for the family is one which doctors should take seriously but it is hard for them to adjust their highly individual medical approach and to develop an understanding of interaction in family groups.

An understanding of family interaction is not the same as the popular idea that parents are to blame for their children's behaviour and that the one who should really be sentenced by the court is the mother, not the child. This is merely to shift the individual focus from child to parent and to see the child as a helpless pawn. A real grasp of interaction precludes blaming since it is based on the assumption that all of us, adults and children, constantly behave as agents for each other. What requires adjustment is the relationship between parent and child rather than the parent or the child himself.

Psychologists who accept learning theory do not consider that there is any need to explore causes of behaviour, since the cause is always that the person has learned maladaptive responses to particular types of situations. What matters is that new learning situations be established and the family helped to stop rewarding responses which might lead into delinquent behaviour.

Delinquency as a process

The shortcoming of sociological and psychological theories is often their static nature. They deal with given environments or past trauma and the links from environment to individual maturation or from past to present are obscure. Some theories do, however, explain delinquency as a process. The accepted version of this process is normally seen as a chain. Members of lower social classes are said not to possess the familial or other resources to acquire cognitive or social skills which lead to success in school. Failure to achieve in school produces strain which is increased if family relationships are unsupportive or broken. Strain consists of a lowered sense of self-worth, alienation and loss of status. Children under strain then turn to deviant peer groups as an alternative means of achieving status and a feeling of belonging.

$$\text{Lower-class membership}$$
$$\downarrow$$
$$\text{Decreased achievement}$$
$$\downarrow$$
$$\text{Increased strain}$$
$$\downarrow$$
$$\text{Identification with delinquents}$$
$$\downarrow$$
$$\text{Delinquent acts}$$

Empey & Lubeck (1973) have tested this process on delinquent and non-delinquent groups. They found that social class was of little explanatory value; a fact which supports a growing belief that middle-class children are also involved in much illegal behaviour but are less likely to be caught. With this exception they found the process did operate in real life. School grades, separation from parents and poor family relationships were all highly predictive of future delinquent acts. They go on to suggest that the process is not a straight chain but involves feedback loops. Children suffering from strain behave in ways which further weaken their position in family and school and so increase the strain. They also suggest that identification may result from, as well as precede, delinquent acts and the stigma which results from prosecution for delinquent behaviour once again increases strain.

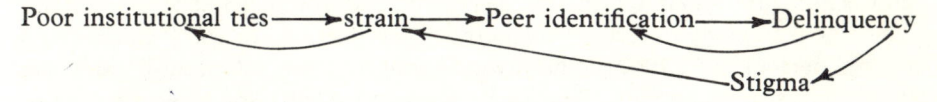

Poor institutional ties ⟶ strain ⟶ Peer identification ⟶ Delinquency ⟶ Stigma (with feedback arrows)

Interactionist theory

So far we have considered explanations of delinquency which take the child as the focus for explanation. The interactionists however are interested in the processes by which society selects, from among the many children who commit delinquent acts, a much smaller group and then processes some of these into the juvenile justice system. Interactionists have studied only parts of the process and the empirical base for their conclusions about processing juvenile delinquents is still rather weak. There have, however, been studies of police practice (Cicourel, 1968) which suggest that in the United States poor black adolescents are more likely to be picked up than other children and that they are also more likely to be referred to the juvenile court from the police station, especially if they are either particularly aggressive or particularly co-operative with the station officer. Once a person has been processed through a court they are much more likely to appear there again. Partly this is because they are now labelled and have attributed to them a master role of juvenile delinquent. Police, public and social workers know this. What is equally important is that somewhere during this process, it is said, the adolescent adjusts his image of himself and begins to see himself as a juvenile delinquent. No longer is he just John who happened to get caught shoplifting—he is John a juvenile delinquent. Once he thus shifts his perception of himself he begins to feel the strains of a poor self-image and to find himself in situations where further delinquency becomes more and more likely. Not only has society labelled him but he has accepted the label and begun to live down to its demands. The process is only a little different from that by which a person acquires the label of doctor and adjusts his self-image and behaviour to fit the expectations which he and others have of a person with this label. The delinquent however lacks the choice which most doctors have had in acquiring their label and 'delinquency' is a negative label entailing stigma, whereas 'doctor' is a positive label giving status.

Treatment measures

With such a range of possible theories and explanations for delinquency and other deviant behaviour, it would be strange if treatment procedures were specific. In fact they are not. Their wide-ranging nature reflects the different theoretical possibilities about causation.

In recent years social planners in Britain and the United States have been influenced by the interactionist approach with its emphasis on society's part in labelling children 'delinquent' and the subsequent problems of managing a spoiled identity. Their response, at least in theory, has been to regard the juvenile justice system as a place of last resort and to emphasize the need to prevent children from entering the system. Children, it is said, should be referred to courts or children's hearings only if there is no other way in which they can get the help they need. This is written into the English law where juvenile courts can take action only if the child's behaviour and status bring him or her within their jurisdiction *and* if the child 'is in need of care or control which he is unlikely to receive unless the court makes an order' (Children and Young Persons Act, 1969). The juvenile courts in most American states act under similar requirements. The Social Work (Scotland) Act, 1968, which contains in Part III the law relating to children in need of compulsory measures of care, does not include such a specific statement. However the whole intention of the Act is that children should receive help on a consensual basis. The law also provides a gatekeeper to the hearing system in the form of a reporter. The reporter has absolute discretion to decide which of the children referred to him by police, social workers, schools and occasionally doctors or members of the public, shall be taken before a children's hearing. The criteria on which reporters make this decision seem to vary but all pay at least some attention to whether or not the child can be helped or prevented from further offences by non-compulsory measures.

In Britain the responsibility for providing help to children in trouble lies with the social work staff of the local authority Social Service department (the Social Work department in Scotland). A child can be referred to the area social work team for the neighbourhood in which he lives by doctors or teachers, or by the police or reporters. He will then be allocated to one of the social workers, who will make an assessment of the child and his family, usually by visiting the home but sometimes by asking the child and his parents to come to the office. Assessment should include discussions with the school and, where there are indications of family health problems, with the family doctor. The underlying assumption on which the social worker operates is one of maximum participation by the child and family in the solution of their own problems. Ideally family and worker together plan what, if any, help is needed. The social worker has three possible ways of helping families:

1. He can provide material help through his own department. Since 1963 local authorities have been authorized to provide financial help to prevent a child being received into care or coming before the juvenile court. Scottish social workers have extended powers under Section 12 of the 1968 Act to give financial help in order to 'promote social welfare'. These financial powers are most frequently used to help families with rent, gas and electricity bills but some social workers also use them to provide holidays or, for example, sports equipment for children in the family. Besides money the Social Service and Social Work departments can provide other 'hard services' such as day care (see Ch. 14).

2. The social worker can act as an advocate or broker for a family with other services. Many families lack the social skills and self-confidence to find their way through the intricacies of the welfare state and as a result get less than their rights. Social workers may help a family to obtain their full entitlements from insurance and supplementary benefits, show them how to make use of medical and dental services or, most frequently, act as advocate for them with the housing department. In acting as an advocate the social worker is seeing

the family as the unit which requires help. Many social workers are beginning to believe that such a piecemeal individual approach is wasteful and stigmatizing for the family. This belief leads them to take a community view of social problems and to work to enable families in a locality with similar situations to come together to solve them. Such social workers see the problem, not as one of family inadequacy, but as political powerlessness. They suggest that what such families need is not advocacy, but power, and the belief that they can change their own situation. Such social workers would help family members to use or to create welfare rights groups, tenants' associations or youth clubs in their neighbourhood and, by uniting, to alter their power base.

This attitude to social problems is more prevalent amongst people who call themselves 'community workers' and who frequently work for voluntary agencies. However some community workers are being appointed to local authority departments and many social workers in their training are exposed to a community work approach and carry this into their local authority jobs.

3. The third area of social work is individual, family or group counselling. Here the emphasis is upon changing attitudes and relationships within and between family members. The social worker may decide that a child referred because of criminal activities needs a caring adult outside the family with whom to talk over ideas about himself and society. On the other hand the difficulty may seem to lie not with the child at all but in the marital relationships of the parents. Here the child may be no more than a pawn in their marital game and counselling is needed with the parents and not the child. Sometimes however a child may have been exposed to his parents' marital problems so long that he has taken them inside himself and acts them out on behalf of the family. Here family group discussions may be the treatment of choice, since members of a group may be able to see how they are using each other and eventually take responsibility for their own behaviour.

This summary of the way social workers can help pre-delinquent children indicates the very general approach which social workers use. They seldom focus solely on the individual child in trouble but are likely to assume that the child's difficulties result from general social or relationship problems in the family. There is however an exception to this rule. Social Service departments have developed intermediate treatment which is intended specifically for children in trouble.

Intermediate treatment
It is easier to name this treatment than to describe it. It is called intermediate because it aims to fill the gap in provision that exists between social work with a child in his own family and removal of a child from his home to some form of residential care. Children who are likely to get into trouble with the law have not usually been able to use traditional youth organizations and so their leisure time is often unorganized. Each area in England and increasingly in Scotland has developed plans for intermediate treatment. For some areas this has meant building a link between the youth service and the social service so that the youth services adapt their programmes to make them more accessible to disadvantaged

children. In addition, however, local authorities and voluntary agencies have developed special programmes for these children. These are usually based on the idea of a club which may meet from one night to every night in the week and may include overnight accommodation or residential periods such as camping or holiday trips. The emphasis is usually upon developing close adult–child relationships and encouraging peer group relationships. Some intermediate treatment schemes have engaged adults from the children's home communities as voluntary workers.

Intermediate treatment schemes are part of an attempt to prevent children entering the juvenile justice system, and they highlight some of the difficulties in preventing delinquency. Most theories agree that one of the best protections against delinquency is to have a non-delinquent self-image and to belong to a non-delinquent peer group. Therefore it would seem logical to try to include in leisure activites, children who have started down the route to delinquency alongside children who do not see themselves as delinquent. Unfortunately delinquent or pre-delinquent children are by definition less likely to be able to make use of such facilities and need special leisuretime activities designed for their particular needs. Once society begins to provide such special facilities it is labelling the children while at the same time attempting to offer ways of decreasing the strain on the child. Intermediate treatment also faces the difficulty of how far a child should or should not have gone along the delinquency road before being allowed to join. At one extreme if the programme is open to all children the disadvantaged ones for whom it is particularly designed may be pushed out. At the other extreme if children who have been before the courts are included or even required to attend, children who are at risk but have not yet come to an official hearing may be stigmatized by association and their delinquent labelling and self-image strengthened.

Similar difficulties confront the Youth Service Bureau which has been established in the United States with the aim, as Norman (1973) says, of 'diverting children from the juvenile justice system'. American local government has no equivalent of Social Service departments carrying ultimate responsibility for children in trouble. Several government departments and many voluntary agencies share the responsibility and children often fall into the gaps between them and get no service. It was concern about such gaps, as well as the acceptance that juvenile court appearances are stigmatizing, which led the federal government to offer part funding of the Youth Service Bureau. Norman suggests that the Bureau should have three functions:

1. Receiving referrals of children from police and probation departments and ensuring that they receive the service they need. The Bureau should preferably not provide service itself but by advocacy or cash payments secure it from other agencies. The Bureau should then follow up and make sure the child has received what he or she needs, be it psychiatric help, family counselling or a foster or group home placement.

2. Developing resources in the community for children in trouble. The Bureau should encourage and enable other agencies to adopt their existing programmes or develop new ones to meet the needs of local youth.

3. Working to change attitudes to troubled youth amongst the public, and particularly amongst groups such as school staff and police who have direct contact with them.

It is interesting to compare the American attempts at diversion with those in Britain. The emphasis in Britain in intermediate treatment is largely upon direct service, although the local authority Social Service departments have an overall obligation to develop resources for children as part of their general responsibility for social welfare and for preventing children appearing before the courts. The idea of changing community attitudes is not so clearly the responsibility of anyone in Britain, although some community workers and social workers define it as a part of their job.

Compulsory measures of care
Once a child has been referred to a court or hearing and found to be in need of compulsory measures, the dispositional alternatives available vary little between England, Scotland and the United States. They can be considered as falling into three groups.

1. *Measures which do not involve any ongoing contact with court or social workers.* All courts and hearings have the option of doing nothing. For some children the appearance itself will have been sufficient to pull them up short and deter any further antisocial behaviour. This is particularly likely with children from relatively stable homes who have become involved in adolescent exploratory behaviour which leads them into conflict with the law. Vaz (1961) has suggested that much middle-class delinquency like shoplifting 'originated as a game played for excitement and novelty'.

If the court or hearing wants to impose some control over a child for a period of time it can, in the United States or Scotland, make use of a deferred decision, and in England of a conditional discharge, which means the case is discharged after a period of time if the child is not involved in further antisocial acts. English juvenile courts also have the power to fine parents and young people. Because fining is regarded as a punishment for a crime, this power is not available to Scottish hearings and American juvenile courts because, unlike English juvenile courts, they have no criminal jurisdiction. Hearings are tribunals outside the justice system and American juvenile courts have only civil jurisdiction.

2. *Measures involving supervision in the community.* The most commonly used measure is to place the child under the supervision of a social worker or a probation officer in England, a social worker in Scotland, or a probation officer in the United States. The supervisor works with the child and family in the ways already described but has a legal right to see the child in the office and in his own home. The supervision order thus includes an element of compulsion and control which is not a part of voluntary supervision. Supervision orders (which may be called probation orders, supervision orders or supervision requirements) may contain specific conditions. For example a child may, with the agreement of the doctor concerned, be required to attend his general practitioner for physical treatment or the child guidance clinic for psychotherapy. He may be required

to attend a club or accept intermediate treatment; or to stop meeting particular friends, going to certain parts of the town or visiting named cafés or drive-in restaurants. Children who break the conditions in their orders or fail to keep in touch with their supervisor can be brought back to the court or hearing for alternative treatment measures.

3. *Measures involving removal from home.* All courts and hearings have powers to remove children from their homes. They can place them in one of two types of care. First, a child can be committed to the care of the local authority by means of a care order (England), residential supervision requirement (Scotland) or committal (United States). The local authority or welfare department social worker then places the child in whatever setting seems most suitable. This may be a private foster home, a small or a large children's home, a residential school or a hostel. In all these situations the child will be with other children and young people who have never been before a court or hearing but whose parents have made voluntary agreements with the authorities for their care. Second, a child may be committed by the court, or placed by the local authority, in an establishment designed particularly for children who have appeared before courts or hearings. In the United States there are State schools run by the Departments of Corrections and juvenile courts can commit either directly to these schools or to the state youth authority, which then decides whether or not to place the child in this type of facility, where there are usually considerable restrictions upon the child's freedom. In Scotland hearings can commit children to List D schools. This curious name comes from a wish to avoid the old name of 'approved school'. They are in fact schools intended to receive children from the hearings which have been put on a list titled 'D' by the central government department known as the Social Work Services Group. In England the courts can no longer commit children to specific institutions. The establishments which used to be known as approved schools and which received children for whom courts made approved school orders are now part of what is known as the community home system. Social Service departments are responsible for maintaining a flexible system of community homes to meet the needs of all children in their care. Courts can only commit children to the care of the local authority and the social worker then makes the decision as to the type of facility needed. This has led to a great deal of discontent amongst juvenile court magistrates, especially when the children are returned to their own homes by social workers after the court has made a care order. Magistrates regret the passing of the old law which allowed them to commit children to approved schools which, they claim, gave the community some protection at least for a while.

All orders which involve a child's being removed from his own home are made for an indefinite period. The time at which a child can return to his home is decided by social workers and residential staff in England and the United States and by the panel members at a follow-up hearing in Scotland. The tendency is for periods away from home to be as short as possible and to be measured in months rather than years.

In England the juvenile court still has powers to give to some young people who break the law, sentences which are clearly punitive in their intention. Had the 1969 Children and Young Persons Act been fully implemented, these powers would have been removed. Since then the climate of opinion has changed and in the late 1970s there is considerable pressure to increase the power of courts to punish young offenders. So far no new Act has been introduced and juvenile courts may only make Attendance and Detention Centre orders. The former involve weekly attendance, often on Saturday afternoons, at a centre (usually run by the police) until a specified number of hours have been served. A Detention Centre order involves three months' residence in an institution run by the prison service. The juvenile court may also refer some young offenders to the Crown Court for consideration of a Borstal sentence. Borstals are also prison service establishments and provide a disciplined regime including work training for an indeterminate period, which is usually about 10 months.

Children's hearings in Scotland and American juvenile courts have no such penal dispositions at their disposal. In Scotland however, some children who commit particularly serious offences are dealt with not by the hearing system but by the sheriff court. The sheriff can sentence the older juvenile offenders to Borstal or to a young offenders institution which is a prison in all but name.

In addition to these committal powers, all three countries make provision under their mental health acts for severely disturbed children to be committed compulsorily to mental hospitals for containment and treatment.

The tensions in the juvenile justice system
Juvenile courts and children's hearings are asked by society to balance a number of conflicting concerns. They are required to consider the welfare of the child but also to protect the community. There is little doubt that from the child's point of view the least harmful thing is usually to do nothing, but the public are said to be unable to tolerate this. In fact the public seldom know much about what happens because hearings are not open to the public and the press are normally forbidden to publish any identifying information. However the magistrates, panel members of hearings and juvenile court judges all interpret their role as that of balancing the child's needs against the protection of the public. This may mean that at times they make orders which are not in the best interest of the child, although this should only happen in cases where a child's antisocial behaviour is serious or particularly dangerous.

This balancing of child's needs against public interest is often confounded by the state of our knowledge about how to change and control behaviour. It is clear that punishing children as an example to other potential wrongdoers, that is, punishment as general deterrence, or punishing children to express society's revenge has no place in the official policy of juvenile justice. However it is much less clear whether punishment in order to deter the individual child from similar future action is acceptable. That depends upon our belief as to how people change. There tends to be a clash of beliefs between people working in the system. Very generally speaking, police, magistrates, panel members and lawyers accept that punishment is a means of altering future behaviour. Social workers have more doubts about this particularly as they are the people who are expected to carry out the punishment, either by making demands on the child while he remains in his own home or by providing a disciplined and controlled environment away from home.

When social workers discuss these issues about their own work, they tend to express them in terms of how far they are willing to act as agents of social control. Most would probably agree that children vary in their need for control, or at least for structure, and that while some neurotic children need a permissive environment in which they may learn that their worst fears are not realized, many delinquent children who act out need an environment where they are controlled, while they gradually learn how to develop controls for themselves.

The tension between caring and punishing and the arguments as to whether punishing is a form of caring run through the juvenile justice system. They are not just apparent between different groups who have different ideologies but can be seen within any one individual. This, however, is not necessarily a cause for concern but for recognition. What society is asking of its juvenile justice system is that it hold a balance between these conflicting forces and not move too far in either direction. A juvenile court should not be a criminal court nor should it be a child guidance clinic.

Concern over caring and punishing is not the only source of tension. Courts and hearings have potentially wide powers over children's lives. In the past these were justified by the argument that since the court's purpose was to meet the child's needs the child did not require protection against the court. This view was more typical of the United States than of England, where the fact that the juvenile court was a criminal court meant that some attention was always given to children's legal rights. The new system of hearings in Scotland, however, denies the possibility of conflicting interests in its emphasis upon discussion with the parents and child with the intention of reaching an agreement about the outcome. Officially children's hearings only deal with situations where parents and child agree with the facts which serve as the reason for the hearing. Where facts are disputed the child must be referred to a sheriff for a decision on the facts. This, however, ignores the possibility that if a lawyer were asked to agree to the facts he would be likely to raise questions such as those of intent, which would not occur to a layman or child but which might lead a judge to decide that the hearing had no jurisdiction.

It is part of the traditional rhetoric of juvenile justice to hold that the court and the child have no conflict of interest and that committal to institutions meets the child's needs. A greater understanding of labelling theories and a more realistic view of many state institutions, List D schools and community homes would suggest a clear conflict of interest. Committal to an institution may be the lesser of the evils or the only solution in a world with few resources to spare for troubled children, but it is seldom in a child's best interest. If one accepts this viewpoint, then children's rights need protecting and the juvenile justice system must open itself to defence lawyers. This is happening in the United States since the Supreme Court in the Gault decision (in re Gault, 1967) stated that children liable to committal were entitled to most of the rights to a trial by due process of law ensured to adult criminal offenders in the constitution. In England there has been some increase in frequency of lawyers appearing in juvenile courts but in Scotland they are virtually unknown in the hearings where they are probably most needed. As well as balancing a child's needs against those of the public, the system must balance a child's needs against his legal rights.

The family doctor and troubled children

General practitioners are often confronted by anxious and confused parents seeking help with their children's social and emotional problems, and the doctor's training makes it natural for him to turn to the medical model. The parents support this because it is what they hope to achieve: parents who consult doctors about children's behaviour do so, in part at least, in the hope that the behaviour can be defined as sickness rather than as badness. Especially amongst middle-class parents sickness provides a more acceptable definition than does badness with its attendant reflection upon themselves as parents.

Sickness, however, may not be the most helpful label from the point of view of future change, since it involves a labelling process and also implies that cure rests with the medical profession into whose hands the family will commit themselves. Probably the most helpful way a doctor can behave is to keep the question an open one allowing the behaviour to be defined as an occasional act, a stage in development, or a piece of exploration. All these allow for ways out of the situation and for seeing it as within the wide range of what comprises normal behaviour. Klein (1973) suggests that 'a concerned policy of doing nothing may be more helpful than active intervention if the long range goal is to reduce the probability of repetition of the acts'. Klein was addressing himself to the police but the same may hold for doctors. It will however be hard for them to reverse their usual procedure and resist the pressure to diagnose. Scheff (1970) has pointed out that with questions of mental illness (and I would add of delinquency), the danger lies in diagnosing rather than in failure to diagnose. This is the reverse of much medical practice where the price of over-diagnosing is no more than some anxiety in the patient. In mental illness and delinquency the price of over-diagnosing may be the beginning of labelling and of an altered self-image for the patient. Because of the doctor's powerful role, a family's perception of a child's stealing may be altered, and the labelling process accelerated, when a doctor diagnoses that a child is stealing and on the way to becoming delinquent. A doctor who listens with concern and does no more may allow child and family to find other ways out of the process.

Sometimes, however, a doctor may have to take some action. This may involve offering some counselling himself and/or referring the child and family for additional help. Where a doctor is well known to the family and trusted by them he has a great advantage over anyone he may call in, because the relationship needed for effective counselling already exists. Doctors may, however, feel reluctant to undertake extensive counselling themselves because in many cases their training will not have prepared them adequately for this role and in addition they may not have, or want to make, the necessary time. Counselling to be useful does take time and a desire to undertake it. Five or even 10 minutes a week squeezed into a busy surgery is not likely to be helpful, however good the doctor–patient relationship. The realities are often such that a doctor needs to refer his troubled child patients.

The choice will often lie between referral to the child psychiatric services and referral to the local authority social workers. After a short while doctors will know their local resources but until they build up this knowledge some general guidelines may be helpful. Referral to child psychiatric services is usually indicated where the doctor thinks the child's problem has an emotional basis. Such a child is more likely to commit offences on his own and often they may have started stealing from home. The parents are more likely to be anxious about their child's problem and must be organized enough to meet the demands of keeping appointments. The doctor may well think there is something unusual about either the child's behaviour or the family relationships.

While social workers are able to help with family relationship problems, they also have access to a wider range of provision for families and children with social and emotional problems. Referral to a social worker seems particularly indicated when the child is involved in group delinquency and is behaving in a way which seems 'normal' for boys in his neighbourhood. It would also be the referral of choice when the family's way of life precludes keeping regular appointments but they would accept home visits and might need financial or material help in addition to family counselling.

REFERENCES

Berlins M, Wansell G 1974 Caught in the act. Penguin, Harmondsworth
Bowlby J 1946 44 juvenile thieves, their characters and home life. Ballière, Tindall, & Cox, London
Cicourel A V 1968 The social organisation of juvenile justice. John Wiley, London
Cloward R, Ohlin L 1960 Delinquent and opportunity, a theory of delinquent gangs. Glencoe Free Press, New York
Durkheim E 1951 Suicide: a study in sociology. Glencoe Free Press, Illinois
Empey L, Lubeck S 1973 Delinquency prevention strategies. In: Adams G B (ed) Juvenile justice management. Thomas, Springfield, Illinois
Fox R G 1971 The XYY offender, a modern myth? The Journal of Criminal Law, Criminology and Police Science 62: 59–64
Glueck S, Glueck E 1968 Delinquents and non delinquents in perspective. Harvard University Press, Cambridge, Mass.
Goring C 1913 The English convict. HMSO, London
Hirschi T 1969 Causes of delinquency. University of California Press, San Francisco
In re Gault (1967) 387 US 1 in US Supreme Court Reports, vol 18L, 2nd ed. The Lawyers' Co-operative Publishing Company, Rochester, NY
Klein M 1973 Issues in police diversion of juvenile offenders. In: Adams G B (ed) Juvenile justice management. Thomas, Springfield, Illinois
Lombroso C 1911 Criminal man. Putnams, New York
Matza D 1964 Delinquency and drift. Wiley, New York.
Merton R 1938 Social structure and anomie. American Sociological Review 3: 672–676
Miller W 1958 Lower class culture as a generating milieu of gang delinquency. Journal of Social Issues 14: No 3, 6–10
Norman S 1973 Youth Service Bureau. National Council for Crime and Delinquency, Paramus, NJ
Reckless W C 1967 The crime problem. Appleton Century Crofts, New York
Scheff T J 1970 Being mentally ill. Aldine Publishing Company, Chicago
Sheldon W 1949 Varieties of delinquent youth. Harper, New York
Vaz E 1961 Middle class juvenile delinquency. Harper Row, New York
Winnicott W D 1963 The mentally ill in your caseload. In: New thinking about casework. Association of Social Workers, London

Part Three:
The Foundations of Child Health

Health education

George Cust

Health education is as old as the practice of medicine. Early attempts were empirical and it is only during the last 30 years that it has developed into anything resembling a scientific discipline. This development has been made possible by the work of the World Health Organization, in whose constitution health education was provided for from the beginning, and by the multidisciplinary professional character of health education in which contributions have been made by behavioural scientists, social anthropologists, educationalists and experts in mass communication. There is a partnership between medical science and social science in the practice of health education and particularly in the research activities which are now an important aspect. For example, for health education purposes epidemiological techniques cannot be confined merely to the plotting of the frequency of events and identifying associations which may or may not be significant. The epidemiological approach must be merged with the behavioural outlook so that we develop an 'epidemiology of behaviour'.

Behavioural basis of health education

A conceptual model can be constructed illustrating the interaction of behavioural patterns with predictable hazards (Fig. 6.1). This model places the behavioural pattern first in the chain of events which can lead from health to disease. Changes in medical thought have resulted from the application of epidemiology to the non-communicable diseases which has enabled us to identify predictable hazards. At the same time there is a growing interest in the idea that the primary cause of some disease is behavioural in character. In this model we are still concerned to identify primary hazards, but we have to go further back than that to identify underlying behavioural patterns that are likely to increase the risk of encounter with such hazards.

The model forecasts a chain of events in which a behavioural pattern increases the chances of meeting a predictable hazard. Ideally health education should intervene at a point where the hazard can be perceived by the individual who, if sufficiently motivated, may then change his behaviour pattern. The sequence of events goes further, however, leading first to a reversible change which may be physiological in character and echoes the observations of Virchow (1858) who drew attention to the fact that pathological and structural changes were preceded by physiological events. For example, changes due to malnutrition are reversible, whether the malnutrition be due to a lack or an excess of food, and so are the early changes due to smoking tobacco. This latter fact has been established by fundamental histological studies (Auerbach et al, 1962) and by observing the beneficial effects of stopping smoking (Doll & Peto, 1976). In infancy and childhood the chances of reversing the physiological or minor pathological departure from the normal are high and it is, in fact, in the field of child welfare that health education has had its most measurable successes. Health education then can intervene even after the encounter with a hazard, with a view to reversing any changes that have occurred. If, on the other hand, the sequence of events leads on to structural and pathological changes requiring medical or surgical therapy, then provided the patient survives this there is still a place for health education in the field of rehabilitation and prevention of the recurrence of the original condition.

Social anthropologists and behavioural scientists have analysed human behaviour to the extent that it is now possible to interpret patterns of behaviour

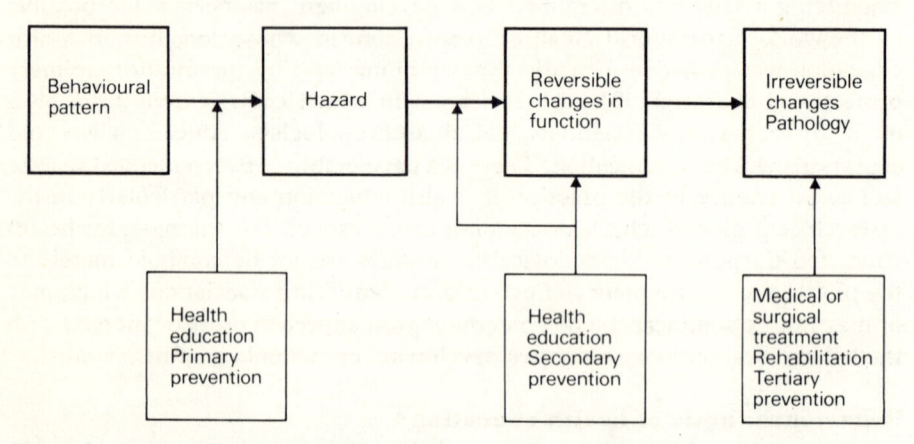

Fig. 6.1 Health education: a conceptual model. Source: Dalzell-Ward A J 1975 A text book of health education, 2nd edn. Reproduced by permission of the Publisher, Tavistock Publications Ltd

in terms of personal motivation. All human beings have an instinctive drive towards the achievement of satisfactions. Davis & Heimler (1967) have been able to assign numerical values to groups of satisfactions, classified variously as financial, sexual, job satisfaction, satisfaction in family life and in children, satisfaction at the expression of personal skills, and satisfaction from relationships in the general community. People vary in their needs to achieve specific satisfactions and in this scheme it is possible to total up an overall score of satisfaction thus providing an index of mental health.

In the drive to achieve satisfaction, however, there may be a conflict with the underlying need to preserve emotional security, and there is thus a rather unstable but dynamic equilibrium between the two drives. It is well recognized that emotional security in the child is derived from quality of affection and parental care which provide a base on which the child can build his personality. It must also be recognized that most older children and adults derive emotional security from membership of a group which is held in high regard. This has a bearing upon health behaviour, particularly in respect of the care of children.

Koos (1954) in the United States observed over 20 years ago that mothers took their small children to 'well baby stations' if this was the acceptable behaviour (social norm) of the group.

This is an example of the favourable effects of group conformity on health behaviour. However, there can be unfavourable effects, particularly in adolescence where the need to conform to the group is pronounced. Thus smoking, the abuse of alcohol, the illicit taking of drugs and sexual promiscuity may be the norm of a group to which the young person wishes to conform.

Identification of the conflict between the drive for satisfaction and the drive to preserve emotional security is a guideline to health education strategies because we can identify target groups and identify their personal goals and ambitions and satisfaction drives. Because the majority of parents have goals, ambitions and satisfaction drives in the interests of their children, health education has had probably the easiest task in this area, certainly in Western Europe and the United States. In developing countries the task is more difficult because group behaviour, as it affects child-rearing practices, is frequently in conflict with what we know about the scientific basis of child development, nutrition and life protection.

Definitions and aims of health education

A section on health education of the public was established by the World Health Organization at its inception, and the first report of an Expert Committee appeared 26 years ago (WHO, 1954). This defined the aims and purposes of health education very simply as: (1) to ensure that communities accept health as a valued asset; (2) to equip the individual with knowledge and to influence his attitudes and promote skills to enable him to solve his own health problems; (3) to promote the development of health services.

This definition held good for many years as it was applicable to all countries in the world, although the emphasis was obviously different in each. However a subsequent report (WHO, 1969) offered a more elaborate definition which indicated the progress in thinking and in the welding together of multidisciplinary professional groups for the practice of health education. The quotation is as follows:

> The term 'health education' has a number of meanings. In its broadest interpretation health education concerns all those experiences of an individual, group, or community that influence beliefs, attitudes, and behaviour with respect to health, as well as the processes and efforts of producing change when this is necessary for optimal health. This all inclusive concept of health education recognizes that many experiences, both positive and negative, have an impact on what an individual, group, or community thinks, feels and does about health; and it does not restrict health education to those situations in which health activities are planned or formal. In the more limited meaning, health education usually means the planned or formal efforts to stimulate and provide experience at times, in ways, and in situations leading to the development of health knowledge, attitudes, and behaviour that are most conducive to the attainment of individual, group, or community health.

Formal efforts in health education, for example health education campaigns using the mass media, are those most recognizable but this statement frees the subject from concentration on formal efforts. There are many inputs into the educational experiences of a child. From the very earliest stages there are the influences of the mother and father. Baric (1979) writing about primary socialization and smoking says, 'This study showed that probably the first year of a child's life is the most sensitive period as far as awareness of the habit, acquisition of manipulative skills, imitation and modelling are concerned. This has been so far disregarded, some health educators and parents alike believed that a child must be capable of "understanding" before it can learn anything.' After the parents come the influences of the rest of the family, grandparents and siblings, and later neighbours and friends. Inputs from the mass media, especially television, come at an early age. The formal education system begins with the nursery school and lasts in Britain until at least the age of 16. With the development of the skill of reading, magazines, comics, newspapers and books become an increasing source of information. Then around puberty the peer group begins to be a powerful influence which lasts until the influence of one special member of the opposite sex becomes of prime importance. Gordon & Dickman (1978) writing about sex education illustrate the power of the informal inputs when they say 'the only way in which parents can be the exclusive sex educators for their children would be to prevent them from having any friends; from talking on the telephone; looking at any but the most carefully censored books, newspapers, or magazines; listening to the radio; playing records or watching TV; and never letting them into a public rest room. The passage of years however might defeat such parental efforts because in adolescence the peer group appears just as influential as parents if not more so.' Into this pattern health care professionals put few but important direct inputs, though the indirect effect of midwife, health visitor and doctor via the parents may play a crucial part in the health of the child.

The main areas of health education
The overall aim of health education is to change health behaviour so that health is promoted and disease prevented. The process of changing health behaviour by health education is to give people new knowledge, helping them to understand this, and to build it into their own knowledge, beliefs and value systems, so that they can make meaningful choices about their health behaviour. It is a truly educational process which involves new knowledge gain, understanding, and the option of choice by the learner. Like all educational processes it often takes time. Health education is different from health propaganda which tells people what they should do without giving them proper explanation, understanding, or the opportunity of choice and decision making for themselves. There are four main areas of health education:

1. *Health promotion.* Such topics as a knowledge of how the body is made and how it works; personal hygiene including oral hygiene; nutrition; exercise; smoking and its effects; use and abuse of alcohol; education in personal relationships; knowledge of family planning; and parent education.
2. *Prevention of specific diseases.* This includes knowledge of and participation in preventive programmes such as early and regular attendance at the antenatal

clinic; bringing the baby to the child health clinic; cervical cytology; immunization programmes.

3. *Self-care.* One of the underlying beliefs of health education is the importance of the role of the individual in his own health. A recent development of this is the role of the individual in his own health care, helping him to distinguish between those signs and symptoms which should be taken early to the general practitioner and those minor self-limiting diseases which he can manage on his own. Included in this must be information about medicines, both prescribed and bought over the counter. How to live with chronic diseases and how to get the best out of the health service are also part of this topic.

4. *Promotion of health knowledge among the public.* There are factors in our society which are anti-health such as the massive promotion of cigarette smoking which may need government action or legislation to control. Some positive health actions, for example fluoridation, need government action before they can take place. There must be a well-informed public to give support on aspects of social policy which affect health and to understand and press for health legislation.

Guidelines to health education needs

Table 6.1 sets out identifiable hazards to health from before birth until the secondary school age. It takes into account the health problems of parents which may affect their emotional capacity to be effective in the care of children. Most middle-class mothers are aware of their role in stimulating the emotional and physical development of their children but they need continual reinforcement of knowledge and confidence by contact with a health visitor who is the primary health educator. Mothers in social classes IV and V (see p. 143) are more likely to consider economic needs first and may find difficulty in understanding the need to achieve primary satisfactions, the need to stimulate the child through language, etc., all of which make inroads into time which has been totally committed to earning wages outside the home as well as domestic duties.

The importance of primary socialization in the establishment of habits and attitudes to health has already been referred to. Up until the age of seven, a child is usually content to accept adults as a reference group and to accede to their demands in respect of behaviour. Thus the attitude of the parents towards health problems, the way in which they handle them, the priority they assign to them in terms of expenditure of time and money, the seriousness with which they accept warnings about their own health, such as the dangers of smoking and unsatisfactory diets, and the attention paid to dental health, all impress themselves on the child's mind and will play a large part in forming his attitudes.

Parental needs

The increasingly high standards now required by our society for the upbringing of children with a view to the development of their potential requires the direct application by parents themselves of concepts of child development which have been formulated and tested during the last 30 years. A list of the knowledge and skills ideally needed by modern parents is now quite formidable, and in

Table 6.1 Guidelines to priorities, prenatal to secondary school periods

Period	Primary health hazards — Physical	Psychological	Present health education — Public authorities	Voluntary organizations
Prenatal	Premature labour due to antepartum haemorrhage; Toxaemia of pregnancy; Low birth-weight —mother smoking; Congenital malformation; Congenital infection	Nothing proven but pregnancy may be rejected by one or both parents which will influence attitude to child. In general, mother should be shielded from stress	Previous immunization against rubella; Antenatal care by Area Health Authority—midwife, GP and consultant obstetrician; Antenatal health education classes (husbands too); Genetic counselling services; HEC/SHEU	NAMCW; Spastics Society; Media—TV, radio, magazines, newspapers
Infant	Low birth-weight; Birth injuries; Respiratory disorders; Hypothermia; Feeding and weaning problems; Infections; Sensory defects detected; Immunization programme commences; First dentition: dental hygiene should commence now; Non-accidental injury	Failure of bonding; Need to achieve primary satisfactions—affection conveyed through physical contact, tone of voice, etc.; Need for continuing and consistent maternal care in order to develop emotional security; Stimulation through play and language	General practitioner; Health visitor; Health education services; Community child health services; Developmental screening by general practitioners and health visitors; HEC/SHEU	NAMCW; NCB; OU Courses; Media
Pre-school	Developmental screening of all children will ascertain sensory and motor defects which may be treated; Accidents in home; Feeding problems; Nutrition—commencement of obesity; Need for play and enjoyment; Respiratory infection and complaints	Bed wetting; Behaviour disorders; Challenge produced by new sibling rivalry; Depression often about death; Sex education should start in home	Health visitor; General practitioner; Community child health services; Psychological services; Hospital paediatric services; Health education services; HEC/SHEU	NAMCW; NCB; ROSPA; Parent education; Media; Pharmacists (advice on medication and prevention of accidental poisoning)

Period	Primary health hazards		Present health education	
	Physical	Psychological	Public authorities	Voluntary organizations
Primary school	Dental health Immunization programme continues Accidents Foot health Personal hygiene Care and use of clothing	Behaviour problems consequent upon adjustment to school Emotional insecurity due to home trouble, aggression or inadequacy Victims of bullying	School Health Service Educational psychologists Child Guidance Clinic Dental clinic Remedial classes in physical education Health education services School health education HEC/SHEU	NAMCW NCB ROSPA Parent education movement Media
Secondary school	Accidents Alcohol Smoking Dental health Sexually transmitted diseases	Problems of developing sexuality Personal relationships Peer group Emotional problems of adolescence Need for preparation for adult parental roles	General practitioner School Health Service Educational psychologists Child Guidance Clinic Dental clinic Health education in schools Counselling services in schools Health education services HEC/SHEU	NAMCW NCB ROSPA Parent education movement Media

NAMCW = National Association for Maternal and Child Welfare
ROSPA = Royal Society for the Prevention of Accidents
HEC = Health Education Council
SHEU = Scottish Health Education Unit
NCB = National Children's Bureau
OU = Open University

a mock advertisement for 'a parent' Shapiro (1979) illustrates these and other aspects of the parents' tasks:

WANTED: responsible persons (m/f) to undertake 20 year project. Candidates should be totally committed, willing to work up to 24 hours daily, including weekends (occasional holidays possible after 5 years' service). Knowledge of health care, nutrition, psychology, child development, the education system essential. Necessary qualities, energy, tolerance, patience, sense of humour. No training or experience needed. No salary, but a very rewarding job for the right person.

MacQueen (1975), referring particularly to genetic counselling in the case of Huntington's chorea, believes that health education should be successful in curtailing hereditary diseases, in promoting early and effective use of health services and in reducing their misuse. Understanding of social and medical services available for the child and the parents, even form-filling and awareness of benefits that are available, must be included in the body of knowledge required by parents today.

The process of education in parenthood, if it can be said to start at any fixed point, should start in a general way in the secondary school. It is picked up in a more specific way during the antenatal period. The primary aims then are to ensure a smooth and happy pregnancy for the couple and eventually a satisfactory labour. There have been criticisms of antenatal classes, viz.

1. Some women fail to recognize the invitation to attend classes. These include a considerable proportion of women in 'at risk' groups who would most benefit by attendance.

2. Most women work until the 28th week of pregnancy; if the course of classes is relatively long, about half the women will be delivered before they have completed the classes.

3. Women are most interested in learning about the labour and some topics taught in classes are not directly relevant.

An early pregnancy meeting of the 'pregnant couples' with midwife, health visitor and doctor and then a shorter course, concentrating upon the delivery and taking place after the woman has ceased employment, is perhaps a better pattern. Education continues after the birth of the baby, first of all by the midwife and then by the health visitor. Further teaching takes place in the child health clinic: many areas have mother/baby clubs, initiated by health visitors, where formal teaching and informal learning take place. Most parents seem to have fewer educational needs as their children get older but appreciate specific sessions at appropriate times on topics such as starting school and facts of life for parents of pre-pubertal children. A few sessions on the physical and emotional problems of adolescence for the parents of older children are usually well attended. These can be organized through the School Health Service.

There is one gap in this continuum which has been explored only by a few health educators and this is for the couple not yet pregnant but thinking of starting a family. Some young couples would welcome a few group discussion sessions on the responsibilities of parenthood and avoidance of hazards in that important first three months of pregnancy.

Development of health education in the United Kingdom and Europe
Development of health education in the United Kingdom has proceeded in parallel with the development of the administration of health and social services. Whereas many pioneers have carried on health education purely by their own initiative, it is a practice which needs the backing of an organization. Health education is not a subject for amateurs and the training needs for professional personnel either to carry out health education as part of their day-to-day duties or to be specialists in the subject are now recognized.

Health education was organized by individual medical officers of health as long ago as 1919 (Daley, 1959). In 1927 the Society of Medical Officers of Health (now the Society for Community Medicine) was responsible for setting up the first independent national body for health education in the United Kingdom, the Central Council for Health Education. This organization continued its work until 1968 when it was taken over by the Health Education Council (HEC). The Central Council for Health Education started from very modest beginnings, aiming at co-ordinating numerous efforts by voluntary bodies and individuals and playing an increasingly active part in the scientific development of the subject. The National Health Service Act of 1946 provided a stimulus to the further development of health education. Section 28 gave Local Health Authorities powers to undertake health education as part of their schemes for the prevention of illness. As regards the care of children, the responsibility for health education was implied in Section 22 and Section 24 of the Act, referring to health visitors. Section 21 provided for the establishment of health centres and indicated that these might be used for health education purposes.

These changes coincided with a new direction in professional education for public health. Training for the Diploma in Public Health (DPH) underwent radical reorganization in 1946 and included studies in Child Development, Psychology, Sociology and Epidemiology which must have fired the imagination of the new generation of medical officers of health. Health education was provided with a scientific basis for the first time and offered the possibility of a practice which could be carried on by any trained people who had been through the necessary preparation and not only by dedicated pioneers. The Central Council for Health Education exploited this situation and in 1948 started a programme of in-service training courses for the medical officers, health visitors, midwives and public health inspectors employed by the Local Authorities. Interest in new methods of communication and learning began to develop and the partnership with educationalists was firmly forged. Certain teachers who left their normal professional environment to work in health education brought with them new skills that were eagerly absorbed by doctors and nurses. It may be said that the impact of education on those professional groups was as exciting as the impact of medicine on teachers. During those formative years teachers, doctors, and nurses created a new inter-disciplinary group.

The development of health education in Continental Europe has been rather different (Federal German Centre for Health Education, 1972). The Netherlands provides services which are closest to those health visiting services which have been the strength of health education in the United Kingdom. In other countries there is a mixture of governmental and voluntary enterprise and the majority have central committees for health education which are responsible for co-ordination, research, training and implementing programmes. In some countries, particularly in Eastern Europe, the tendency has been for the development of health education and its control to be in medical hands, while in others educationalists or behavioural scientists have taken the lead. In the Federal Republic of Germany and in Italy there are central research institutes which act as power houses of new information and for training. Development of health education specialists has proceeded in many countries and some have extremely ambitious programmes, using television and radio on a scale not yet found possible in the United Kingdom. In several countries studies have been made of people's attitudes to their health problems, motivation for health behaviour, reasons for 'anti-health' behaviour and the like. Research activities were slow to develop in the United Kingdom but in recent years the HEC and the Scottish Health Education Unit (SHEU) have earmarked funds for research and evaluation projects, including grants to academic researchers, provision of lectureships at universities and market research.

There are several international health education agencies. Apart from WHO there is the International Union for Health Education of the Public (founded in 1952), a non-governmental organization in official relationship with WHO. The International Union, through its triennial conferences held in different centres of the world and through its regional meetings, makes it possible for health education specialists from all countries to meet regularly, to correspond with each other and, through the medium of the International Journal for Health Education, to exchange ideas and to be stimulated to apply them in their own countries. Of particular interest to child health is the International Federation for Parent Education, founded in 1965.

The Cohen Committee
The next stage in development in the United Kingdom is marked by the report of the Cohen Committee (HMSO, 1964), a joint committee of the Central and Scottish Health Services Councils under the chairmanship of Lord Cohen of Birkenhead. The report made a number of important recommendations. There should be an enquiry into the various factors influencing mothers in the way they bring up their children. High priority should continue to be given to the health education of mothers. This is a pressing need to educate mothers and children in dental care and to cultivate a public opinion favourable to fluoridation. More education about the emotional needs of parents and children is desirable. Careful consideration should be given to the time spent by health visitors in educating mothers.

The major recommendations, however, concerned the future development of health education in the United Kingdom. The government should establish a strong 'Central Board in England and Wales' which would promote a climate of opinion generally favourable to health education, develop 'blanket' programmes of education on selected priority subjects and secure support from all possible national sources, commercial and voluntary as well as medical. The training of specialist health educators should be fostered and there should be promotion of training in health education of doctors, nurses, teachers and dentists. Evaluation of the results achieved by health education was considered a high priority. It was recommended that in Scotland there should be a parallel board absorbing the health education functions of the Scottish Home and Health Department and the Scottish Council for Health Education. In the event, the Scottish Council for Health Education survived and continues to function, complementary to the Scottish Health Education Unit which was set up by the Home and Health Department following the report of the Cohen Committee.

Recommendations were also made regarding the practice of medicine and nursing. Health visitors should be attached to general practitioners and health education should be regarded as an important subject in the undergraduate medical and dental curriculum. More provision should be made for postgraduate medical and dental instruction in health education and general dental practitioners should carry out more dental education at the chairside.

Certain recommendations were made regarding health education in schools, including greater attention to health education in colleges of education and the allocation of periods of health education in the schools' syllabus. Co-operation between Education and Public Health departments of Local Authorities and Central Government in the field of health education was urged. Regarding the content of the school health education syllabus, the report recommended that this should be broadly based, aimed at giving the child such knowledge as will equip him to face the social and health problems he will meet in later years.

The Health Education Council
The setting-up of the HEC in 1968 was a direct result of the recommendations of the Cohen Committee. The new Council was able to invest in mass communication on a scale that had not previously been possible, and to initiate research into such aspects as attitudes, motivation, levels of knowledge, and effectiveness of communication.

The Council has also been concerned with the development of health education as a profession. This has been pursued in a number of ways. One way is through masters degree courses at universities such as Manchester, Nottingham and Chelsea College, aimed at producing graduate specialists equipped with the techniques of evaluation and research as well as organizing ability. The aim of these courses is to extend the range of academic knowledge about health education. The HEC also encourages courses leading to the Diploma in Health Education, such as those at the University of Leeds and at the Polytechnic of the South Bank in London. These courses are undertaken mainly by people who intend to be health education officers working in the National Health Service. The students mainly come from nursing and teaching. The courses are full-time, last one academic year and can take altogether 42 students each year. To help health workers, whether in the health service or local authority service, to learn more about the methods and practice of health education, the Council has set up a network of courses in polytechnics and colleges of technology which lead to a Certificate in Health Education. These courses are part-time (whole-time equivalent of 36 days) and are held each year in about 14 colleges, training some 140 health professionals each year.

In the field of school health education, the HEC is active in curriculum development, and maintains a close association with the Schools' Council. Curriculum development implies a study of the educational needs of children of different age groups and, with the co-operation of teachers, the selection and testing of materials that can supply these needs and the investigation and testing of methods of teaching.

Health education in the reorganized National Health Service
Since the reorganization of the National Health Service, health education has been officially recognized as part of the scheme for general health care (NHS circular HRC (74) 27, 1974) and is now the responsibility of Area Health Authorities. It is also recognized as a fundamental component of the preventive health services. In England and Wales, the Area Medical Officer is responsible to the Area Health Authority for health education. The Area Health Education Officer is responsible to the Area Medical Officer for the day-to-day management of the health education services. Resources given to health education vary considerably between Areas but on the whole considerable progress has been made

and there are several Area Health Authorities with large units and with budgets which allow progressive planning. There are (June 1979) 343 health education officers in post in Britain, though two thirds of these do not have a diploma in health education, and there is a requirement in 10 years for about a thousand health education officers.

The administrative provisions for Scotland are set out in a memorandum by the Scottish Home and Health Department (1974). Each Health Board is expected to make specific provision for the organization of health education in its area. An Area Health Education Officer is appointed to each Board under the general authority of the Chief Administrative Medical Officer. In consultation with officers of the Board (particularly the community medicine specialist, nursing adviser and dental adviser) he is the source of health information for the Health Board. The central body is the Scottish Health Education Unit which was transferred from the Scottish Home and Health Department to the Common Service Agency and is thus now part of the National Health Service.

The development of health education in Britain has benefited considerably by the government's policy of giving high priority to prevention. This has been clearly expressed in its publications such as *Prevention and Health, Everybody's Business* (1976); *The First Report of the Expenditure Committee, Preventive Medicine* (1977); *The White Paper—Prevention and Health* (1977); and in the series of prevention guidance booklets such as *Reducing the Risk: Safer Pregnancy and Childbirth* (1977).

An important aspect of the reorganization of the National Health Service is that, whereas health education was formerly confined almost entirely to the practice of preventive medicine, it can now be included in the activities of general family practice and hospital practice. The attachment of health visitors to general practices was the first step in this direction, but now the Health Education Officer and his team of experts can work with all three branches of medical practice. Already many general practitioners have taken an interest in health education and some have evolved elaborate schemes of their own. Many of these place the necessary emphasis on child care, particularly the scheme evolved by Hasler (1968) who organized a health education team which would give advice to the parents of young children in a group practice or to those married couples who were about to have children. Pike (1979) has developed a leaflet which is given to the parents of new babies in his practice. It contains information about prevention such as immunization and about illnesses early in life.

Parentcraft and parent education

Parentcraft is a basic subject and it is one of the oldest topics in health education. For many years it was confined to the conventional tasks of child rearing concerned with nutrition, hygiene and protection from common dangers, but it has now broadened its scope. There has been increasing interest in the emotional life of the child and in the inculcation of skills in handling children through various stages of development. Such skills are more often expressed by attitudes than by any particular actions. Since the time when parentcraft was established as the grassroots of health education, the clinical science of developmental paediatrics has produced new knowledge which should be of great use to parents.

There is also need to give information and guidance about the diagnosis and management of sick children. It is the mother who makes the first diagnosis when she decides that the child's illness is beyond her competence and that medical help is needed.

Two particular schemes in the United Kingdom should be mentioned. The National Association for Maternal and Child Welfare (1973) operates a scheme for parentcraft teaching in schools. The Gloucestershire Family Life Association (1966) has brought together various disciplines and interests concerned with developing effective parents who can give their children emotional satisfaction as well as physical and social care. Attention is paid to emotional maturity, social responsibility and responsibility to oneself. Innovations in this scheme include the introduction of discussions on the theme of cruelty. The topics of sexually transmitted diseases and contraception respectively are introduced from about the age of 14 years. Increasing interest in parent education on lines advocated by the International Federation of Parent Education has led recently to further interest in the setting up of a British Association for Parent Education.

Health education in schools

The importance of formal health education in schools has always been more clearly recognized by health workers than by educationalists. A recent report on health education by the Welsh General Medical Services Committee (1978) recommended 'An integrated Health Education programme in the schools combined with the teaching of human biology in order that basic health measures and facts on the basic human anatomy and physiology become common knowledge among the school leavers.'

There are a number of difficulties in the way of the quicker development of health education in schools. At central level there are two separate departments—the Department of Education and Science (DES) for education and the Department of Health and Social Services (DHSS) for health. During the 1950s and 1960s, the importance of health education in schools (except for sex education) was not reflected in any of the major reports on education at this time. The publication of *Health Education in Schools* by the DES (1977a) was therefore welcome and the Departmental Memorandum 15/77 (DES, 1977b) commended this publication to local education authorities and pressed schools and those responsible for teacher education courses to take health education seriously.

Health education has never been a separate public examination subject and schools have never been stimulated by the examination motive to put health education on the curriculum. School staff—and the head teacher in particular—have the responsibility of planning the curriculum in their own schools and need not teach health education if they do not wish to do so.

A postal survey of the 100 secondary school head teachers in Nottinghamshire (Burrows & Small, 1975) showed that about half of them had positive attitudes to health education and believed that the effects of health education in schools are advantageous and that schools should pay more attention to health education. Younger, newly trained teachers with enthusiasm for teaching health education may meet with considerable frustration when they find there is no place for health education in their school because of negative attitudes of some head teachers.

Difficulties arise in the actual teaching of health education because of problems in teaching methodology. There are parts of health education for which every teacher is not equipped, either because of lack of knowledge or because of personality. There is no health education department within a school, no specialist adviser in health education at the local education authority to stimulate development or act as a centre of advice and no obviously vacant spot in a busy timetable. Health professionals often underestimate the pressure on the school timetable. However, there is considerable health educational content in some curricula, in the form of health education, social studies, education in personal relationships or teaching of parentcraft, and in subjects such as biology or home economics. In a survey of 15–16-year-olds in Northern Ireland, McGuffin (1978) reported that children who had taken courses such as biology or home economics had better health knowledge than those who had not. Those with better health knowledge had better health behaviour. The days are past when the visiting doctor or health visitor went into a school to give a one-off lecture on smoking/drugs/contraception in response to a head teacher's request (stimulated by a child having been found smoking in the lavatory, in possession of pep pills or pregnant). Health education needs to be integrated into the curriculum and though health workers can give great help to teacher colleagues, either with some special lesson in the curriculum or by helping the teacher to learn about a health topic, this aspect of education is a job for the teachers. They are trained in teaching children and there are 424 000 of them compared with 7500 health visitors and 22 000 general practitioners.

A great step forward for school health education has been curriculum development. This started with mathematics in 1950 and then spread to science with the Nuffield Science Courses. All these curriculum projects are teacher-oriented and a lot of the learning is through experiment and discovery. In 1964 the Schools' Council was set up with a majority of teacher members. It is supported by the DES and local education authorities. It has carried out research into curricula, teaching methods and examinations over many school subjects. Four of the earlier topics contained some health education—*Schools' Council Humanities Project* (1970) for children aged 14–16; *Nuffield Secondary Science* (1971) for children aged 13–16; *Schools' Council Moral Education Project, Lifeline* (1972) for ages 13–16; and *Schools' Council General Studies Project* (1972) for young people aged 15–19.

With financial support from the HEC there have been specific health education projects; *The Schools' Council Health Education Project* (1977)—*All About Me (Ages 5–8)* and *Think Well (ages 9–13)*—and a project which began its investigation phase in 1977—*The Schools' Council Health Education Project ages 13–18*.

The HEC has supported two projects of its own. *Living Well* (1977) aimed to promote healthy living by helping young people to cope with and approach positively the challenges, complexities and anxieties of everyday life. The second project—*Your Body 10–12* (Wilcox et al, 1978)—with a structured approach, community participation (especially by parents), extensive use of resources and group work, is undergoing evaluation in a group of Sheffield schools. The health aim of this project, in which primary schoolchildren learn about their lungs and respiratory system, is to reduce the numbers of these children who start to smoke as they get older.

Important work is therefore taking place but in the words of Sutherland (1979), 'Health education may well succeed in improving its status in schools and in the training of teachers as time goes by, but it would be unreasonable to expect changes to be either rapid in taking place or dramatically effective in altering the health of the nation quickly for the better.'

Defining targets

There is a growing tendency to define targets for health education activities rather than to adopt the general 'blanket' approach which was characteristic of this field 25 years ago. The definition of targets depends upon epidemiological patterns and studies undertaken as to the feasibility of health education. For example, there must be a well-defined epidemiology and this must be related in turn to environmental or personal factors with a certainty that personal or group behaviour is involved. It is also necessary to study the characteristics of the target group which is defined according to age, sex, occupation, social class or geographical location. Social survey studies designed to reveal what people know and understand about the particular health problem, and their attitude towards it, are necessary before projects are designed. Evaluation procedures are built into every project now, so baseline observations are essential, although it should not be assumed that these will always provide a basis on which to measure progress.

As an example, when health education is concerned with child-rearing practices it is important to obtain a picture of parental attitudes. Information should be obtained on how far child-rearing practices are merely a continuation of practices of a former generation, on who has the most influence in the family, and on attitudes to the three basic aspects of life—nutrition, excretion and sex. Studies carried out in primitive communities in developing countries have revealed attitudes to child rearing which are considered bizarre in the West, and these have their counterpart in the highly developed countries.

Health education designed to deter expectant mothers from smoking during pregnancy is another example of the integration of epidemiological and behavioural concepts. Studies have been undertaken first to establish how many expectant mothers smoke and secondly to identify special characteristics which would then suggest a target group. A study of smoking habits in pregnancy (SHEU, 1975) showed that there was a relationship between social class and smoking, for example 66 per cent of women in social class I were non-smokers, but only 29.7 per cent in social class V did not smoke. There was also an association with husbands' smoking. Women of low parity were more likely to stop smoking during pregnancy.

It is also necessary to ascertain the attitudes of professional attendants. The response to a circular sent to all general practitioners and consultants in England and Wales in 1974 indicated that a campaign against smoking in pregnancy had the wholehearted support of the medical profession. It was necessary, however, to ensure that midwives were also fully in the picture regarding this problem and were sympathetic to efforts to stop mothers from smoking. The HEC arranged a series of seminars to cover all the branches of the Royal College of Midwives in England and Wales over a period of two years. Basic scientific information was derived from a number of authorities who have studied the subject, in particular Butler et al (1972). Motives for smoking, and in particular the influence of husbands and people at work, were also discussed.

Another example of fundamental research to produce guidelines for campaigns is a study of 1069 home accidents to children under the age of five years (de Fonseka et al, 1974). It was found that the bedroom, lounge and staircase presented the greatest risk to children under five years of age, and that fractures and concussion accounted for the majority of severe injuries.

Use of mass media

All the health campaigns and health educational programmes directed at the general public have been made possible by the availability of far greater financial resources for television and other advertising. The HEC and the SHEU carry out campaigns regularly on a number of topics, the priority for which is decided on the grounds of importance to the community and feasibility. Communications research is undertaken to ascertain the level of knowledge and attitudes of the target group and to pre-test materials that have been designed for publicity purposes on representative samples of the target group. When the theme has been defined from a medical and scientific brief, various concepts are worked out by advertising and communications experts and those which have most impact on a sample audience are then put into production.

In the field of child health, the HEC has conducted national television campaigns on the prevention of accidental child poisoning, smoking and primary socialization, and smoking in pregnancy. At a regional level the Council has used television for a campaign on family planning. These campaigns are invariably supported by posters and leaflets which are distributed to Area Health Authorities for use in their areas and to individuals. Considerable local work by the health education officers, including the use of local radio and press and meetings with groups, takes place to support these campaigns. Support by health care professionals is important. Television 'spots' are very short, lasting at the most $1\frac{1}{2}$ minutes, and they often make use of some dramatized incident. Surveys following a campaign measure its effectiveness. The Open University has designed two eight-week courses for young parents using television, radio and printed material. The 1977–8 presentations of *The First Year of Life and the Pre-School Child* had 14 000 students and 1500 self-help groups were set up to support the programmes.

Group health education

Projects such as those mentioned above are useful when we are faced with matters of public concern and where there is firm support. Day-to-day health education, however, is carried out on a personal basis, at its best in small groups. The aim is that small numbers of people take an active part in the learning process and that the subject is presented to them in such a way that they have an understanding of their own motivations and attitudes.

Health visitors were the first health workers in this country to take up group health education in the field of child health and they will always be valuable primary health educators. Midwives too are concerned with antenatal health education (Royal College of Midwives, 1966). There is scope for social workers who so far have not played a prominent part in health education but whose particular interest in group dynamics and the behavioural sciences would fit them for further training in health education practice.

Health education groups have been formed from mothers making use of the child health services and to a certain extent from parents who are members of Parent Teacher Associations at schools. The incentive has been to become more effective in their role as parents and health education has been seen in the context of some tangible service such as the supervision of child health by clinical techniques and the giving of individual advice on nutrition, clothing and general care.

The technique of group discussion requires some training and experience which is not easy to acquire: the best technical manual on the group method so far is that by Thompson & Kahn (1972).

The development of educational technology has given us a rich supply of interesting and diverting methods of communicating ideas and facts by visual and auditory reinforcement. The experienced health educator will make use of all of them, selecting an appropriate method and medium for the task. There was a time when health educators could get by on improvisation, but they are now in competition with the skilled television professionals. It is therefore necessary for a health education officer when equipping his department to include the whole range of visual aids, if the budget allows. Health education officers are in a position to advise their professional colleagues on the availability and suitability of audio-visual aids. Discrimination and skill are most needed in the use of film, for the era of the conventional didactic documentary on health education is over. Film is the most expensive and sensitive medium we use and it is best reserved for tasks which cannot be satisfactorily undertaken by other media. It is most valuable in the field of human relations and emotional health. Ideally it should be so visual in character that a commentary or captions are virtually unnecessary. Film is useful as a stimulus to thought and discussion leading to those increased powers of deduction which should be the aim of every educational process. The way in which the film is presented and the conduct of the discussion afterwards are therefore as important as the quality of the film itself.

Broadcast television programmes now frequently include items about health and in particular about children, for example the BBC series *Parents and Children*. Although designed for the home circle, they are useful for discussion by groups under the control of trained health educators.

Appendix

Some useful addresses
The Health Education Council,
78 New Oxford Street,
London, WC1A 1AH.

International Union for Health Education,
9 rue Newton,
75116 Paris,
France.

National Children's Bureau,
8 Wakley Street,
London, EC1V 7QG.

Oral Hygiene Service,
Hesketh House,
Portman Square,
London, W1A 1D7.

Scottish Health Education Unit,
Health Education Centre,
21 Lansdowne Crescent,
Edinburgh, EH12 5EH.

National Association for Maternal and Child Welfare,
1 South Audley Street,
London W1Y 6JS.

General Dental Council,
Dental Health Education Section,
37 Wimpole Street,
London, W1M 8DG.

REFERENCES

Auerbach O, Stout A P, Hammond E C, Garfinkel L 1962 Bronchial epithelium in former smokers. New England Journal of Medicine 267: 119–125
Baric L 1979 Primary socialisation and smoking. Health Education Council Monograph Series No 1. Health Education Council, London
Burrows L, Small S D 1975 Health education in Nottinghamshire Secondary Schools. Occasional Paper No 1. Leverhulme Health Education Project, University of Nottingham
Butler N R, Goldstein H, Ross E M 1972 Cigarette smoking in pregnancy: its influence on birth weight and perinatal mortality. British Medical Journal ii: 127–130
Daley A 1959 The Central Council for Health Education—the first twenty-five years, 1927–52. Health Education Journal 17: 24–35
Dalzell-Ward A J 1975 A text book of health education. 2nd edn. Tavistock Publications, London
Davis H, Heimler E 1967 An experiment in the assessment of social function. Medical Officer 117: 31–32
de Fonseka C, Roberts J L, Simpson D, Knight M, Dale J W 1974 Studies of home accidents—injury to children in home accidents. Health Education Council, Medical Research Division Report, No 86, London
Department of Education and Science 1977a Health education in schools. HMSO, London
Department of Education and Science 1977b Administrative Memorandum 15/77. HMSO, London
Doll R, Peto R 1976 Mortality in relation to smoking: 20 years observation on male British doctors. British Medical Journal 4: 1525–1536
Federal German Centre for Health Education 1972 Health education in Europe. International Journal for Health Education (Geneva) vii: 137

Gloucestershire Family Life Association 1966 Education in personal relationships and family life, 2nd edn. Gloucester
Gordon S, Dickman J R 1978 Sex Education. The parents' role. Public Affairs Pamphlet No 549. Public Affairs Pamphlets, New York
Hasler J C 1968 Health education by community health team. British Medical Journal iii: 366–367
HMSO 1964 Report of a Joint Committee of the Central and Scottish Health Services Councils on Health Education (Cohen Report). HMSO, London
Koos E L 1954 The health of Regionville: what the people thought and did about it. Columbia University Press, New York
McGuffin S J 1978 The health knowledge and related behaviour of 16-year-olds in Northern Ireland. Research Report to the Health Education Council
MacQueen I A G 1975 The challenge of health education today. Public Health (London) 89: 93–96
National Association for Maternal and Child Welfare 1973 Revised syllabus of examinations. London
Pike L 1979 Report on the use of a booklet for parents. Report to the Health Education Council Research Committee. London
Royal College of Midwives 1966 Preparation for parenthood. London
Scottish Health Education Unit 1975 Smoking in Pregnancy. Edinburgh
Scottish Home and Health Department 1974 Health education in Health Boards: a memorandum by the Consultative Committee of Medical Officers of Health. HSR (74) M.1. HMSO, Edinburgh
Shapiro Jean 1979 Tomorrow's parents. Good Housekeeping Magazine (March)
Sutherland I. (ed) 1979 Health education: perspectives and choices. George Allen & Unwin, London
Thompson S, Kahn J H 1972 The group process as a helping Technique. Pergamon Press, Oxford
Virchow R 1858 Cellular pathology. Hirschwald, Berlin
Welsh General Medical Services Committee 1978 Report of a working party on health education in Wales. British Medical Association, London
Wilcox B, Engel E, Reid D 1978 Smoking education in children. UK trials of an international project. International Journal of Health Education 21: 236–244
World Health Organization 1954 Report of Expert Committee on Health Education of the Public. Technical Report Series, No 89. WHO, Geneva
World Health Organization 1969 Research in health education—Report of a WHO Scientific Group. Technical Report Series, No 432. WHO, Geneva

I. D. Gerald Richards

The epidemiology of disease in childhood

Epidemiology (*epi* upon, *demos* the people) is the study of the determinants and distribution of health and disease in populations. The health problems of children have been more extensively studied by epidemiological methods than have those of any other age group. Many of these investigations have been into perinatal and infant mortality but, as death-rates have fallen, increasing attention has been paid to specific problems such as the congenital malformations, low birth-weight, malignant disease, injury and respiratory tract infection. Much of this research has been in search of causes but epidemiological information is now being used increasingly in determining the needs of populations for health services and in examining their effects (the process of evaluation).

This chapter considers secular trends in the health of Britain's children, the present dimensions of ill health in childhood and the contribution of epidemilogy to our understanding of the causes of selected common diseases.

Demographic and health trends

Marriages
Since the Second World War there has been a trend towards earlier marriage so that now one third of brides are aged less than 20 years. Alongside this trend, there has been a very rapid increase in the divorce rate. It is highest in those marriages in which the wife was aged less than 20 at the time of marriage; for example, of such marriages occurring in 1951, 20 per cent had been dissolved by 1976 (Office of Population Census and Surveys, 1979). This is a trend which must have a profound effect on child health in this country, since two thirds of the couples divorcing have children; moreover it represents only the tip of a large iceberg of marital disharmony and breakdown of family life.

Births
The birth-rate has almost halved since the turn of the century. After a peak in 1964, the rate has declined rapidly due to postponement of starting a family and a fall in fertility* affecting women of all ages and parities. The most likely reasons for this trend are economic (such as the cost of housing) and the greater availability and efficiency of contraceptives. The birth-rate is highest in the less favoured social groups.

---

* Fertility rate = number of births per 1000 women aged 15 to 44 years.

Two other significant trends have occurred. The percentage of infants born illegitimate has doubled since the early years of the century, the present rate being 10 per cent; about one third are to women aged less than 20. A rapid increase has occurred in the proportion of births taking place in hospital so that by 1976 only 2.5 per cent were occurring at home compared with 33 per cent in 1961.

Mortality

Because the causes of still-birth* and death in the first week after birth are similar, it is convenient to consider such perinatal deaths together. During the years of the great industrial depression in Britain (1929–33), perinatal mortality rates were high but, as economic conditions improved between 1934 and 1940, mortality began to fall. Due to an improvement in maternal health and nutrition and in obstetric care, rates then fell sharply with the exception of the years between 1948 and 1957 when changes associated with the introduction of the National Health Service (the increase in general practitioner antenatal care) halted the decline in the still-birth rate in England and Wales (Richards & Lowe, 1966).

The average life expectation for a girl at birth is now 75 years but, because of higher male mortality at all ages, it is only 69 years for a boy. These figures are appreciably greater (by 12 years and 10 years respectively) than for children born in 1931 and are an indication of the improvement that has taken place in the health of Britian's population.

Mortality in infancy (the first year after birth) is now only one tenth of the level in the early years of the century when the rate was about 150 deaths per 1000 live births. For statistical purposes, infancy is divided into the neonatal period, comprising the early neonatal period (first week) and late neonatal period (remainder of the first four weeks), and the post-neonatal period (from four weeks to one year). Mortality has decreased less in the neonatal period than in the remainder of the first year. This difference is a reflection of the causes of mortality in the two periods, deaths in the neonatal period being mainly due to causes associated with low birth-weight, abnormalities of pregnancy and delivery, and congenital malformation, while in the post-neonatal period many deaths are due to diseases, such as infections, which are related to environmental conditions.

The great reduction which has occurred in childhood mortality has been due very largely to a fall in deaths from infectious disease. Several factors have been responsible for this change: a falling birth-rate, the control of adverse environmental influences by improvements in sanitation, housing and nutrition and, from the second quarter of this century, specific medical measures (immunization and treatment). The virtual elimination of diphtheria, smallpox and poliomyelitis in Britain is almost certainly due to immunization against these diseases. For three diseases, tuberculosis, whooping cough and measles, immunization procedures were introduced too late to have much influence on the downward trend of mortality.

* Still-birth refers to a child which has issued forth from its mother after the 28th week of pregnancy and which did not breathe or show any other sign of life.

Mortality in some handicapping conditions has fallen considerably. In Down's syndrome this has been due largely to the decline in the prevalence of tuberculosis in the community while in spina bifida it is the result of more active treatment. In the latter condition, survival now appears to be falling again due to more selective surgery (DHSS, 1974; Weatherall & White, 1976).

The incidence of mental and neurological handicap in low birth-weight infants has decreased markedly over the past 20 years due, probably, to improvements in neonatal care. A striking example of this change is seen in the studies conducted by Drillien (1969, 1974). At the age of 11 to 13 years, nearly half the Edinburgh children of birth-weight 1500 g or less born in 1953–60 had moderate or severe handicaps (being educationally subnormal and/or suffering from cerebral palsy and epilepsy). Children of similar birth-weight born in 1966–70 and examined two to three years after birth were found to have a much lower prevalence (22 per cent) of moderate or severe handicap.

The improved nutrition of children, which has been an important factor in lowering mortality from some infectious diseases such as tuberculosis, has also resulted in the virtual disappearance of severe nutritional diseases, for example infantile rickets, and in the increased stature of children and earlier puberty. Nevertheless, cases of rickets still occur in some deprived areas and in certain immigrant communities (Richards et al, 1968; Goel, 1979). Malnutrition in another form—obesity—is becoming increasingly common, especially among girls.

The dimensions of ill health in childhood

A composite picture of the extent of childhood illness can be obtained only by bringing together mortality data and such information on morbidity (*morbes* = disease) as is available from population surveys, records of hospital in-patient care, school medical examinations, registers of handicapped children and schemes for the notification of certain conditions such as the infectious diseases, congenital malformations and child battering. Valuable compilations of such data have been published by Franklin (1976) and in the Report of the Committee on Child Health Services (Court, 1976).

Mortality

Of every thousand babies born alive, 14 die in infancy (1977 rate). One third of such deaths occur on the first day and a further third during the remainder of the first month, mainly in the first week. The principal causes of infant mortality are complications of pregnancy and delivery (accounting for 45 per cent of the deaths), congenital anomalies (22 per cent) and respiratory infection (8 per cent).

In contrast, the remainder of childhood is a time of low mortality. For every 10 deaths in infancy, there are only four in the whole of the period between the first and the fifteenth birthdays, almost half of these being before the age of five. Between one and five years, a quarter of the deaths are due to injuries. The other common causes are, in descending order, congenital anomalies, respiratory infection and neoplastic disease. From five to 14 years, injuries again head the list and account for almost two thirds of the deaths, but neoplastic disease replaces respiratory infection as the second commonest cause of death.

Morbidity

Four large British studies have provided a considerable amount of information of the extent of ill health in childhood and on its causes. Three are investigations of national samples of children and the fourth is a study of a thousand families in Newcastle upon Tyne.

Children under five

Douglas & Blomfield (1958) studied the health in the first five years of life of 5386 children born in 1946, the information being specially collected by health visitors, school doctors and school nurses. Thirty-seven per cent of the children had at least one infectious disease and 8 per cent had two or more. In the first two years of life, 29 per cent had at least one lower respiratory tract infection and, in the first four years, discharging ears were reported in 7 per cent. A quarter had significant accidents.

The National Child Development Study (1958 Cohort)

In the first British Perinatal Mortality Survey (Butler & Bonham, 1963; Butler & Alberman, 1969) information was collected on virtually every birth in Britain during one week in March 1958. This group of children, numbering some 17 000 births in all, has been investigated throughout childhood.

When studied at the age of seven years (Pringle et al, 1966) many children had a history of significant illness, the most frequent being earache without running ears (32 per cent), bronchitis with wheezing (18 per cent), periodic vomiting or bilious attacks (17 per cent), speech defect (16 per cent), periodic abdominal pain (15 per cent), recurrent ear or throat infections (13 per cent), nocturnal enuresis after the age of five (11 per cent), hearing difficulty (10 per cent), recurrent mouth ulcers (10 per cent) and running ears (9 per cent). On medical examination, the defect found most often in these seven-year-old children was dental caries—teeth were decayed, missing or filled in 88 per cent—but visual defects (14 per cent), squint (6 per cent) and hearing impairment (5 per cent) were also common.

The British Births Child Study

The British Births Survey took place during one week in April 1970 throughout the United Kingdom (Chamberlain et al, 1975; 1978); from this cohort of 16 000 births a 10 per cent sample was taken and the children were traced and examined at the ages of 22 months and $3\frac{1}{2}$ years. A study of the prevalence of illness in these early years of life has been published by Chamberlain & Simpson (1979). By the age of $3\frac{1}{2}$ years, half the children had attended hospital (either as an out-patient or an in-patient) because of an accident or for an illness requiring specialist attention.

The study of a thousand families in Newcastle

This is a unique study of children from birth to their fifteenth birthday. The original group of 1142 was representative of all families with infants born in

Newcastle in 1947 and the findings have been published as three books (Spence et al, 1954; Miller et al, 1960; Miller et al, 1974).

Four fifths of all recorded illnesses before five years of age were infective in origin, with respiratory illnesses predominating. Accidents were responsible for nearly half of the non-infective episodes. In the school years, illness was much less common. Although declining in frequency and severity with age, respiratory infection still accounted for a large proportion (two thirds) of the episodes of illness; next in frequency were the acute infectious fevers. About 40 per cent of the children caused anxiety to their parents because of emotional disturbance and nearly one in five were considered maladjusted.

At a special school medical examination at the age of 13 years, the conditions found most often were teeth decayed, missing or filled (over 90 per cent of children), visual acuity less than 6/6 in one or both eyes (22 per cent), headaches (23 per cent), abdominal pain (19 per cent) and enuresis at 13 (5 per cent).

General practice

To meet the need for information on illness as seen in general practice, two national studies based on selected practices have been carried out by the Royal College of General Practitioners in association with the General Register Office

Table 7.1 Childhood illness in general practice. Source: Office of Population Censuses and Surveys (1974)

Diagnosis	Episodes in a year (per 1000 population) Age (years) 0–4	5–14
Diseases of respiratory system	1009	521
Acute nasopharyngitis	470	152
Acute pharyngitis and tonsillitis	213	186
Acute bronchitis and bronchiolitis	185	73
Catarrh	48	22
Symptoms and ill-defined conditions	343	168
Cough	113	49
Acute vomiting and/or diarrhoea	112	31
Infective and parasitic diseases	209	160
Measles, rubella, chickenpox, whooping cough	84	51
Intestinal infectious diseases	63	17
Viral warts	5	42
Diseases of nervous system and sense organs	312	161
Acute otitis media	186	83
Conjunctivitis and ophthalmia	70	19
Diseases of skin and subcutaneous tissues	214	150
Eczema and dermatitis	100	30
Infective conditions	55	60
Accidents, poisonings and violence	92	113
Lacerations, abrasions and superficial injuries	49	58
Sprains	10	28
All episodes	2873	1505

(the 1955/56 study) and the Office of Population Censuses and Surveys and the Department of Health and Social Security (the 1970/71 study).

Table 7.1 shows some of the findings from the more recent survey. The childhood illnesses coming to the attention of the general practitioner most often are respiratory tract infections, with particularly high rates in children of pre-school age. Also common are the communicable diseases, acute otitis media, eczema, and injuries. The study shows that 20 per cent of all general practitioner consultations are in the age group 0 to 14 years.

School medical examinations

Children are routinely examined in school at five years of age and again at 13. The main defects recorded are shown in Table 7.2. In school entrants, dental

Table 7.2 Defects found at routine school medical examinations, Scotland, 1977. Source: Scottish Home and Health Department (1979)

Diagnosis	Entrants Boys	Entrants Girls	Leavers Boys	Leavers Girls
Dental caries	12 729	12 991	6633	5260
Refractive error	4800	5082	11 595	13 314
Strabismus	2789	2863	889	994
Enuresis	5569	5135	604	311
Speech disorder	4897	2405	565	208
Verruca	742	847	1392	1381
Pediculosis	154	247	313	349
Colour blindness	313	25	4206	222
Asthma	1328	603	2074	1012
Disease of tonsils	8176	8317	1599	2168
Diseases of respiratory system	4871	4349	2216	1946
Eczema	1169	1141	688	777
Inflammatory condition of ear	1175	1008	443	463
Impairment of hearing	1792	1622	1237	1245
Obesity	677	1314	2311	3852

Rate per 100 000 examined

caries is the most common condition but the prevalence rate shown (approximately 13 per cent) is probably very far short of the true position: data for England and Wales show that just over half of all children having their first dental inspection at school or in a clinic are found to require dental treatment (DHSS, 1974). Also common are disease of the tonsils, disease of the respiratory system (mainly coughs and colds), refractive errors, enuresis and strabismus.

In 13-year-old children, dental caries is again the defect recorded most often, followed by refractive errors. Other common defects are colour blindness in boys, obesity, disease of the tonsils and respiratory system, pediculosis and verruca.

Hospital in-patients

Each year in Britain there are almost a million hospital admissions under the age of 15 years, a rate of approximately seven admissions per hundred children. The most common cause of admission is injury, followed by perinatal morbidity and then hypertrophy of the tonsils and adenoids (mainly for operative

Table 7.3 Hospital in-patients in England and Wales aged 0 to 14 years. Sources: Department of Health and Social Security and Office of Population Censuses and Surveys (1978)

Diagnosis	Percentage of all discharges, 0–14 years
Injury	14
Causes of perinatal morbidity	9
Hypertrophy of tonsils and adenoids	8
Congenital anomalies	7
Respiratory tract infection	6
Infectious diseases	5
Poisoning	5
Appendicitis	3
Strabismus	2
Otitis media/mastoiditis	2

treatment) (Table 7.3). Unfortunately, there are no national statistics on out-patient or casualty department attendances.

Congenital malformations

A congenital malformation is defined as a 'macroscopical abnormality of structure attributed to faulty development and present at birth' (McKeown & Record, 1960). Since the causes of most malformations are unknown, some arbitrary classification has to be devised and this is usually by anatomical system. In determining the prevalence of these conditions at birth, the notification of birth form (suitably modified) is a valuable source of information. However, some defects may not be apparent at birth and so reasonable completeness of ascertainment can be assumed only when all possible sources of information have been tapped. These include registrations of still-birth and death, notifications from clinicians, health visitors and pathologists, registers of handicapped children and hospital diagnostic indices.

Three large population studies have been conducted in Britain covering the whole range of malformations. These investigations show that between 2 and 4 per cent of infants are malformed at birth, the most common defects being

Table 7.4 Prevalence at birth of certain congenital malformations. Sources: Birmingham—Leck et al (1968); Liverpool—Smithells (1968); S. Wales—Richards & Lowe (1971)

	Prevalence per thousand births		
Type of defect	Birmingham 1950–4 94 474 total births	Liverpool 1960–4 91 176 total births	S. Wales 1964–6 90 921 singleton births
All malformed infants	23.1	23.9	35.7
Anencephaly	2.0	3.1	3.1
Spina bifida (without anencephaly)	2.2	3.4	3.9
Cardiac malformation	4.2	5.0	4.4
Talipes	5.7	2.7	3.4
Dislocation of hip	0.9	0.7	0.9
Cleft lip and/or palate	2.0	1.5	2.1
Down's syndrome	1.6	1.4	1.0

those of the central nervous system (mainly anencephalus and spina bifida) and of the heart (Table 7.4).

The handicapped
Statistics published by the Department of Education and Science (1974) show that, in England and Wales, more than 150 000 pupils either require or receive special education on account of a handicap. This represents 18 per 1000 of the school population.

Two thirds of these handicapped children are educationally subnormal and it has been estimated by the Department of Health and Social Security (1971) that about four children per 1000 are severely mentally handicapped. The second largest group are maladjusted children, that is those with emotional instability or psychological disturbance. In a study of handicapped children in the Isle of Wight, 6.8 per cent of 10- and 11-year-old children were regarded as having a psychiatric disorder (Rutter et al, 1970) and in a national study of seven-year-old children as many as 14 per cent were judged to be maladjusted (Pringle et al, 1966). Children with physical handicaps comprise the next largest group, about a third being cases of cerebral palsy.

About one child in every 1000 is born profoundly deaf but the number born with moderate or lesser degrees of deafness is several times greater than this. The prevalence of hearing defects among school entrants in 1964–65 was 7.9 per 1000 children examined (Central Health Services Council, 1971), while a further 18.3 per 1000 required observation with regard to their hearing ability (DHSS and Welsh Office, 1971).

The reported prevalence of epilepsy varies widely from 2.1 per 1000 schoolchildren in Scotland (Scottish Home and Health Department, 1968) to 7.2 per 1000 in the Isle of Wight (Rutter et al, 1970). The variations in the rates obtained from such studies are likely to reflect differences in the completeness of the ascertainment of cases. It has been estimated that in England and Wales about 100 000 children under the age of 17 have epilepsy (DHSS, 1969).

Communicable diseases
Certain infectious diseases are notifiable to the local authority; they are prescribed by the Health Services and Public Health Act 1968. Notifications show that much preventable infectious disease still occurs among children in Britain. For example, 154 000 cases of measles were notified in 1973, 11 000 cases of food poisoning and dysentery, and 2500 cases of whooping cough. Deaths from infectious diseases are mainly due to diarrhoeal diseases and meningococcal infection, with the highest mortality in the first year of life.

Child abuse
There are several difficulties in assessing the true incidence of child abuse.

1. The term 'child abuse' refers to a much greater dimension of maltreatment than non-accidental physical injury (the 'battered child syndrome') and there is no generally accepted definition of the term.
2. A large number of cases—possibly the majority—do not come to official notice. Even if reporting were compulsory, a high level of ascertainment would

be dependent on the medical profession's awareness of the problem and on its co-operation.

3. The incidence of child abuse in various sections of the community can be determined only by studies of large populations; investigations based on hospital or agency information are not necessarily representative.

Kempe (1971) has estimated that the incidence of child abuse in the United States is about six per 1000 live births, half of which suffer significant injury and half serious deprivation. More recent estimates put the figure much higher, especially if all forms of abuse are included (Solomons, 1979). On the basis of Kempe's estimate, there would be about 4800 cases per annum in the United Kingdom: Hall (1975) has calculated that there are almost four and a half thousand children being treated annually in accident and emergency departments with injuries of an inadequately explained nature. The National Society for the Prevention of Cruelty to Children (1977) estimates that nearly 8000 children sustain such injuries each year in England and Wales.

Recorded fatality rates for battered children vary between 1 per cent and 17 per cent but these are based mainly on hospital cases (and hence on children with severe injuries): the true figure in Britain may be about 3 per cent (Mac Keith, 1975). Kempe et al (1962) estimated that 15 per cent of survivors were left with 'permanent brain damage' while Martin (1972) reported that as many as a third were mentally retarded.

The search for causes
The health of a population is determined by five groups of factors:

1. Its genetic constitution.
2. Its age and sex structure.
3. The physical environment, for example hazards at home, at work or school, on the roads and in leisure activities, atmospheric pollution, food and water supplies and sanitation.
4. Personal behaviour, for example sexual behaviour, child-rearing practices, malnutrition, smoking, abuse of drugs and alcohol, and the use made of the health services.
5. The availability and quality of health and social services.

Epidemiology examines these factors in order to identify causal agents, paths of transmission of communicable diseases and the conditions predisposing to the occurrence and continuation of the disease process. The knowledge thus gained can lead to:
1. The introduction of new preventive measures;
2. The control of environmental hazards;
3. The identification of 'high-risk' groups requiring special care;
4. Changes in the health services.

Perinatal mortality
Much of our understanding of this subject is derived from the first British Perinatal Mortality Survey which covered a national sample of over 17 000 births

in 1958 as well as 7000 additional perinatal and late neonatal deaths (Butler & Bonham, 1963; Butler & Alberman, 1969). Valuable information has also been provided by the second survey of British births (Chamberlain et al, 1975, 1978).

Mortality is higher in the first pregnancy than in the next two or three, after which the hazard rises with increasing parity. Maternal age has an independent effect on reproductive efficiency, the general trend being a rise in perinatal mortality with increasing age. The basis of these trends is little understood. Perinatal mortality is higher in illegitimate than in legitimate births. Low socio-economic status and short stature are both associated with an excess of mortality, suggesting that poor general health and malnutrition in childhood and during pregnancy impair reproductive efficiency.

Perinatal mortality rates are higher in Wales, the North of England and the industrial belt of Scotland than in the remainder of Britain. Reasons for this geographical pattern are complex and include the socio-economic status (both past and present) of the mothers, and differences in birth-rates; variation in the quality of health services and the extent to which they are used may also be important factors.

Some women have a poor reproductive pattern which may be repeated in a series of pregnancies. The risk of perinatal death is raised if there has been a previous premature delivery, abortion, still-birth or neonatal death. Harmful factors in the current pregnancy include blood group incompatibility, chronic hypertension, renal disease, diabetes, multiple pregnancy and malpresentation. Butler & Alberman (1969) have shown that the mean birth-weight of infants born to smokers is about 170 g lower than to non-smokers and that still-birth rates are about 40 per cent higher in smokers. They conclude that smoking in the latter part of pregnancy is prejudicial to the growth and survival of the fetus.

The causes of perinatal death fall into two broad categories (Baird et al, 1954). The first group are obstetric causes (toxaemia, mechanical causes, unexplained deaths of mature babies and Rhesus incompatibility) which are capable of being reduced by high standards of obstetric care. The second group (unexplained prematurity, fetal defects and antepartum haemorrhage) is less amenable to obstetrical intervention, being related to the effects of unfavourable environmental influences on the mother's reproductive function. Although levels of perinatal mortality in Britain have fallen strikingly during the past 40 years, there is still considerable room for improvement (DHSS, 1977): as many as a third of the deaths in one area have been shown to be from causes which are capable of being reduced by high standards of obstetric care (McIlwaine et al, 1974). Substantial progress might be made if a greater proportion of births were to occur at the optimal maternal age (20–29 years), if fewer mothers had more than two children and if the rates experienced in social classes I and II* could be extended to all babies (Lambert, 1976).

Infant mortality
The geographical pattern is similar to that described for perinatal mortality and rates are highest in areas of overcrowding, poor housing and high birth-rates (Richards, 1971). The infant mortality rate in social class V is twice the rate

*See appendix.

in social class I, the difference between the classes being greater in the post-neonatal period than in the neonatal. Social class differences in mortality are greater for infections (mainly pneumonia and gastroenteritis) and accidental suffocation than for congenital anomalies and perinatal causes. In discussing such gradients, Kincaid (1965) remarked that 'what we are dealing with are not isolated factors but whole patterns of behaviour. And in so far as these factors vary between the various social classes, what are in question are differences between the whole way of life of different sections of the community.'

The social class differences in neonatal and post-neonatal mortality have remained consistent over a long period. This is surprising since welfare legislation has undoubtedly been of more benefit to the poorer sections of the community than to the well-to-do and there has been more scope for the reduction of mortality from infection and other preventable causes in the poorer classes. McKeown & Lowe (1974) have suggested two possible reasons for this paradox: 'the better educated and well-to-do parents have earlier access to and make better use of social and medical advances; and there is more social mobility now than formerly, so that those in class V today are more likely to be there because of ill health or lack of ability than those in class V forty years ago'.

Cot deaths

About half the post-neonatal deaths occur at home as unexpected cot deaths. At autopsy, there is evidence of a definite disease state in a third of cases; this may be a severe acute disease such as meningitis, acute obstructive tracheobronchitis or gastroenteritis with hypernatraemia or a chronic condition such as a congenital malformation (Protestos et al, 1973). The factors leading to these deaths appear to lie in a general lack of ability of some parents to recognize the importance of symptoms, their unwillingness or inability to avail themselves of health services, and the amount of drive and persistence required to obtain general practice services in some areas. There is also failure on the part of some practitioners to recognize severe illness in the children (Richards & McIntosh, 1972; McWeeny & Emery, 1975).

However, in a third of cot deaths there are no features of acute disease at autopsy and in a further third a lesion that would be expected to cause minor illness (Protestos et al, 1973). These two groups together constitute what is usually referred to as the sudden infant death syndrome (SIDS). The peak age incidence of SIDS occurs at 12 to 16 weeks and it is uncommon after nine months. The incidence of these deaths is highest in socially deprived families characterized by low parental intelligence, poor maternal efficiency and a multiplicity of problems—illegitimacy, cohabitation or a tense marital situation (Vaughan, 1968; Richards & McIntosh, 1972; Richards, 1974). In this group, too, there is evidence of failure by the parents to recognize serious illness in their baby. A study of the obstetric and perinatal histories of babies dying of SIDS has shown that the most powerful criterion for identifying high risk children is failure of the mother to bring the baby to the first follow-up clinic after discharge from hospital (Protestos et al, 1973).

The seasonal incidence and social class pattern favour an infective cause for SIDS; overlaying, suffocation from bedclothes or a soft pillow, and inhalation of regurgitated milk are now believed to be uncommon causes of cot death. All the common respiratory pathogens have been isolated in SIDS and it has been suggested that a high proportion of these deaths is due to a fulminating infection of the lower respiratory tract (Johnstone & Lawy, 1966). Attempts at virus isolations have been disappointing (Valdes-Dapena & Hummeler, 1963; Urquhart & Grist, 1972) and there is no evidence that overwhelming virus infection is a common feature in SIDS. Many other causes have been suggested for these unexplained deaths, including nasal obstruction in those infants who are unable to substitute oral breathing if the nose is obstructed, and hypoglycaemia due to nocturnal fasting or to an excess of protein in the feeds. But we are probably not considering a single disease entity, and all that can be said at present is that the characteristic age range suggests that 'while passing through this period of increased physiological vulnerability, some critical combination of intrinsic and extrinsic factors proves lethal' (Froggatt et al, 1971).

Low birth-weight
Babies who weigh 2500 g or less at birth constitute in Britain only 7 per cent of the newborn, yet over half of all neonatal deaths occur in this group. Two thirds of these births are truly premature, i.e. the babies are born before 37 completed weeks from the first day of the mother's last menstrual period. In most cases, the cause of the early onset of labour is unknown. The babies' problems are those of immaturity and the major cause of death is hyaline membrane disease which occurs with increasing frequency and severity at decreasing gestational ages. The other group of low birth-weight babies are those who are light for the gestational age at which they are born, either because of poor growth potential (including fetal malformation and intrauterine infection such as rubella) or a growth-restricting intrauterine environment. In the latter group, maternal factors have an important influence on fetal growth, especially poor socio-economic status. The problems occurring in light-for-dates babies are intrauterine hypoxia, birth asphyxia and symptomatic hypoglycaemia.

There is a much higher incidence of neurological handicap—especially cerebral palsy, mental retardation, epilepsy and learning difficulties—in children of low birth-weight compared with the general population. The incidence of neurological disorder is highest in children of birth weight less than 1500 g. Preterm babies are more likely to develop cerebral palsy and light-for-dates babies to be mentally retarded or have fits. There have been many enquiries into the effect of low birth-weight on intelligence but the evidence is contradictory (McKeown & Record, 1971). Mean birth-weight is undoubtedly low in mentally subnormal children and McDonald (1964) found in a study of infants of less than 4 lb birth-weight that, after exclusion of those with cerebral palsy, blindness, deafness and intelligence quotients (IQ) below 50, the IQ of the remainder was about the same as for normal births. Verbal reasoning scores in the school examination at 11+ years have been found to increase with increasing birth-weight (Record et al, 1969); both shortening and prolongation of the duration of gestation have an adverse effect on measured intelligence (Record et al, 1969; Neligan et al, 1974). IQ and birth-weight are both lower in the children of poor families than in the more privileged and it is not known to what extent social class is responsible for the associations described above.

In the first two years of life, low birth-weight babies are more liable to colds and coughs and to have an excess of hospital admissions for lower respiratory infections (Douglas & Blomfield, 1958).

Congenital malformations
Since Hale's observation in 1933 that sows on a diet deficient in vitamin A produce piglets without eyeballs, very many physical and chemical agents have been shown to be teratogenic in the animal laboratory. The search by epidemiological methods for environmental components in the aetiology of human malformations has been less rewarding. There is good evidence that environmental influences are involved, for the incidence rates of various defects show geographical, secular and seasonal fluctuations and social class, maternal age and parity differences. In addition, the concordance rate for identical twins is well below 100 per cent for most malformations, although higher than for fraternal twins of like sex. Discordance in identical twin pairs is almost the rule in some malformations, for example anencephaly (Penrose, 1961).

While some of the marked international differences in the incidence of congenital malformations (such as the low rate of neural tube defects in negro populations) are likely to be largely genetic in origin, the geographical variations within the British Isles in malformation incidence remain unexplained. Most prominent among these are the high incidence of anencephaly in Northern Ireland (Elwood, 1970) and of anencephaly and spina bifida in South Wales (Richards & Lowe, 1971).

Many congenital malformations are more common among first births but anencephaly and spina bifida show a U-shaped trend with parity. Two conditions are known to be age-dependent, Down's syndrome which is related to maternal age (Penrose, 1934; Carter & MacCarthy, 1951) and achondroplasia related to paternal age (Penrose, 1955). The incidence of most congenital malformations is higher among male infants than among female: a small number, for example anencephaly and congenital dislocation of the hip, show a female preponderance.

Several studies have shown that neural tube defects have a higher incidence among poorer families (Rogers & Weatherall, 1976), the social class difference being greatest in anencephaly (Edwards, 1958; Wilson, 1971). In South Wales, there is a dichotomy rather than a gradient with an appreciably higher incidence of anencephaly and spina bifida among births to wives of manual workers (Lowe, 1972). There is no evidence of an increased incidence of malformations among illegitimate births.

Seasonal variations in incidence have been reported for some malformations, for example an excess among winter births for anencephaly (McKeown & Record, 1951; Edwards, 1958)—although much of this seasonal pattern has now disappeared (Leck & Record, 1966)—and for congenital dislocation of the hip (Record & Edwards, 1958).

Women who have given birth to children with malformations of the central nervous system have a raised miscarriage rate among earlier pregnancies

(Malpas, 1937; Record & McKeown, 1950; Smithells & Chinn, 1965) and in one study (Richards et al, 1972) it was found that in these mothers more than 40 per cent of all known pregnancies ended in either miscarriage or the birth of a child with a congenital defect. Studies of other pregnancy factors, such as illnesses and drugs, have not been very fruitful, with the exception of a small number of uncommon conditions such as the embryopathy due to rubella and thalidomide. It now seems likely that, although environmental influences are undoubtedly important, they will prove to be much more subtle and much less accessible to control than was at one time hoped.

Handicapping conditions

More than a century ago, Little (1843–4) described the range of handicapping conditions of the central nervous system which could be caused by adverse factors acting before, during, or soon after a child's birth. In recent years, a considerable amount of epidemiological research has been devoted to unravelling the relationship between antecedent factors and the subsequent development of children. Although much remains to be discovered about the aetiology of most handicapping conditions, these investigations have already made a valuable contribution to our understanding of the problem.

There is no evidence that complications of delivery (Drillien, 1969) or birth injury (Kushlick & Cox, 1973) are important causes of severe mental subnormality. Neligan et al (1974) have shown that for both the severely and educationally subnormal groups there is an excess of babies of low birth-weight as compared with groups of mentally normal children. They have also shown that in the educationally subnormal and borderline subnormal groups (but not in the severely subnormal) there is a great excess of social class IV and V children and that this is related to the quality of the mother's care of her child and the number of her previous pregnancies.

Several large retrospective studies of cerebral palsy have been reported (e.g. Asher & Schonell, 1950; Lilienfeld & Parkhurst, 1951; Skatvedt, 1958; Henderson, 1961; Ingram, 1964; Griffiths & Barrett, 1967) but, in some, information on antecedent factors has been derived from the mother's history (which may not be reliable) or from incomplete clinical records. The factor which features consistently in most studies is low birth-weight. Lilienfeld & Parkhurst (1951) also reported an excess of breech deliveries compared with the total survivors of the neonatal period in the same population. There is evidence that improvements in perinatal care have been followed by a diminution in the prevalence of cerebral palsy (Hagberg et al, 1975).

In the Newcastle study of a thousand families (Miller et al, 1974), disturbed children tended to be below average in height, weight, intelligence and educational attainment. The parents were younger, and more recently married: many of the mothers were mentally ill and their own childhood had been unhappy. Separation of the child from the mother for longer than a month, separation from father before the age of two, and admission to hospital without the mother, were all judged to be important factors.

Respiratory disease

Infection of the respiratory tract is important as a cause of morbidity and mortality in childhood and an association has been demonstrated between a history of lower respiratory tract disease in early childhood and respiratory symptoms in early adult life. The evidence, though incomplete, does suggest that the 'chesty' child may become the adult chronic bronchitic (Colley, 1971).

The incidence of lower respiratory tract infection is highest in the poorer families (Grundy & Lewis-Faning, 1957; Douglas & Blomfield, 1958: Colley & Reid, 1970). Overcrowding in the home is one of the factors that might be responsible for this association and it has been shown to increase the risk of transmitting respiratory infection within the family (Brimblecombe et al, 1958). Children who smoke have a higher prevalence of respiratory symptoms (cough and phlegm) than non-smokers (Holland et al, 1969) and smoking in the family is significantly associated with lower respiratory tract infection in childhood (Chamberlain & Simpson, 1979).

Although asthma appears to be more common in children from better-off families (Logan, 1960; Graham et al, 1967), there is evidence that the prevalence of severe asthma is greatest in the children of semi-skilled and unskilled workers (Mitchell & Dawson, 1973). Between 1960 and 1965 there was an eight-fold increase in the death-rate from asthma among children aged 10 to 14 years, probably due to greater use of pressurized bronchodilator aerosols containing sympathomimetic amines (Inman & Adelstein, 1969).

Communicable diseases

Social group differences in the incidence of communicable diseases are small but poorer children tend to catch these diseases earlier in life and the presence of a schoolchild in the family makes infection more likely (Douglas & Blomfield, 1958). The risk of death from infection is highest in the later-born children of large families because of their higher susceptibility to infection and higher case-fatality (Lowe & McKeown, 1954).

Accidents and injuries

Information about accidents which cause death is much more reliable and complete than it is concerning injuries not resulting in death. Accidental deaths are subject to scrutiny by coroners (procurators fiscal in Scotland) and the circumstances are recorded in Registrar General reports. For the (much more numerous) injuries not causing death, there is no standard system of recording.

Most accidental injuries in children are related to domestic life or road transport; a smaller number are due to recreational accidents, falls in the street or drowning. In infancy, accidental death is usually due to suffocation or respiratory obstruction by inhalation of milk or stomach contents. Once a child starts to crawl and walk, he encounters dangers associated with domestic processes and objects leading to burns, scalds, falls from furniture and injuries from sharp objects. Poisoning is not a significant cause of accidental death in childhood (Table 7.5).

Accidents are an important cause of admission to hospital in childhood, with the highest admission rates for burns and poisoning in the age group one to four years and for fractures and dislocations between five and 14 years. Boys are more liable to injury than girls and their injuries tend to be more severe (Douglas & Blomfield, 1958: Miller et al, 1974). Accidents are more common and more severe in the poorer families, especially where maternal care is unsatisfactory or where they are living in blocks of flats or overcrowded dwellings. They are also more common in children whose mothers go out to work (Chamberlain & Simpson, 1979). Less intelligent children, who fail to learn by experience, have an increased risk of multiple accident.

Table 7.5 Deaths from accidents, violence and poisoning (England and Wales 1976). Source: Office of Population Censuses and Surveys (1978)

	Sex	0–4	5–9	10–14	Total
All deaths due to accidents, poisoning or violence	M	407	259	247	913
	F	241	135	112	488
Motor vehicle transport accidents	M	89	138	116	343
	F	48	73	49	170
Drowning	M	38	39	26	103
	F	17	13	7	37
Inhalation and ingestion of food	M	88	3	7	98
	F	34	1	1	36
Falls	M	31	18	21	70
	F	14	7	4	25
Accidental mechanical suffocation	M	23	3	24	50
	F	25	1	1	27
Homicide	M	35	1	3	39
	F	27	10	9	46
Poisoning	M	11	5	4	20
	F	6	3	4	13

Deaths by age group (years)

Non-accidental injury
Since Wooley & Evans suggested in 1955 that previously unexplained fractures might have been inflicted intentionally, much research has been made into the characteristics of the parents and the reasons for the child abuse. Although it can occur to children of any age, non-accidental injury is more often reported in children under three years of age, and from poor socio-economic backgrounds. Infants of low birth-weight appear to be at particular risk, suggesting that impaired mother/infant bonding is a factor.

Battering parents tend to be young and socially isolated (Skinner & Castle, 1969). It has been suggested that they were deprived of mothering in their own childhood (Steele & Pollock, 1968; Galdston, 1965). Some authors have reported a high frequency of illegitimate pregnancies (Birrell & Birrell, 1968; Simons et al, 1966). However, most parents in deprived sections of the community do not batter their children and the relevance of these personal characteristics and environmental factors can only be determined by controlled studies.

One such investigation has been conducted in Birmingham (Smith et al, 1973, 1974; Smith & Hanson, 1974; Smith, 1975; Hanson et al, 1977). It confirmed that battering is associated with youthful parents, predominantly in social classes IV and V. Lack of family cohesiveness (e.g. an absent father or cohabitation), early marriage, premarital conception, short acquaintance before marriage, a negative attitude towards contraception and disharmony in child rearing formed the typical background to baby battering. Only a minority of battering parents were obviously mentally ill but nearly half the mothers were of subnormal intelligence. One third of the fathers were psychopaths and three quarters of the mothers had an abnormal personality. Many of the parents had criminal records.

Illegitimate children and one-parent families
One in 12 of all children are in families in which one of the parents raises the family without a partner, either through illegitimacy, death, divorce or separation. Illegitimate births are distributed fairly evenly throughout the different sections of society and at least a quarter are to married or cohabiting women (Illsley & Gill, 1968); a third are to women aged less than 20 years. Follow-up studies of illegitimate children are often difficult because of the desire on the part of the parents to remain anonymous and also the high degree of mobility of these families.

In a detailed study of unmarried mothers and their children in the Edinburgh area, Weir (1970) found that the mothers came from intact homes and from broken homes, with a slight preponderance of homes broken by separation or divorce. Many of the mothers had known the baby's father well and, for some, the relationship had been a very long-standing and deep one. The majority did not appear to be promiscuous. The group of mothers who kept their infants were shown to be less favoured economically and more likely to have moved away from their parents, so lacking parental support.

Crellin et al (1971) have studied the 679 illegitimate children in the National Child Development Survey (1958 cohort). The risk of an illegitimate pregnancy was found to be high in young women whose own father had been frequently away from home or had died. The home environment of the illegitimately born children was more unfavourable than that of the legitimate or of the illegitimate who were subsequently adopted. The latter group grew up under the most favoured conditions and there was a marked degree of downward social mobility among the families who had not given up the illegitimate child for adoption. In ability and attainment, the latter group did less well than legitimate children or those that were adopted.

Conclusion
This review of the contribution of epidemiology to our understanding of child health problems has, of necessity, been confined to selected common conditions. It must be mentioned, however, that much epidemiological research has also been devoted to other important conditions such as dental caries, the childhood malignancies and urinary tract infection.

From an examination of the dimensions of ill health, it will be concluded that childhood is a time of high morbidity, much of it potentially avoidable, with high mortality in infancy. When the epidemiology of individual conditions is studied with a view to defining vulnerable groups of children, it is clear that much of this unnecessary illness and death occurs in the less privileged sections of the community and in those families where parental care is inadequate. These are the groups which require special preventive care, especially by health visitors and general practitioners (Richards et al, 1979). However, mortality studies have also shown that many deaths could be avoided by higher standards of medical care—obstetric, paediatric and general practitioner. There is, therefore, need for constant monitoring of the state of child health in the community so that deficiencies can be identified and then corrected.

Appendix

Social classification used by the Registrar General
Classification of Occupations, 1966, published for the General Register Office by HMSO.

I Professional, etc. occupations
II Intermediate occupations
III Skilled occupations
IV Partly skilled occupations
V Unskilled.

REFERENCES

Asher P, Schonell F E 1950 A survey of 400 cases of cerebral palsy in childhood. Archives of Disease in Childhood 25: 360–379
Baird D, Walker J, Thomson A M 1954 The causes and prevention of stillbirths and first week deaths. Journal of Obstetrics and Gynaecology of the British Empire 61: 433–448
Birrell R G, Birrell J H W 1968 The maltreatment syndrome in children: a hospital survey. Medical Journal of Australia 2: 1023–1029
Brimblecombe F S W, Cruickshank R, Masters P L, Reid D D, Stewart G T, Sanderson D 1958 Family studies of respiratory infection. British Medical Journal i: 119–128
Butler N R, Alberman E D 1969 Perinatal problems. Livingstone, Edinburgh
Butler N R, Bonham D G 1963 Perinatal mortality. Livingstone, Edinburgh
Carter C O, MacCarthy D 1951 Incidence of mongolism and its diagnosis in the newborn. British Journal of Social Medicine 5: 83–90
Central Health Services Council 1971 Memorandum on deafness in early childhood. HMSO, London
Chamberlain G, Philipp E, Howlett B, Masters K 1978 British births 1970. Vol 2. Obstetric care. Heinemann, London
Chamberlain R, Chamberlain G, Howlett B, Claireaux A 1975 British births 1970. Vol 1. The first week of life. Heinemann, London
Chamberlain R, Simpson R 1979 The prevalence of illness in childhood. Pitman Medical, Tunbridge Wells
Colley J R T 1971 Respiratory disease in childhood. British Medical Bulletin 27: 9–13
Colley J R T, Reid D D 1970 Urban and social origins of childhood bronchitis in England and Wales. British Medical Journal ii: 213–217
Court S D M (chairman) 1976 Fit for the future: Report of the Committee on Child Health Services. HMSO London
Crellin E, Pringle M L K, West P 1971 Born illegitimate. Social and educational implications. National Foundation for Educational Research in England and Wales, London
Department of Education and Science 1974 The health of the school child 1971–72. HMSO, London
Department of Health and Social Security 1969 People with epilepsy. HMSO, London
Department of Health and Social Security 1971 Better services for the mentally handicapped. HMSO, London
Department of Health and Social Security 1974 On the state of the public health. HMSO, London

Department of Health and Social Security 1977 Prevention and health: reducing the risk. HMSO, London
Department of Health and Social Security and Office of Population Censuses and Surveys 1978 Report on hospital in-patient enquiry for the year 1975. HMSO, London
Department of Health and Social Security and the Welsh Office 1971 Deafness in early childhood. HMSO, London
Douglas J W B, Blomfield J M 1958 Children under five. George Allen & Unwin, London
Drillien C M 1969 School disposal and performance for children of different birthweights born 1953–1960. Archives of Disease in Childhood 44: 562–570
Drillien C M 1974 Prevention of handicap in infants of very low birth weight. In: Woodford F P (ed) Prevention of handicap in infants of low birth weight. Institute for Research into Mental and Multiple Handicap, London
Edwards J H 1958 Congenital malformations of the central nervous system in Scotland. British Journal of Preventive and Social Medicine 12: 115–130
Elwood J H 1970 Anencephalus in the British Isles. Developmental Medicine and Child Neurology 12: 582–591
Franklin A W 1976 Widening horizons of child health. MTP Press, Lancaster
Froggatt P, Lynas M A, MacKenzie G 1971 Epidemiology of sudden unexpected death in infants ('cot death') in Northern Ireland. British Journal of Preventive and Social Medicine 25: 119–134
Galdston R 1965 Observations on children who have been physically abused and their parents. American Journal of Psychiatry 122: 125–130
Goel K M 1979 Nutrition survey of immigrant children in Glasgow. Scottish Home and Health Department, Edinburgh
Graham P J, Rutter M L, Yale W W, Pless I B 1967 Childhood asthma: a psychosomatic disorder? British Journal of Preventive and Social Medicine 21: 78–85
Griffiths M I, Barrett N M 1967 Cerebral palsy in Birmingham. Developmental Medicine and Child Neurology 9: 33–46.
Grundy F, Lewis-Faning E 1957 Morbidity and mortality in the first year of life. The Eugenics Society, Cardiff
Hagberg B, Hagberg G, Olow I 1975 The changing panorama of cerebral palsy in Sweden 1954–70. Acta paediatrica Scandinavica 64: 187–200
Hale F 1933 Pigs born without eyeballs. Journal of Heredity 24: 105 ff
Hall M H 1975 A view from the emergency and accident department. In: Franklin A W (ed) Concerning child abuse. Churchill Livingstone, Edinburgh
Hanson R, McCulloch J W, Hartley S A 1977 Key characteristics in child abuse. In: Franklin A W (ed) Child abuse: prediction, prevention and follow-up. Churchill Livingstone, Edinburgh
Henderson J L (ed) 1961 Cerebral palsy in childhood and adolescence. Livingstone, Edinburgh
Holland W W, Halil T, Bennett A E, Elliott A 1969 Factors influencing the onset of chronic respiratory disease. British Medical Journal i: 205–208
Illsley R, Gill D 1968 Changing trends in illegitimacy. Social Science and Medicine: An International Journal vol 2, No 4
Ingram T T S 1964 Paediatric aspects of cerebral palsy. Livingstone, Edinburgh
Inman W H W, Adelstein A M 1969 Rise and fall of asthma mortality in England and Wales in relation to use of pressurised aerosols. Lancet ii: 279–285
Johnstone J M, Lawy H S 1966 Role of infection in cot death. British Medical Journal i: 706–709
Kempe C H 1971 Paediatric implications of the battered-baby syndrome. Archives of Disease in Childhood 46: 28–37
Kempe C H, Silverman F N, Steele B F, Droegemuller W, Silver H K 1962 The battered-child syndrome. Journal of the American Medical Association 181: 17–24
Kincaid J C 1965 Social pathology in foetal and infant loss. British Medical Journal i: 1057–1060
Kushlick A, Cox G R 1973 The epidemiology of mental handicap. Developmental Medicine and Child Neurology 15: 748–759
Lambert P 1976 Perinatal mortality: social and environmental factors. Office of Population Censuses and Surveys. HMSO, London
Leck I, Record R G 1966 Seasonal incidence of anencephalus. British Journal of Preventive and Social Medicine 20: 67–75
Leck I, Record R G, McKeown T, Edwards J H 1968 The incidence of malformations in Birmingham, England, 1950–1959. Teratology 1: 263, 280

Lilienfeld A M, Parkhurst E 1951 A study of the association of factors in pregnancy and parturition with the development of cerebral palsy. American Journal of Hygiene 53: 262 ff
Little W J, 1843–4 Lecture VIII in 'Course of lectures on the deformities of the human frame'. Lancet i: 319
Logan W P D 1960 Morbidity statistics for general practice. Studies in Medical and Population Subjects, No 14, vol. 2. HMSO, London
Lowe C R 1972 Congenital malformations and the problem of their control. British Medical Journal iii: 515–520
Lowe C R, McKeown T 1954 Incidence of infectious disease in the first three years of life related to social circumstances. British Journal of Preventive and Social Medicine 8: 24–28
McDonald A D 1964 Intelligence in children of very low birth weight. British Journal of Preventive and Social Medicine 18: 59–74
McIlwaine G, Macnaughton M C, Richards I D G 1974 A study of perinatal deaths in Glasgow. Health Bulletin 32: 103–105
Mac Keith R 1975 Speculations on some possible long-term effects. In: Franklin A W (ed) Concerning child abuse. Churchill Livingstone, Edinburgh
McKeown T, Lowe C R 1974 An introduction to social medicine. Blackwell, Oxford
McKeown T, Record R G 1951 Seasonal incidence of congenital malformations of the central nervous system. Lancet i: 192–196
McKeown T, Record R G 1960 Malformation in a population observed for five years after birth. In: Wolstenholme G E W, O'Connor C M (eds) CIBA Foundation Symposium on Congenital Malformations. Churchill, London, p 21
McKeown T, Record R G 1971 Early environmental influences on the development of intelligence. British Medical Bulletin 27: 48–52
McWeeny P M, Emery J L 1975 Unexpected postneonatal deaths (cot deaths) due to recognizable disease. Archives of Disease in Childhood 50: 191–196
Malpas P 1937 The incidence of human malformations and the significance of changes in the maternal environment in their causation. Journal of Obstetrics and Gynaecology of the British Empire 44: 434–453
Martin H 1972 The child and his development. In Helping the battered child and his family. Lippincott, Philadelphia
Miller F J W, Court S D M, Knox E G, Brandon S 1974 The school years in Newcastle upon Tyne 1956–62. Oxford University Press, London
Miller F J W, Court S D M, Walton W S, Knox E G 1960 Growing up in Newcastle upon Tyne. Oxford University Press, London
Mitchell R G, Dawson B 1973 Educational and social characteristics of children with asthma. Archives of Disease in Childhood 48: 467–471
National Society for the Prevention of Cruelty to Children 1977, Child victims of physical abuse. NSPCC, London
Neligan G, Prudham D, Steiner H 1974 The formative years—birth, family and development in Newcastle upon Tyne. Nuffield Provincial Hospitals Trust. Oxford University Press, London
Office of Population Censuses and Surveys 1974 Morbidity statistics from general practice. Second national study 1970–71. Studies on Medical and Population Subjects, No 26. HMSO
Office of Population Censuses and Surveys 1978 Mortality statistics: cause. Review of the Registrar General on deaths by cause, sex and age in England and Wales 1976. HMSO, London
Office of Population Censuses and Surveys 1979 Demographic review 1977. HMSO, London
Penrose L S 1934 A method of separating the relative aetiological effects of birth order and maternal age with specific reference to mongolian imbecility. Annals of Eugenics 6: 108–122
Penrose L S 1955 Parental age and mutation. Lancet ii: 312–313
Penrose L S 1961 Recent Advances in Human Genetics. Churchill, London
Pringle M L K, Butler N R, Davie R 1966 11,000 Seven-year-olds. Longman, London
Protestos C D, Carpenter R G, McWeeny P M, Emery J L 1973 Obstetric and perinatal histories of children who died unexpectedly (cot death). Archives of Disease in Childhood 48: 835–841
Record R G, Edwards J H 1958 Environmental influences related to the aetiology of congenital dislocation of the hip. British Journal of Preventive and Social Medicine 12: 8–22
Record R G, McKeown T 1950 Congenital malformations of the central nervous system. II. Maternal reproductive history and familial incidence. British Journal of Preventive and Social Medicine 4: 26–50
Record R G, McKeown T, Edwards J H 1969 The relation of measured intelligence to birth weight and duration of gestation. Annals of Human Genetics 33: 71–79

Richards I D G 1971 Infant mortality in Scotland. Scottish Health Service Studies, No 16. Scottish Home and Health Department, Edinburgh
Richards I D G 1974 Unexpected deaths of babies. Nursing Mirror 138: no 7, 53–55
Richards I D G, Lowe C R 1966 Changes in the stillbirth-rate in England and Wales. Lancet i: 1169–1173
Richards I D G, Lowe C R 1971 Incidence of congenital defects in South Wales, 1964–6. British Journal of Preventive and Social Medicine 25: 59–64
Richards I D G, McIntosh, H T 1972 Confidential inquiry into 226 consecutive infant deaths. Archives of Disease in Childhood 47: 697–706
Richards I D G, McIntosh H T, Sweenie S 1972 A genetic study of anencephaly and spina bifida in Glasgow. Developmental Medicine and Child Neurology 14: 626–639
Richards I D G, McIntosh H T, Sweenie S 1979 A hundred vulnerable families. Public Health, 93: 16–24
Richards I D G, Sweet E M, Arneil G C 1968 Infantile rickets persists in Glasgow. Lancet i: 803–805
Rogers S C, Weatherall J A C 1976 Anencephalus, spina bifida and hydrocephalus: England and Wales 1964–72. Studies on Medical and Population Subjects No 32. Office of Population Censuses and Surveys. HMSO, London
Rutter M, Tizard J, Whitmore K 1970 Education, health and behaviour. Longman, London
Scottish Home and Health Department 1968 Medical care of epilepsy in Scotland. HMSO, Edinburgh
Scottish Home and Health Department 1979 Scottish health statistics 1977. HMSO, Edinburgh
Simons B, Downs E F, Hurster M M, Archer M 1966 Child abuse: epidemiological study of medically reported cases. New York State Journal of Medicine 66: 2783–2788
Skatvedt M 1958 Cerebral palsy: a clinical study of 370 cases. Acta Paediatrica Scandinavica 46: Suppl 111
Skinner A E, Castle R L 1969 78 Battered children: a retrospective study. National Society for the Prevention of Cruelty to Children, London
Smith S M 1975 The battered child syndrome: some research findings. Nursing Mirror 140: no 22, 48–53
Smith S M, Hanson R 1974 134 battered children: a medical and psychological study. British Medical Journal iii: 666–670
Smith S M, Hanson R, Noble S 1973 Parents of battered babies: a controlled study. British Medical Journal iv: 388–391
Smith S M, Hanson R, Noble S 1974 Social aspects of the battered baby syndrome. British Journal of Psychiatry 125: 568–582
Smithells R W 1968 Incidence of congenital abnormalities in Liverpool, 1960–64. British Journal of Preventive and Social Medicine 22: 36–37
Smithells R W, Chinn E R 1965 Spina bifida in Liverpool. Developmental Medicine and Child Neurology 7: 258–268
Solomons G 1979 Child abuse and developmental disabilities. Developmental Medicine and Child Neurology 21: 101–108
Spence J C, Walton W S, Miller F J W, Court S D M 1954 A thousand families in Newcastle upon Tyne. Oxford University Press, London
Steele B F, Pollock C B 1968 A psychiatric study of parents who abuse infants and small children. In: Helfer R E, Kempe C H (ed) The Battered Child. University of Chicago Press, Chicago and London
Urquhart G E D, Grist N R 1972 Virological studies of sudden, unexplained infant deaths in Glasgow, 1967–70. Journal of Clinical Pathology 25: 443–446
Valdes-Dapena M A, Hummeler K 1963 Sudden and unexpected death in infants. II Viral infections as causative factors. Journal of Paediatrics 63: 398–401
Vaughan D H 1968 Families experiencing a sudden unexpected infant death. Journal of the Royal College of General Practitioners 16: 359–367
Weatherall J A C, White G C 1976 A study of survival of children with spina bifida. Studies on Medical and Population Subjects No 31. Office of Population Censuses and Surveys. HMSO, London
Weir S 1970 A study of unmarried mothers and their children in Scotland. Scottish Health Service Studies, No 13. Scottish Home and Health Department, Edinburgh
Wilson T S 1971 A study of congenital malformations of the central nervous system among Glasgow births 1964–1968. Health Bulletin 29: 79–87
Wooley P V, Evans W A 1955 Significance of skeletal lesions in infants resembling those of traumatic origin. Journal of the American Medical Association 158: 539–543

Nutrition and nutritional disorders of children

In present-day Britain children are as well nourished as at any time in our history. This is illustrated by the fact that the average height of schoolchildren has increased by nearly one centimetre every 10 years since 1870. Gross undernutrition due to lack of availability of food is seen in many developing countries, leading to kwashiorkor and marasmic malnutrition, but these conditions are very rare in Britain. Occasionally examples of nutritional marasmus due to neglect are seen in the children of mothers with gross psychosocial problems and indeed marasmus and failure to thrive constitute one variant of the syndrome of child abuse. Such cases are exceptional but even so certain problems of nutrition do arise amongst our children, some common and some unusual but more serious.

Nutritional disorders of children in Britain may be divided into two categories: those conditions which have a wide distribution amongst the child population without a marked relationship to ethnic factors; and those which show a predilection for certain ethnic groups. In the first category are included complications of the artificial feeding of infants in the first few months of life, and such conditions as obesity and dental caries; in the second are diseases such as rickets and certain forms of anaemia.

Early infant feeding

For many centuries attempts have been made to use the milk of other mammals for the rearing of human babies. The results were usually disastrous but when the role of infection became known and techniques of sterilization became available, the modification of cow's milk for feeding human infants assumed new importance. Within the last 40 years, the commercial preparation of baby milk feeds has developed enormously. The danger of contamination of bottle feeds has largely been overcome and so modern mothers have had available for years artificial milk feeds which have been apparently safe and which have been widely advertised, their use being supported and encouraged by the nursing and medical professions. In the nineteenth century the artificial feeding of babies was accompanied by appalling death rates: for example, in some orphanages the infant mortality was over 900 per 1000 (Levin, 1963). During this century mortality rates have fallen progressively so that by 1978, when about 70 per cent of all babies received no breast milk at all, the infant mortality rate was only 17.0 per 1000. Until recently, therefore, it seemed that the artificial feeding of babies with dried or modified cow's milk had become completely safe and so breast feeding became more and more unpopular.

Dangers of cow's milk
A number of disorders affecting infants in the first few weeks of life have been shown to be directly or indirectly due to feeding unmodified cow's milk.

Hypernatraemia. Cow's milk contains about four times the amount of sodium that is found in human milk (cow's milk 88 mg sodium per dl, human milk 23 mg sodium per dl). The sodium present in milk feeds in excess of the baby's own needs must be excreted by the kidneys. In the early weeks of life the concentrating power of the kidney is completely adequate for excreting the excess sodium obtained from human milk. In the case of cow's milk, however, the excess is so great that in some small babies all the sodium cannot be excreted and the plasma sodium rises to levels which can be dangerous. Even in bigger babies, if some minor illness such as diarrhoea or respiratory infection leads to excessive loss of water from the intestine or by evaporation from the lungs, the reduction in water available for urine formation results in retention of sodium. This leads to the dangerous condition of hypernatraemia in which sodium can pass into intracellular fluid and, in the case of the brain, cause convulsions and brain damage. The number of children who become ill from hypernatraemia or who develop brain damage is not known and may be small, but very many infants fed on unmodified artificial feeds do have an abnormally high plasma sodium even when appearing to be well. For instance, apparently healthy babies so fed may have plasma sodium levels of over 155 millimole per litre, compared with the average normal level of 140 (Davies, 1973). These babies may become ill if they develop any condition leading to fluid loss. In Britain today those most at risk are the babies of the least well educated or illiterate mothers. It is known that dangerous hypernatraemia has been caused by using more scoops of unmodified dried milk per feed than the instructions indicate, by packing milk into the scoop, and by using heaped instead of level scoops. It is therefore very important that community health personnel should understand this condition and be meticulous in instructing or supervising mothers who decide to feed their infants 'on the bottle' in the early months of life. It has recently been suggested that hypernatraemia could be the cause in some cases of 'sudden infant death'.

Hypocalcaemia. Cow's milk also contains much more phosphate than does human milk (cow's milk 145 mg phosphate per dl, human milk 22 mg per dl). This enormous difference results in babies fed on cow's milk absorbing much more phosphorus than babies who are breast-fed. This leads to phosphate retention in the blood and the high blood phosphate causes a lowering of the blood calcium level. This in turn may cause fits and so in small infants the feeding of cow's milk can actually cause convulsions due to hypocalcaemia.

New milk preparations
The commercial manufacturers of baby milks have endeavoured to lower the concentration of sodium and phosphorus in the newer special baby milks and the concentration of sodium in such milks is much nearer the concentration

in breast milk. However, these ultra-modified milks are expensive and the ordinary baby milks are all very high in sodium content. A government report (HMSO, 1975) on the feeding of babies recommends that artificial milk feeds 'should contain a concentration of phosphorus, sodium and protein which is lower than that of cow's milk and nearer to that of breast milk'.

With the general rise in the cost of food, modern modified milks are becoming expensive and therefore mothers who do not wish to breast feed may well be tempted to use liquid cow's milk, which is subsidized and therefore relatively cheap, although no longer recommended for infant feeding.

Advantages of breast milk

In the world in general, the most important characteristic of human breast milk is the protection it affords against infection and against gastroenteritis in particular. The reasons for this are not merely that the milk as produced is sterile but that, in addition, there are present in human breast milk many factors which combine to prevent the infant's alimentary tract from being infected with pathogenic viruses or bacteria.

Immune globulins, mainly IgA, are secreted in the breast milk and these are effective against viruses and against pathogenic *Escherichia coli* which cause gastroenteritis. The IgA is actively secreted by the breast and is absent from commercial cow's milk. Lactoferrin is a protein which is present in human breast milk and which has the property of combining with iron. It has recently been demonstrated that iron is necessary for the multiplication of pathogenic *E. coli* in the infant intestine and lactoferrin in milk so effectively fixes the iron that none is available for metabolism by the *E. coli* (Bullen, 1975). It has also been shown that the effects of immune globulins and lactoferrin are synergistic so that each enhances the protective activity of the other.

Other intrinsic protective properties of human breast milk include active phagocytic cells in the milk and lysozymes which are effective against staphylococcal infections. In addition to these intrinsic factors, breast milk has properties which result in a more acid type of stool and also predispose to the growth in the infant intestine of *Lactobacillus acidophilus*, which organism appears to inhibit the growth of pathogenic *E. coli*.

It is apparent, therefore, that human breast milk has many advantages over commercial baby feeds which are made by modifying cow's milk. In the world at large there is no doubt that the major advantage is protection against gastroenteritis and many thousands of babies die each year in the tropics because mothers are persuaded to abandon the traditional method of rearing their children by breast feeding. In addition, there are certain theoretical advantages which have to do with the biological nature of the protein in human breast milk. However cow's milk is modified, its protein can never be changed into human protein by industrial processes. In the first few months of life the level of circulating immune globulins in the blood is very low and it seems that the human baby has become adapted in the course of evolution to receiving nothing but human protein until he is about four or five months old. It has been suggested that exposure of human babies to foreign protein in the alimentary canal before they have developed higher levels of immune globulins can predispose to the development of eczema and asthma, especially in families with a strong history of allergic disorders. In some children allergy to cow's milk can be a serious illness (though in this country such cases are rare) and there have been suggestions that allergy can be incriminated in some instances of sudden infant death.

Other advantages of breast feeding, which are perhaps not quite so well documented, include the emotional bonding of infant and mother by the satisfying relationship of breast feeding, as compared with the less intimate process of bottle feeding. It has been noticed by some research workers that enamel hypoplasia of the teeth is seen almost entirely amongst babies who have been fed on cow's milk from the time of birth (Stimmler et al, 1973). It is very unusual for a baby to become obese in the first year of life if he has been breast fed and this may turn out to be one of the biggest advantages of breast feeding.

Breast feeding has become so unusual in Britain that many mothers have no idea how to perform this natural function. They therefore require help from a very early stage and staff at the antenatal clinic must make sure that every mother has been told of, and understands, the advantages of breast feeding her child. During the past few years, there has been a slight resurgence of breast feeding and interest in breast feeding but in our experience this has been largely amongst mothers in social classes I and II and amongst those who have had advanced secondary or university education. In some inner-city areas with a high proportion of immigrant mothers there has also been a change in the pattern of feeding. This is particularly so amongst West Indian mothers, more of whom are becoming converted to bottle feeding. In south-west London, breast feeding is now more common amongst Caucasian mothers than amongst their West Indian counterparts.

Throughout pregnancy, the mother must be given a good diet and supplementary vitamins, while when the breasts begin to enlarge the mother must be taught proper care of the nipples. The use of nipple shields in particular, with light massage of the nipple, may well make breast feeding easier after the child is born. In the postnatal wards it is of utmost importance for staff to realize that many mothers require privacy in order to breast feed their child happily. It is probable that emotional tension, anxiety, and sometimes embarrassment are major causes for failure of breast feeding.

Obesity

Obesity is one of the major nutritional diseases of the developed world and is the cause in adult life of increased morbidity and mortality. It has been shown that children who are obese in childhood have an 80 per cent chance of becoming obese adults. What is less certain is whether obesity in childhood due to overnutrition is one cause of the increased incidence of obesity in later life. We do know that the incidence of childhood obesity—and of infant obesity in particular—has been increasing.

The most accurate way of defining obesity would be in terms of the normal and abnormal percentage of body fat in an individual but such measurement is extremely difficult. Skinfold thickness has been used and is easier to measure if accurate skin calipers are available. Most workers use the definition that a child is obese if his weight exceeds by 20 per cent the mean weight for height and sex of children of his own age (Lloyd et al, 1961).

Obesity in infancy
Shukla et al (1972) found that 17 per cent of 300 Birmingham children under the age of one year were obese and a further 28 per cent were between 10 and 20 per cent overweight. If this is a true prevalence it means that a survey of our present infant population would not give accurate normal values of weight for age because obesity is so common that the average values would be increased above the physiologically normal averages. For workers in the field of preventive medicine two questions need to be asked—whether adult obesity has its origins in the methods of feeding used during infancy and whether obesity can be prevented by control of infant weight gain.

Increase in total body fat can be due to increase in the number of fat cells or increase in the amount of fat in each cell. It has been suggested that if a baby becomes obese in the first year of life, the absolute number of fat cells is increased. This hypothesis was originally based on the work of Hirsch & Han (1969) who showed that in rats overfed at an early stage of life the absolute number of cells is increased, whereas later on the increase in fat in an overfed animal is due to increase in cell size without increase in cell numbers. It has also been suggested that obese children who were obese as infants have a greater number of fat cells than children whose obesity was of later onset. The implication is that control of weight gain in the first year of life may be of use in preventing adult obesity. This has not been proven, however, and Mellbin & Vuille (1973) found in a survey of seven-year-old children in Sweden that overfeeding in the first year of life was not a factor in the development of obesity.

The work of Poskitt & Cole (1978) suggests that a familial tendency to be overweight, perhaps genetically determined, is more important than early overfeeding. Jean Meyer (1975) showed that if neither parent is obese the chance of their child being obese is only 7 per cent, if one parent is obese the risk for the child is 40 per cent, and if both parents are obese the child has an 80 per cent chance of being obese himself. In the case of adopted children, there was no significant relationship between adoptive parents' weights and the child's weight. Thus whatever the genetic factors are, they may be more important than the nutritional environment in determining the risk of long-term obesity.

Nevertheless in the early years of life obesity is on the increase and, since obese infants are known to be at greater risk from respiratory disease and infantile obesity is certainly related to adult obesity, every effort must be made to prevent the condition. This is especially so when, from the dietary history of the infant, obesity is clearly associated with an abnormally high intake of food. It is very unusual for an infant wholly breast fed to be obese. The danger points during the first year of life are therefore likely to be the too early introduction of solid food and the use of sucrose as a sweetener in the infant diet.

Childhood obesity
Obesity in the older child is a complex problem, with hereditary and psychological factors playing an important role. Some facts about childhood obesity which

have relevance to therapy should be noted. The activity of fat children is very much less than the activity of normal children in the same environment. Thus Meyer (1975) found that obese girls eat up to 400 calories (1.7 MJ) per day less than the non-obese, but the time they spend in activity is only one third as much as the time spent in activity by their non-obese colleagues. Obese children are usually taller than average for their age and they develop the changes of puberty about one year earlier than non-obese children. The psychological effects of obesity are complex and are usually maximal at or about puberty, when children are most sensitive about their appearance. Psychological disturbance can cause compulsive overeating which may lead to obesity, while obesity not related to overeating can itself lead to deep emotional and psychological stress. All these factors mean that control of diet alone cannot be adequate therapy for obesity in childhood, and attention must be given to exercise as well, especially in the teenager. Moreover, amongst girls in particular, one must be aware of the danger of inducing anorexia nervosa if too much emphasis is laid on diet as a means of controlling body size. Anorexic drugs are of no long-term use and some, such as amphetamines, must never be used because of the dangers of addiction. Indeed, there seems little indication for drug therapy in the management of obesity.

Adolescence is a time of increased growth and it is probably not safe to aim for impressive weight loss by dieting at this time. It has been shown that, at the time of adolescent growth spurt, considerable dietary restriction for obesity inhibits linear growth but more moderate restriction allows normal growth to take place (Heald, 1975).

Conclusion
It seems probable that infantile obesity is one of the aetiological factors in adult obesity. If possible, therefore, babies should be entirely breast fed in the early months of life. Sucrose should not be given in artificial feeds and there is no need to introduce mixed feeding before the age of four months. The calorie intake of obese infants should be checked and reduced if possible.

In older children the use of anorexic drugs is not advised. In addition to dietary control, all obese children should be encouraged to take exercise. Strict dieting should be employed only for those children whose food intake is excessive. In adolescence too much emphasis on relieving weight loss by dieting increases the risk of anorexia nervosa, especially in girls.

Dental caries

One of the diseases uncommon in many developing countries but rife in Europe and North America is dental caries. The enamel of teeth is hard and when smooth and intact is resistant to cariogenic bacteria. In an acid environment, erosion of the enamel surface takes place and the teeth become vulnerable to bacterial action. It is known that very quickly after the ingestion of sugar, and sucrose in particular, the pH of the saliva or fluid between the teeth falls to as low as 4.0 and can still be at this level 20 minutes after the sugar has been eaten, especially if there is marked plaque formation on the teeth (Bowen, 1972). Such a pH rapidly erodes enamel. The fall in the pH is due to the production of acid by bacteria acting on carbohydrate and so reduction in sugar intake and the cleansing of teeth by brushing after eating food or drinking sugar-containing drinks can reduce the incidence of dental decay. However, to alter cultural behaviour in order to achieve good dental hygiene is very difficult, and the introduction of 'blanket' measures which cover the whole population, for example, fluoridation of water supplies, is more feasible and therefore likely to be successful.

Fluoridation
The enamel of teeth consists of a very hard material called hydroxy-apatite. If fluoride is available during the development of the enamel, it is incorporated into the crystalline structure forming fluoro-hydroxy-apatite. This material is even harder than ordinary enamel and is much more resistant to acid erosion and bacterial invasion. The source of fluoride for most people is the drinking water and a level of one part per million is needed to afford good protection against dental caries. The fluoride content of water varies from one part of the country to another and in areas with a natural level below one part per million, fluoride can be added at the reservoir source of drinking water to achieve a safe and protective level.

Murray (1969) compared two areas—York, which has a very low fluoride content in the drinking water, and West Hartlepool, which has a level of over one part per million of fluoride. In York only 22.4 per cent of five-year-old children were caries-free, compared with 51.2 per cent in West Hartlepool. In Anglesey and Watford in 1969, after seven years of fluoridation, caries in the primary teeth of children from three to seven years old was reduced by over 50 per cent, compared with the incidence before fluoridation. In the same population, the number of children with 10 or more carious teeth fell by 80 per cent. During the same period in Kilmarnock, fluoridation had been discontinued in 1962 and by 1968 the prevalence of tooth decay had increased and had reached the level in non-fluoridated areas.

Thus the fluoridation of water supplies to raise the level of fluoride to a minimum of one part per million has been shown to have a direct beneficial effect on the incidence of dental caries. Fluoridation is carried out only in areas where the fluoride content is low: many areas of the country have naturally high levels of fluoride, for example Burnham-on-Crouch and Braintree, and here the children are protected against caries by natural fluoridation. The supposed dangers of fluoridation have never been proven and the prevention of dental caries is one of the most important health measures we can undertake. This must be impressed on local authorities who should understand that fluoridation means increasing the fluoride in water to a safe level which is the same as, or less than, that in many areas of the country where the fluoride in the water occurs naturally. Attention to this problem in childhood will eventually be of immense value to the nutritional health of the geriatric population 70 years from now.

Handicapped children
Until recently the care of the teeth of handicapped children has been neglected and indeed the number of dentists available for community work is so small

that many centres for handicapped children are still without proper dental care. It is an essential part of nursing and medical care that the teeth should be cleaned whenever a handicapped child is fed. Especially is this the case in those handicapped children who suffer from epilepsy and who are treated with phenytoin, because this drug in the presence of poor dental hygiene leads to gum hypertrophy with consequent increased risk of gingivitis.

Also important is the ability of doctors and nurses to recognize children with malocclusion or overcrowding of teeth so that proper orthodontic care can be organized before irreversible malocclusion or crowding states are reached, for these predispose to caries.

Nutritional rickets

One hundred years ago, rickets was rife among children in Britain. In 1868, Gee found that 30 per cent of children under two years of age at the Hospital for Sick Children in London were suffering from rickets (Starr, 1895). Until the Second World War, rickets continued to be seen not uncommonly in paediatric departments but after 1945, with widespread use of supplementary vitamins, nutritional rickets became very rare. In the late 1950s, however, rickets again made its appearance in Britain. It occurred mainly in the children of immigrant communities, although Arneil & Crosbie (1963) found that in Glasgow, in addition to babies of immigrant mothers, some indigenous babies developed rickets, probably due to the feeding of liquid cow's milk. Since that time, rickets in children and osteomalacia in young adults have been reported as relatively common in immigrant people, especially those of Asian origin.

Aetiology of rickets

Nutritional rickets is primarily due to dietary deficiency of vitamin D. The recommended daily intake of the vitamin for infants and children is 400 international units (10 µg of cholecalciferol). Few common foods are good sources, for only egg yolk, fatty fish and fortified foodstuffs such as margarine contain significant amounts. Cow's milk contains only about 10 to 30 units of vitamin D per litre. Until recently it was believed that human milk also contained very little but it is now known that, where a healthy mother is not herself deficient in the vitamin, vitamin D activity is present in her milk as a water-soluble conjugate with sulphate (Lakdawala & Widdowson, 1977). This accounts for the earlier observation that rickets was less common amongst breast-fed babies than amongst those fed artificially. It may also explain why Mellanby, in his original work on rickets, found it impossible to produce the disease in rats unless the mother had been deprived of vitamin D during pregnancy. Nevertheless, the breast-fed baby of a poorly nourished mother, like the baby fed on liquid cow's milk, may receive very little vitamin D. Many immigrant mothers breast feed their infants and many, perhaps because of language difficulties, do not attend child health clinics, consult a doctor for advice on feeding, or understand advice that is given.

Ultraviolet light has the property of converting certain sterols in the skin into 25-hydroxycholecalciferol, which is the active circulating form of vitamin D. Thus deficiency is especially likely to arise if a diet low in vitamin D is consumed by an individual whose exposure to sunlight is inadequate. Blood levels of vitamin D have been shown to vary with the season, being lowest at the end of winter and highest at the end of summer. The same fluctuation takes place in European, Asian and African people, so that the role of skin pigmentation is not as important as was once thought. It seems likely that the contribution of sunlight has been underestimated in this country, for it has recently been shown (Lawson et al, 1979) that elderly people depend greatly on the ultraviolet light to which they are exposed during the summer months. The variation of vitamin D levels in their blood appears to be related to the amount of time spent out of doors. However, it is very difficult to alter behaviour and for large sections of our population vitamin D deficiency must be countered by the addition of vitamin D to the diet.

Cholecalciferol in food or formed by the action of ultraviolet light on the skin sterols is hydroxylated in the liver to form 25-hydroxycholecalciferol, which can be measured in the blood. Further hydroxylation takes place in the kidneys to form dihydroxycholecalciferol. Thus liver and kidneys are both involved in the internal metabolism of vitamin D. The effect of the vitamin is to increase the absorption of calcium from the intestinal tract and to facilitate its deposition in the bones. It is, therefore, essential for the calcification of cartilage and for normal ossification.

The effects of vitamin D deficiency are greatest at those times of life when rapid growth is taking place, such as in the first few years, just before puberty and during pregnancy. In the adult, when growth has ceased, lack of vitamin D causes decalcification of the skeleton, producing osteomalacia. Vitamin D deficiency especially affects immigrant women, because their traditional dress shields a large part of their skin from ultraviolet light and dietary deficiency is therefore not compensated for by irradiation of the skin. When such women become pregnant, the vitamin deficiency can affect the fetus and recently fetal and neonatal rickets have been reported in babies of mothers who were themselves vitamin D deficient (Ford et al, 1973).

Clinical features
In very severe cases of fetal rickets, the bones may be so decalcified that fractures occur and a mistaken diagnosis of osteogenesis imperfecta may be made. At birth the diagnosis of rickets is often missed but can be suspected when the bones of the skull are so thin that the physical sign of craniotabes can be demonstrated. If pressure is applied over the occipital bones and behind the ears in a baby with craniotabes, it is possible to indent the bones very easily with the fingertips, giving rise to a sensation rather like pressing a table-tennis ball. Neonatal rickets may present as convulsions, because in severe vitamin D deficiency the blood calcium level tends to fall and sometimes reaches such a low level that hypocalcaemic fits occur.

As the child grows and particularly when weight bearing begins around the age of one year, the clinical picture of nutritional rickets becomes increasingly obvious. The baby may show beading of the costochondral junctions, swelling of the wrists and ankles, and bowing of the legs, particularly the lower part of the legs, i.e. the lower tibia.

Prevention of rickets
Fetal and neonatal rickets are easily prevented by making certain that all pregnant women, and especially those of Asian origin, receive supplementary vitamin D. Infantile rickets is also readily preventable and all nursing and medical staff working in the child health service, especially those in areas with many immigrants, must ensure that infants and children receive adequate supplements of vitamin D. Care must be taken, however, that the intake is not excessive, because the vitamin can cause hypercalcaemia, in which the level of plasma calcium rises well above normal and may damage the brain, kidneys and other organs.

An important step in the prevention of rickets is the identification of the 'at risk' groups in the community. No firm policy has yet been reached about the method of ensuring an increased intake of vitamin D by these groups. Some research projects have shown that rickets can be controlled in an Asian community by fortifying Chapatti flour, but no widespread use of fortified foodstuffs has as yet been instituted. It is not legally possible to fortify liquid milk and there is also doubt as to whether such fortification would be safe for all children. For the present, therefore, the objective must be supplementary prescription of vitamin D for all infants and for all 'at risk' adolescents and pregnant women. Above all, health staff must be aware that human breast milk and raw cow's milk, as well as butter and cream, do not contain enough vitamin D to ensure an adequate daily intake by all children. The problem of rickets in Britain today appears to be mainly amongst the immigrant community but, with the rising cost of fortified dried milks, there may be a general trend towards the use of raw cow's milk for infant feeding, in which case we can expect cases of rickets to occur amongst the indigenous population as well as in the children of immigrants.

Recommended daily intake

Most countries provide tables of recommended daily intakes of food substances and in the United Kingdom details are published by Her Majesty's Stationery Office (HMSO, 1979). Recommendations vary from country to country and the difference in the case of some substances is substantial. The main reason for this is that methods of working out recommended allowances also vary. Moreover, the needs of different individuals vary with occupation and sex as well as with body size and the efficiency of physiological processes such as digestion, absorption and utilization. Usually the minimum requirement is worked out by calculating the amount of a food substance which is necessary to maintain the body in balance, adding to this the amount required for growth and then adding on percentages which represent the efficiency of absorption and utilization and a further percentage to make allowance for the variation from one individual to another. This means that most of the recommended intakes are well above the minimum requirement and that the intakes of some children, even in social classes I, II and III, may be less than the recommended intake according to the official tables. However, the importance of recommended intakes is that they represent a nutritional intake which will not lead to deficiency and which will not lead to overnutrition in the average person, although there is still a suspicion that the recommended energy intake may be at a level which for some individuals could lead to obesity.

In the report of the government Committee on Medical Aspects of Food Policy (1969) it was stated that the average daily energy intake of 64 per cent of British schoolchildren was below that recommended for the age. This at first sight appears to suggest a degree of undernutrition but the vast majority of the children with supposedly inadequate intakes of energy were from the more affluent social classes. It is therefore likely that the recommended intakes of energy are too high and that other factors, perhaps including exercise, are the major ones in determining the intake of energy by individual children. Indeed, the report shows that the intakes of most dietary constituents are in excess of the recommended daily intakes and only vitamin D and iron appear to be at an inadequate level. This is of interest when we know that some children do in fact develop rickets but neither this disease nor anaemia is widespread in the general childhood population. Similarly the data on protein intake were reassuring in that it was above the recommended level and indeed was higher in the lower social groups than in the higher social groups, though the protein was largely of vegetable origin in the former.

Thus it is seen that by all methods of investigation—measurement of size, identification of cases of nutritional disorder and survey of levels of intake—the children of the United Kingdom appear to be in a good nutritional state. There are, however, some groups particularly 'at risk', such as Asian children who have a predisposition to specific deficiencies, and these groups must be identified. There are also without doubt some families with psychosocial problems who are 'at risk'. Another important group comprises those children who are 'at risk' of overnutrition, particularly of salt and calories, which can lead to disease. These groups must be searched for in the community and when identified their nutritional behaviour needs to be altered, while both parents and children must be educated to understand the simple facts of nutritional well-being.

REFERENCES

Arneil G C, Crosbie J C 1963 Infantile rickets returns to Glasgow. Lancet ii: 423–425
Bowen W H 1972 Dental caries. Archives of Disease in Childhood 47: 849–853
Bullen J J 1975 Iron-binding proteins in milk and resistance to *Escherichia coli* infection in infants. Postgraduate Medical Journal 51 (Suppl 3): 67–70
Committee on Medical Aspects of Food Policy, Report No 122 1969 HMSO, London
Davies D P 1973 Plasma osmolality and feeding practices of healthy infants in first three months of life. British Medical Journal ii: 340–342
Ford J A, Davidson D C, McIntosh W B, Fyfe W M, Dunnigan M G 1973 Neonatal rickets in Asian immigrant population. British Medical Journal iii: 211–212
Heald F P 1975 In: Childhood obesity. Wiley, New York
Hirsch J, Han P W 1969 Cellularity of rat adipose tissue. Journal of Lipid Research 10: 77–82
HMSO 1975 Present-day practice in infant feeding. Report on Health and Social Subjects, No 9. HMSO, London
HMSO 1979 Recommended daily amounts of food energy and nutrients for groups of people in the United Kingdom. HMSO, London
Lakdawala D R, Widdowson E M 1977 Vitamin D in human milk. Lancet i: 167–168
Lawson D E M, Paul A A, Black A E, Cole T J, Mandal A R, Davie M 1979 Relative contributions of diet and sunlight to vitamin D state in the elderly. British Medical Journal ii: 303–305

Levin S S 1963 A philosophy of infant feeding. Thomas, Springfield, Illinois
Lloyd J K, Wolff O H, Whelen W S 1961 Childhood obesity. British Medical Journal ii: 145–148
Mellbin T, Vuille J C 1973 Physical development at 7 years of age in relation to velocity of weight gain in infancy with special reference to incidence of overweight. British Journal of Preventive and Social Medicine 27: 225–235
Meyer J 1975 In: Childhood obesity. Wiley, New York
Murray J 1969 Caries experience of 5-year-old children from fluoride and non-fluoride communities. British Dental Journal 126: 352–354
Poskitt E M E, Cole T J 1978 Nature, nurture and childhood overweight. British Medical Journal i: 603–605
Shukla A, Forsyth H A, Anderson C M, Marwah S M 1972 Infantile overnutrition in the first year of life. British Medical Journal iv: 507–515
Starr Louis 1895 An American textbook of the diseases of children, part 4. Redman, London
Stimmler L, Snodgrass G J A I, Jaffe E 1973 Dental defects associated with neonatal symptomatic hypocalcaemia. Archives of Disease in Childhood 48: 217–220

Part Four: Health and Social Services

Ross G. Mitchell

Community child health services

Planning and funding of health care
In many parts of the world, resources for modern health care are very deficient. Two thirds of the services available are bought by the relatively wealthy one tenth of the population. The few doctors work mainly in the cities, serving the rich and devoting only a small proportion of their time to the pressing needs of the majority. In rural areas care is provided largely by traditional healers in the villages, while in the peri-urban shanty towns there are often no services at all. If health care is to be improved in these poor countries, there is no real alternative to a structured public health service, giving high priority to sanitation and housing, nutrition, health education and the control of common infections.

In more affluent countries, there are several options. Health care may be left almost entirely to the influence of the open market, with little or no central control. In these circumstances, multiple programmes evolve, financed by fee-for-service payment, public subscription or philanthropy. Such a free enterprise system harnesses creative energy and promotes excellence but services tend to go to those with greatest purchasing power and the general standard fluctuates according to supply and demand.

In the so-called 'welfare' state, characteristic of some western European countries, much of the service may still be provided from private and voluntary sources but distribution and costs are subject to supervision by government, which assumes responsibility for ensuring that there are services to meet the needs. In the fully socialist health services of eastern Europe, all planning and the use of resources are centrally controlled.

The provision of any service which is not self-financing requires the allocation of funds. The proportion of the national resources devoted to health care depends on the importance which the government of the day attaches to the health of the nation and on the pressures of other demands. Once the allocation has been decided, the health service itself must make a secondary distribution and this requires decisions on priorities. These are often determined by the interplay of individual value judgements and competing interests rather than according to a rational policy: yet with a limited budget the need to consider the purpose and objectives of a health service becomes urgent.

If it is to survive, a society must be reasonably efficient and productive. This economic view will stress the need to maintain the maximum number of working adults and so will advocate expenditure on the perinatal and infant services (laying a sound foundation) and on acute medicine (keeping the working population in good health) at the expense of the chronic sick, the handicapped and the elderly (unproductive liabilities). On the other hand, the humanitarian view of 'each according to his need' will allocate resources to those most requiring them—and large sums will go to the psychiatric and geriatric services and to the care of the handicapped. If the conceived purpose of a health service is the satisfaction of consumer demand, then priorities will be determined by popular opinion, influenced by the mass media and by vested interests. Thus the amount of money available for child health services will depend on the view that society itself takes about the importance of children.

Programmes of child health care

In most countries, health services for children have developed irregularly in response to evident need and the pressure of demand. Though the health of newborn infants and children in schools usually receives special attention, and in some cities there are hospitals catering specifically for the young, the bulk of health care for children is generally provided as an integral part of services for the community as a whole. In the absence of organized provision for all children, there is often an unstructured mixture of partial facilities, with many gaps and overlaps, and with confusion over aims and responsibilities. Deficiencies are remedied by a patchwork of local and voluntary endeavour, initiative being taken in communities where the need is least, for they are likely to be most concerned and to command the necessary resources. People living in deprived areas tend to be inactive from poverty, indifference and apathy.

Increasing awareness of these consequences of failure to plan and provide has led to action in many countries to improve the organization and integration of health services for children. In the United Kingdom, in the United States and in some European countries, steps have been taken towards establishing comprehensive child health services available to all children and directing effort to where it is most needed (Wallace, 1971; Mitchell, 1976). The creation of a health service on a national scale necessarily implies the attempt to achieve a uniformly high standard of service throughout the country. This ideal is probably unattainable because of differing environmental circumstances and different degrees of ability, industry and enthusiasm amongst those who staff the service. Nevertheless, at least minimal levels should be attained in every area, with concentration of further resources where the need is greatest. Thereafter the aim should be a gradual and uniform raising of standards. Such a global approach is open to the objection that it tends to stifle local initiative and enterprise and to prevent the emergence of centres of excellence, but these and other disadvantages can be countered by planned experiment and evaluation. The American pattern of multiple sources of delivery of health care undoubtedly gives greater opportunity for innovation and encourages advances by the method of trial and error, but the penalty that may be incurred is that the quality of care will be very uneven and many children may not be reached at all. Thus in some communities excellent services for the white majority co-exist with neglect of the needs of minority groups and in general the operation of a free market has created gaps in the availability of services (Kerr, 1975; Schorr, 1978).

A child health service should be not only available to all children but also used by all. The effectiveness of the health programmes in Finland and Sweden has been due to the very high coverage of all infants and young children. This has been achieved by the concerted effort of a number of institutions acting in a favourable social environment, by providing sufficient numbers of health workers and by intensive health education (Wynn & Wynn, 1974a; Petersson, 1978). A different approach has been adopted in France, where the proportion of children reached has been increased by a system of financial inducements to use the services and penalties for failing to do so: new legislation introduced in 1970 aims to give all children an equal right to health care (Wynn & Wynn, 1974b).

In the Soviet Union and the People's Republic of China, well-established health services provide for all children, giving special priority to preventive paediatrics and to the health of children in rural communities (Mellander, 1973; Hyde, 1974). The importance of child health in Soviet policy is manifest by the large proportion of doctors practising paediatrics, the official recognition of a wide range of paediatric specialties and the existence of many hospital units and dispensaries catering solely for child patients (Ryan, 1978). In Soviet institutes of medical education there are separate Faculties of Paediatrics training the many thousands of paediatricians required to staff the children's polyclinics which are the basis of the child health services (Butrov, 1974): in China, on the other hand, training in paediatrics is part of general medical education and specialist paediatricians work mainly in large hospitals and medical schools. Both countries make much use of medical auxiliaries, including 'feldshers' in the Soviet Union and 'barefoot doctors' in China. The latter receive a short task-orientated training in medical care and public health and then work closely with the peasants in rural communes. In Chinese cities, the health of children is supervised in local health stations and organized nurseries by neighbourhood health workers and 'Red Guard Doctors' (Rudolph, 1974).

Among the most comprehensive systems of health care is that in the United Kingdom: here for 20 years from the inception of the National Health Service in 1948, general medical practitioners and hospital boards provided medical care for adults and children in common, while preventive health measures for infants and children were largely undertaken by local authorities (town and county councils) as part of their general responsibility for the health of their communities. Although the intention was to meet all health needs, there were many gaps and remarkable variations in expenditure on health between different parts of the country. In 1974, the separate services were merged under Health Authorities, each providing total health care for a defined geographic area. With this integration of health services, the opportunity was taken to redesign the arrangements for the care of infants and children. The foundations of a comprehensive child health service were laid in England in 1974–5, although the Committee on Child Health Services did not report until 1976 (Court, 1976: see p. 176). In Scotland, a comparable service was instituted in 1974, following publication of the Brotherston report *Towards an Integrated Child Health Service* (Scottish

Home and Health Department, 1973). Similar arrangements were made in Wales and Northern Ireland, although the latter went a stage further by unifying health and social services in a single framework.

In some countries, attention has been directed less to comprehensive programmes than to identifying and making special provision for certain categories of children who are unable to take advantage of health services, for example children in the care of public agencies, in remote areas, or isolated by racial or religious segregation. In yet other lands, action has simply consisted of better co-ordination of existing government and voluntary services.

While these moves towards integration of child health services have been taking place, the whole idea of separate services for children has been challenged by some on economic or holistic grounds (Bhatia, 1973) or from a desire to organize the health services on different lines, for example, into mental health services and physical health services or into preventive and therapeutic services. It is necessary therefore to consider the case for a clearly identifiable child health service as part of the total provision for the health of a community.

Rationale of a child health service

In large parts of the world, such as India, Africa and Latin America, there are nearly as many children as adults. For example, in Dahomey, West Africa, and on the mainland of Middle America (including Mexico) 46 per cent of the total population are under 15, in India 44 per cent and in Ethiopia 42 per cent. In such countries, a universal health service is in effect a child health service, since nearly half of the patients are children. By contrast, in most industrial countries the number of children is substantially less than that of adults. For example, in the United Kingdom and the United States there are approximately three adults to every child, children under 15 years of age constituting 24 per cent and 28 per cent of the population respectively. In consequence of this numerical inferiority, health services tend to be designed primarily for adults and aimed at the massive geriatric and psychogeriatric problems. Provision specifically for children is often made grudgingly because it is inconvenient and may involve costs out of proportion to the numbers expected to benefit. Moreover, because the administration is largely in the hands of people concerned mainly or wholly with adults, the interests of children are often under-represented or even unrepresented in planning and management. As a result, the necessary arrangements for children may not be made, since those responsible either do not know or are unwilling to admit that children's needs are different from those of adults (Forfar, 1973). Even people who recognize the differences are sometimes reluctant to concede that they are sufficiently important to warrant special provision. Thus, for example, the needs of school health and educational medicine, which have no close parallel in the adult health service, may be ill-understood. In the most favourable circumstances, children in a service designed for adults generally come off second best because of their minority status in the eyes of those who wield power. In the economic climate of western countries today, increasing costs cause parents and society to view childbearing and child rearing as a liability, competing with other values. In the words of Brim (1975), 'When things get tight, children are the first to go.'

These policies are shortsighted. The aged and the mentally ill must be provided for and a civilized society will do the best it can. Yet they are a noncontributory liability and there is a limit to the burden which can be borne by a diminishing number of young adults. By contrast, children are the future workers, the creators of wealth. Nurture and protection in the early years lay the foundations of health throughout adult life and ensure a new generation of strong young men and women. This goal will not be reached if it is a secondary objective to which a health service fashioned for adults is merely adapted. Nor will it readily be achieved if it is combined with other aims, as in maternal and child health, for the interests of the two, though often the same, may sometimes conflict.

Children are a vulnerable section of the community and cannot articulate their own needs. Moreover, these needs are greatest amongst the poorest families, yet their ability to pay is least. No matter how health care for children is funded, financial barriers to full use by all children are unacceptable. Since the money allocated for child health care depends on society's views about children, it will clearly be advantageous if the child health service constitutes a single, distinct and large part of the total health services, rather than being fragmented and submerged throughout them. Such a clearly identifiable service should be carefully designed to reach all children and flexible enough to respond promptly to changing needs. Forward planning and a workable strategy of implementation are therefore essential features. A service of this kind, which is manifestly well organized and achieving its objectives, is the one most likely to attract the resources it requires.

There is thus philosophical, organizational and financial justification for establishing a health service specifically for children, with a programme aimed at promoting the health and well-being of infants, children and adolescents. Although such a child health service should have a manifest identity and authority to make and implement decisions, it ought not to be seen as a service in isolation, for a child's needs must be related to those of his family and of the community in which he lives. Plans may have to be modified if children's interests conflict with those of others and it is a responsibility of a child health service not only to co-ordinate the work of all those concerned with children but also to ensure that the provisions made are properly integrated with those for the community as a whole. Nevertheless, a service in which children come first, organized by people who understand children and have their welfare at heart, is mandatory if optimum health care for all children is to be assured.

Objectives of a child health service

When a new service is established, it is essential for all concerned and for the general public to be clear about its purpose. Objectives must be defined and subsequently analysed in terms of what must be done to achieve each objective, what staff and resources will be required, and how success will be measured. While the detailed objectives of a child health service will vary from country to country, the fundamental purpose is the same—to ensure optimum mental, physical and emotional development of all children so that they are capable of achieving their full potential in adult life: with the corollary that childhood itself should be a time of happiness and health as well as a preparation for the future. This being the ultimate goal, the immediate priorities depend on the state of advancement of the health services and the resources available. The general aims are to ensure that all professional workers are well trained and have a thorough understanding of normal child development and its variants: to promote good health among all children by comprehensive preventive measures; to provide effective and universally available therapeutic services which are continuously improving as medical technology advances; and to direct effort where it is most needed.

A child health service which sets out with these aims should include the following:

1. The machinery for identifying, keeping contact with and recording the progress of every child.
2. Comprehensive care for all newborn infants and collaboration with the obstetric services in ensuring optimum fetal health.
3. A programme of preventive measures, including protective immunization; health education and advice to parents; genetic counselling; and supervision of the environment, for example nurseries and crèches, schools, recreational areas.
4. Screening for the early detection of disease and for deviations from normal development.
5. Prompt and efficient medical and nursing care for the child who is mentally or physically ill, meets with an accident, or otherwise needs treatment.
6. A diagnostic and assessment service for children with chronic disability, intellectual, physical or emotional, including adequate and appropriate provision for all the requirements of the handicapped child.
7. A preventive and therapeutic dental service.
8. Supervision of the health of the adolescent by collaboration between general practitioner, paediatrician, adult physician and psychiatrist, with the aim of promoting health and well-being in adolescence and early adult life, ensuring that the parents of the next generation are as well prepared as possible for their new role, and effecting a smooth transition from the child health service to the adult health service.
9. A consultative service for teachers, social workers, and all other professions concerned with children and adolescents, including agencies responsible for vocational training and later employment.
10. A system for continuously evaluating the efficiency and quality of the service and sufficient flexibility to change in response to demonstrated deficiencies or new requirements.
11. An advisory structure to give professional advice on the planning, policy and management of the service.
12. A programme of clinical and operational research, with adequate financial and other resources which cannot be diverted to meet service needs.
13. A programme of continuing postgraduate education for the professional staff of the service.
14. Participation in the professional education of medical, nursing and social work students and any other trainees whose later work will be with children.

15. The giving of advice and, where appropriate, direct help to other services for children, especially those in developing countries and special relief services organized to deal with large-scale disasters, such as famine, epidemic disease, or floods.

While this list outlines the main components of a child health service, it is not exhaustive and is likely to vary in detail from country to country according to the economic and educational status of the population, the resources allocated to the service and the quality of professional staff available. These, and other factors, will also determine priorities within the list and the proportion of money and materials which can be devoted to each. A wealthy country like the United States can contemplate a comprehensive programme of health care including medical, dental, social, emotional, educational, vocational, recreational, nutritional, housing and environmental aspects as well as day care, homemaking, babysitting and transportation (Wallace, 1971). A country with slender resources must often choose between various objectives, all of them desirable. Thus, for example, it may not be feasible to provide the standard of care for the severely mentally and physically handicapped which modern medicine makes possible and which professional workers demand. Humanitarian considerations dictate that at least the minimal needs of every handicapped child be met but, although 'the least they should have is the best' is a laudable precept, its implementation when resources are limited would mean less for other children. Optimum provision for the handicapped may then have to take second place to more pressing needs.

A really poor country may find that a large part of the money allocated to child health is absorbed by combating malnutrition and gastrointestinal disease alone, and that provision of such things as child psychiatric and preventive dental services is far beyond its resources. In such a country, preventive measures, health education for self-help, and primary care will properly take precedence over new hospitals with advanced therapeutic technology.

Every country must thus determine its own policy and priorities; once these have been agreed, much detailed work is required to break down each objective into its component parts and to translate these into day-to-day requirements.

In countries where the great majority of children attend school throughout childhood, many of the activities listed above will take place in the context of a school health service, for example screening for abnormality, assessment of disability causing educational difficulty, participation in the provision of special educational measures, consultation with teachers, and so on. However, any tendency for school health work to become isolated from the main stream of paediatrics must be resisted, and there should be close co-operation between the school doctor, other paediatricians in the child health service and general practitioners. The general aims of health staff working in schools are to promote the health and well-being of all schoolchildren, to ensure that children ill at school receive proper attention, to recommend suitable provision for children with learning and other difficulties, to participate in the care of children with disabilities of all kinds, and to co-operate in identifying and meeting their special educational needs. It is the expertise required for these latter activities that constitutes the science of educational medicine. While an effective school health service is highly desirable, in some developing countries the traditional western emphasis on school health may result in an over-concentration of resources in the schools, to the detriment of the many children who never attend school or only attend for short periods.

It is important to establish the age ranges of child and adult health services, so that responsibility for providing health care is clear. In practice any such ruling must not be interpreted too strictly, for the optimum time for transfer will vary according to need and individual choice. Nevertheless, past failure to define responsibility has often meant a serious lack of facilities for school-leavers, in health care as well as in other fields such as vocational training and social support. This has been especially depriving for the handicapped adolescent and a child health service should accord a high priority to this group. Social and further educational services for the young usually have a continuing commitment to the age of 18 years or later and, although child health provision has tended to cease earlier, there is much to be said for extending it to 18 years as well, while recognizing that the adolescent will often prefer to make use of services for adults.

Evaluation of services

It is not easy to evaluate a programme of health care because objectives cannot readily be defined and measured nor is there a simple relationship between action and outcome. Nevertheless, the great expense of modern medical care demands that the effectiveness, efficiency and cost of services be assessed as accurately as possible and be kept under continuous review. Among the criteria appropriate to such an evaluation, vital statistics such as perinatal mortality or child morbidity rates have some value, though they are indirect and rather crude indices. Moreover, it may be misleading to attribute improvement in these rates to better health care, since social changes, such as a rising standard of living, may be the real reason. However, a decline in morbidity may sometimes be clearly due to a health measure: for example, the virtual eradication of diphtheria and poliomyelitis in Britain by immunization.

Parental satisfaction must be one criterion of the value of child health services, since these are aimed at meeting their needs and expectations. Yet some parents may be too easily pleased while the vociferous demands of others may mislead and indeed may have to be resisted in order to meet unexpressed and perhaps hitherto unidentified needs. It has been said that when demand has been met, subsequent use is a good indication of the real need. This is not entirely true and especially not in the case of child health services, for the needs of children may not be recognized even by their parents and some families have to be educated and stimulated to use new services.

Satisfaction expressed by professional staff is another yardstick but potentially fallacious, since staff may be too complacent or may set their sights impossibly high. Nevertheless, it is probably true that a service which is praised by both parents and staff is likely to be a good one, whereas general dissatisfaction should be taken as grounds for radical review.

The ultimate criterion of an effective service is the benefit conferred on the child himself. However, such things as promotion of health, freedom from disease, relief of suffering and reduction of disability are not easily assessed quantitatively. Moreover, although they are admirable objectives, the role played by the health services cannot readily be separated from other influences.

Various ways of evaluating child health care have been proposed and in some instances tried out. The numbers of 'items of service' and the extent of access and use have been combined into a 'quality-index' as a means of comparing health services but this can only be a very superficial assessment of their worth (Petersson, 1978). The method of Project Systems Analysis (Scottish Home and Health Department, 1974b) holds promise of a more systematic approach as does the risk strategy which aims at identifying and measuring the factors which render children vulnerable to ill health, intervening in order to reduce the risk, and monitoring the effects of that intervention (WHO, 1978a). These and similar ways of trying to evaluate and improve services are of interest but they require sustained effort and are demanding of staff and resources, so that their application is by no means simple.

Proof of the value of child health services is thus not easy to obtain but the lack of scientific evidence should not be used to justify failure to establish and maintain services or as a reason for resisting change (Mitchell, 1977). In the words of Schorr (1978) we must not 'exclude from our health system those services whose effectiveness we have not yet learned how to quantify and those which involve human values that cannot be reduced to equations'. A child who suffers permanent disability as a result of preventable disease represents a human tragedy and a loss of potential as well as a financial burden on society which will far outweigh the original cost of effective care. Cuts in services which seem appropriate in the short term may thus prove to be false economies, for cost/effectiveness in child health services can only be judged over a long-time scale (Forfar, 1979).

Staffing of a child health service
When the objectives of a child health service have been agreed and the ways of achieving them defined, it is necessary to identify the professional workers who will undertake the work. The role of each profession tends to become established by custom, and may not always remain the most appropriate as circumstances change. It is desirable, therefore, that practice should not become fixed and inflexible but should vary depending on who at the time will be most efficient and acceptable to children and their families. Relative cost and availability of professional workers will also materially influence the roles they play.

The principal professions concerned are doctors, nurses, psychologists, therapists, social workers and teachers. While each of these have their own expertise, the contributions they make complement one another and to some extent overlap. For example, all may give advice on health matters to children and their parents; social workers, nurses and doctors may all go into the home to provide what is essentially social support to families in difficulties; teachers and psychologists may both undertake remedial education with handicapped children. When two or more workers are concerned with the same child it is important that they define their respective roles, co-ordinate their activities and avoid conflicts of advice. A single child health service greatly increases the ability to achieve such co-operation because the means of communication and of allocating resources are readily available as part of the service.

The pattern of professional work varies in different countries according to the organization of society, the supply of skilled professional workers, and the traditional practices which have developed over the years. For example, in the United Kingdom, general practitioners undertake most of the primary medical care of children, working increasingly with nurses trained as health visitors, and consulting with paediatricians or other appropriate specialists when further advice is required or when hospital care is indicated. In the United States there are both general and paediatric practitioners, but the predominant pattern is for a paediatrician to undertake preventive and curative paediatrics both in and out of hospital, in consultation, where necessary, with system specialists. In European countries the practice of child health care varies between these two models, that in the Netherlands being closest to the British pattern. In the USSR paediatric specialization begins during undergraduate training, and much of the health care of children is undertaken by district paediatricians, each responsible for 900 to 1000 children in a 'microdistrict' (Bamford & Mitchell, 1976). In India, with its huge population and relatively meagre resources, basic child care is undertaken mainly by auxiliary nurse midwives who are often poorly trained and equipped for the task (Ghai, 1973).

Failure to define the roles of different professional workers, disparity in their numbers and changing status in the community may lead to conflicts of interest. Thus in the United Kingdom social support is sometimes given to families by health visitors in situations more appropriate to the casework skills of the social worker, and this may lead to duplication of effort and conflicting advice. Shortage of child psychiatrists has forced the assumption of a quasi-medical role by some psychologists. The rising professional standing of social workers and psychologists *vis-a-vis* the traditional professions of medicine and nursing has been the source of tensions and in some instances competition to provide services. In all such inter-professional disputes, it is the child and his family who are liable to suffer and a child health service should seek to reach agreement on professional roles and establish a review mechanism whereby practice can be kept under continuous scrutiny and changed as necessary.

The growing complexity of child health care and the need to provide for all the child's requirements have led increasingly to teamwork between different professional workers and here a rigid demarcation is unnecessary and indeed undesirable. While it is clearly important to discuss the way in which each member contributes, experience has shown that, in a closely knit team, workers become so familiar with one another's views and methods that when necessary they can assume other workers' roles by mutual agreement. The membership of a multidisciplinary child health team will vary according to its particular purpose, but is likely always to include a paediatrician, who is usually the best person to act as co-ordinator. It does not follow that he must always be chairman or spokesman for the team, but he should be responsible for its successful working, ensuring that communication is rapid and effective, that differences in aims and priorities are reconciled and that tasks are clearly assigned and understood. An authoritarian approach and any belief or suggestion that it is 'the paediatrician's team' or that he is the dominant member should be eschewed: nevertheless, it is a sound and widely approved principle that in health matters the doctor retains the final responsibility.

New roles in clinical child health care

The world shortage of doctors, their maldistribution and the increasing need for teamwork is resulting in the emergence of new health professions and new roles for existing personnel. In the long-established professions of medicine and nursing, the tasks undertaken by each have been precisely delineated by long usage, but they are not as immutable as some would believe. Experience shows that nurses can undertake many of the tasks traditionally regarded as the doctor's, including technical procedures in the surgical theatre, developmental diagnosis in population screening programmes, and emergency treatment such as resuscitation. In some respects nurses may perform better than doctors, as has been demonstrated in the case of nurse practitioners in the United States. In many countries, including the USSR and China, auxiliary medical workers acting as doctor's assistants provide a large part of the health care of children. Whatever the training of such auxiliaries and whatever they are called—medical orderlies, health technicians, feldshers or 'barefoot doctors'—they play a central and indispensable role in large parts of the world where the population is expanding rapidly and the number of doctors is seriously inadequate. In rural areas, they may be supported by part-time primary health workers recruited from the community itself, trained locally and combining health work with their normal occupations (Morley, 1978).

The shortage of doctors is accentuated by the great cost of medical education to western standards, by emigration of doctors to wealthier countries to obtain higher incomes, better facilities and freedom to practise without political interference (Senewiratne, 1975) and by the reluctance of most doctors to practise outside large towns. Even in the United States, the population has been increasing more quickly than the medical manpower available for child health care. In response to this relative lack of doctors, new kinds of health professional are being evolved. Where services are considered inadequate, traditional practices have been changed or adapted to allow these new workers to participate in improving the quality of health care for children. The ways in which this is being achieved inevitably vary by country and community according to local needs and the resources available (Elliott, 1979).

Specially trained nurses are assuming many responsibilities in child health care formerly considered the prerogative of physicians. The first paediatric nurse-practitioners graduated in Denver, Colorado, in 1965. After four months' special post-registration training, these nurses are capable of taking histories; performing physical examinations; evaluating hearing, speech, vision and developmental status; managing common problems of healthy children and some of the minor disorders; and counselling parents. It has been shown that paediatric nurse-practitioners can, by themselves, care for approximately three quarters of all children attending ambulatory centres for paediatric care: usually, however, they work in collaboration with doctors, so increasing the contribution which both make to total child health care (Silver et al, 1968).

In the schools, similarly trained school nurse-practitioners can considerably expand the traditional role of the school nurse. They can assume responsibility for identifying and managing many of the health problems of schoolchildren, carry out routine health examinations, assess and co-ordinate the evaluation of learning disorders and other psycho-educational problems, counsel parents and make home visits (Silver, 1971).

The Child Health Associate is an entirely new type of health professional, introduced in an attempt to improve the child health services and capable of providing even broader health care to children than nurse-practitioners. The three-year training programme in Colorado concentrates on the practical application of paediatric knowledge and on experience of child care in wards, nurseries and health centres (Silver & Ott, 1973). The Child Health Associate has abilities to solve problems and make decisions approaching those of physicians and is trained to give comprehensive primary care to children, including both diagnosis and treatment. Working principally as colleagues and associates of doctors, Child Health Associates are said to have the knowledge and skill to care for 80 to 90 per cent of the patients seen in a typical American paediatric practice.

Other developments in Colorado and elsewhere in the United States have included the training of primary care physicians, with less extensive knowledge and skill than the fully qualified doctor but the ability to practise independently within a clearly defined and limited area of medicine, such as ambulatory child care: and the use of family health workers, who are assistants partially trained in nursing, social and advisory techniques and who act principally as links between health teams and families.

It is not yet clear whether the introduction of such well-trained health workers will be as successful in other states and countries as in Colorado. It is evident that suitably trained nurses can, and many would say should, provide a larger part of the health care of children, but in some countries the shortage of nurses is as acute as that of doctors. Whatever new health professionals are introduced, they cannot and are not intended to supplant the fully trained paediatrician, but they may be seen as a threat to standards of excellence in paediatric practice, as attacking the exclusiveness of the medical profession, or as a means of exploiting highly motivated people as cheap labour. At the very least, however, such experiments do show what can be done when vigorous efforts are made to identify and meet health needs without the shackles of traditional concepts and legal restrictions (Paxman et al, 1979).

So far there has been no widespread movement in the United Kingdom towards greater use of nurses and auxiliaries or the training of new health professionals, but our heavy reliance on overseas medical graduates makes us very vulnerable to sudden changes in the movement of doctors, and the child health service may come to depend increasingly on doctors' assistants of various kinds.

Doctors in a child health service
It is obviously to the advantage of the child and his family if one doctor who

knows them well has continuing responsibility for all ordinary care, both preventive and therapeutic. Unfortunately this ideal can seldom be achieved for a number of reasons. In many countries, doctors are tending more and more to work in groups and are less willing to be continuously available to families in the way that a wholly personal service demands. Thus responsibility inevitably becomes diffused among a number of doctors, though any adverse effect of this can be reduced by close co-operation and a good records system.

The question arises whether all primary care for children should be undertaken by general practitioners or by paediatricians. While opinions and needs vary from country to country, it is clear that truly *general* practice demands a very wide and relatively superficial knowledge and that all general practitioners may not be sufficiently interested in paediatrics to acquire the degree of skill necessary for comprehensive child care. The formal recognition of certain family doctors as having such special expertise has been proposed in Britain (Court, 1976) but has been rejected as a policy. Nevertheless, there are increasing numbers of family doctors with special interest and training in paediatrics, mainly in group practices and health centres. In the USSR and to a lesser extent in the United States, primary care is undertaken by paediatric practitioners. In the latter country, a prestigious national 'task force' (Kempe, 1979) recently affirmed its support for the primary paediatrician. It rejected the principle of general practitioner care for children, believing that adherence to this concept is the reason for unsatisfactory standards in Britain, rather than that British family doctors currently in practice have had little paediatric training, are few in number where the need is greatest, and are motivated towards treatment of disease rather than the promotion of health (Court, 1976).

Other countries have adopted various patterns of care between these extremes and in many there is shared responsibility for the primary care of children, as indeed there is in Britain itself. Shared care developed in this country because prevention and treatment were the responsibility of two different services until the recent integration. At present, primary contact with the child for ordinary medical care is made by the general practitioner: primary contact for developmental screening and immunization is made either by the general practitioner who agrees to undertake these measures or by the doctor in the child health clinic: and primary contact in the school is made by the school doctor.

Responsibility for school health is a controversial subject. Some believe that there is a component consisting of health surveillance, immunization and the like which is part of primary care and should therefore be undertaken by the primary care team: that specialized clinical work relating to children who have difficulties in adaptation at school because of disability or for other reasons should be undertaken by specialist paediatricians trained in educational medicine: and that health matters which concern the school population and the organization and evaluation of school health work are the province of the specialist in community medicine. This broadly was the proposal of the Court Committee (1976) and one advantage claimed was that these doctors working together within the school health service would promote the unity of prevention and treatment. However, others consider that the primary and specialist elements of school health work are not so easily separated: for example, that the ability to recognize the early features of maladaptation or learning difficulty in any child requires expertise beyond that of the primary care doctor. The truth is probably that there is no 'right' pattern. In some circumstances—for example, In the rural or small urban school—an interested family doctor may effectively take on the role of school doctor: in large schools and special schools for the handicapped, paediatric staff with special training and experience in educational medicine will be necessary.

The specialist in this field requires many attributes, including a sound knowledge of paediatrics and developmental neurology, an understanding of the educational system and its resources, the ability to co-operate with colleagues from other disciplines, and an appreciation of the special approaches and methodology of psychology, education and social work. A high level of skill in all these areas demands outstanding professional qualities and long training and can only be expected of a small number of specialists. However, all doctors working in schools should have some level of competence in educational medicine, even although their work is largely restricted to the primary care element of school health. The greater expertise of an experienced specialist should always be available for advice on request and for the maintenance of overall high standards of clinical practice in the service. There are thus considerable implications for postgraduate medical education in the growth of this specialty, which has been defined as 'the study of children in the school environment, of the pressures they meet and their reactions to them, of the diseases which interfere with their capacity for learning, and of the special needs of those who are handicapped' (Scottish Home and Health Department, 1974a).

Constraints on the development of services

Despite increasing professional recognition of children's needs, there is widespread reluctance to provide health services for them in appropriate ways. In the world as a whole, better perinatal care, better nutrition, and the eradication of infection would do more to improve child health than all the investigative and therapeutic technology of modern medicine. Yet many developing countries still squander their meagre resources on expensive hospitals, lavishly equipped and staffed by highly qualified personnel, in the belief that this enhances national prestige. Such policies, modelled on those of the rich industrial West, have failed to meet the real needs of children. Only in a few countries has a realistic response to the challenge been made. Thus the self-help community programmes established with limited resources in the Chinese People's Republic are increasingly being acknowledged as more suitable for developing societies than western systems based on high-cost technology. The 'Under Fives Clinic' concept developed in Nigeria may well have relevance to areas other than rural Africa (Cunningham, 1978).

In wealthier countries which have the means to provide optimal health services for children, there is more talk than action. Expenditure on military services still far outstrips expenditure on health care. It has been estimated that for the cost of one intercontinental ballistic missile, 50 million undernourished children could be adequately fed, and 65 000 day-care centres and 34 000 primary schools could be built (Henderson, 1978). In virtually all such countries there is resistance to deploying resources in more effective and equitable ways. Thus in Britain, for example, the Court Report (1976) set out in great detail the inadequacies and requirements of the health services for children but met with only a lukewarm response from an apathetic public, government officials unwilling to be convinced, and a medical profession preoccupied with its own affairs.

Clearly it is a matter of urgent and world-wide importance to make a fresh examination of priorities, define aims and redesign child health programmes accordingly. This is by no means a simple task. Even with careful planning, change is likely to be resisted, for people are often satisfied with inadequate but familiar services if they have no experience of anything better. They may be reluctant to lose facilities which have apparently served them well, even though these have failed to meet their real needs and ought to be replaced by more effective services. Adaptation to new circumstances requires the co-operation of many and much goodwill on the part of the community. These will only be gained by meticulous groundwork, including explanations to staff and preparation of the general public to accept the unaccustomed arrangements (Madeley & Latham, 1979). Professional workers must be re-educated for their new roles and established patterns of behaviour must be modified. Care should be taken that the transition is not accompanied by even a temporary deterioration of services.

At present there is some national and international pressure for innovation in national policies of providing health care for children. A WHO/UNICEF report speaks of 'a world-wide strategy which should ensure health for all the world's peoples by the year 2000' (WHO, 1978b). The International Year of the Child (1979) stimulated much discussion about the objectives of child health programmes (WHO, 1979). Yet despite the optimism, the outlook for the world's children seems sombre. On current trends, four out of five people in the world at the turn of the century will live in deprived rural areas or urban slums with little or no access to health care—and 35 per cent of them will be children. Half of the 1000 million people in India will be absolutely poor by any standards. The best that their illiterate and malnourished children can expect will be continuing existence at a subsistence level.

These dire prophecies need not be fulfilled if health and social objectives were to change radically and if the basic needs of food, clothing and shelter were accorded the highest priorities in economic planning. Unfortunately, there is little real evidence that governments do intend to spend less on armaments and industrial technology and more on agriculture, housing and education. Only a small proportion of the gross national product is spent on health services—less than 6 per cent in the United Kingdom and less than 1 per cent in many developing countries. The future does not augur well for children, whose condition will only improve when there is universal recognition that they represent our most valuable economic asset which must be safeguarded from the earliest stage.

Child health services in Britain

It has been shown repeatedly that the healthier, better-nourished children in Britain, as in most other countries, receive the lion's share of health care, while those who need it most get least. Thus West & Lowe (1976) reported that regions of high need in England and Wales have low provision of child health services and make less use of them. The reasons are complex and include greater demand and capacity for self-help among parents whose standard of living is high, apathy with low expectations among the underprivileged, reluctance of professional staff to work in deprived areas and lack of imaginative planning. There is growing realization that any general improvement in the major indices of health in childhood can only be achieved by reorganizing and redistributing services according to the real needs of children and their families. Moreover, health services cannot be considered in isolation: family support is a co-operative endeavour and we must clearly plan in terms of social, educational, housing and other services as well. Committee structures in which the health, education and social work professions interchange ideas and participate in planning have been established in England and Wales and in Scotland: although far from perfect, these multidisciplinary committees are helping to bring the different disciplines together and so to achieve greater co-ordination of services for children. More research is needed into criteria for identifying vulnerable families: techniques of health education more effective than the present ones: methods of stimulating self-help in apathetic communities: and new ways of bringing resources and services directly to those who require them.

The move towards redesigning and integrating the child health services was accelerated by publication of the Brotherston Report in Scotland (1973) and the Court Report in England and Wales (1976): both deplored the fragmented nature of the health care hitherto available to children and advocated integration into a single comprehensive service. The new child health services gradually taking shape in the United Kingdom are designed to take account of the interdependence of environmental control, preventive medicine and patient care, recognizing that failure of any one of these will affect all the rest. However, it takes time to change patterns of practice and even more to change attitudes. It would be over-optimistic to hope that even the main proposals of the Court and Brotherston Committees could all be implemented forthwith, especially in the present economic climate, but it is not unreasonable to anticipate a progressive evolution of services along the lines they recommend. A synopsis of the Court Report is given here but the original reports themselves should be read to appreciate their breadth of vision and their full implications.

The Court Report

The Report of the Committee on Child Health Services was published in 1976 under the title *Fit for the Future*. It is in two volumes, the main report (comprising the introduction and four parts) in Volume I and tables of statistical data in Volume II.

Part I reviews the changing pictures of family life and of child health: the health services at present available: and the ways in which children's needs could be met more effectively, both in Britain and in other countries. Part II considers the perinatal period, early development, health at school and in adolescence, illness in childhood, dental health and handicapping and psychiatric disorders. It ends with a review of the need for advocacy of children's interests. Part III examines in detail the changes required in the organization of child health services in England and Wales and their priorities.

In Part IV the major recommendations are summarized. There are 232 of these, all directed at achieving the objective of a new integrated child health service, described in the following words:

> We want to see a child- and family-centred service; in which skilled help is readily available and accessible; which is integrated in as much as it sees the child as a whole and as a continuously developing person. We want to see a service which ensures that this paediatric skill and knowledge are applied in the care of every child whatever his age or disability and wherever he lives, and we want a service which is increasingly orientated to prevention.

The Court Report contains a great deal of interest and importance, with valuable guidance on many aspects of child health care. Almost every paragraph contains some memorable phrase or informative statement. The reader will make his own selection and the following are simply a few of those that especially caught this author's eye. They give a flavour of the whole report but clearly they can only be illustrative of some 400 pages.

Introduction	Our proposals aim at a child-centred service which looks at the needs of children and their parents in the family and educational setting, combines all aspects of medicine and offers access through a single door.
4.5	One of the first criteria for measuring the success of a child health service must be the extent to which it is readily accessible and comprehensive to those who have to use it.
4.6	Many parents have a strong feeling that they are regarded as passive bystanders rather than active partners in the health care of their children.
5.6	The need is for a service that is geared to ensuring that parents are well informed and increasingly involved in their children's development and health.
5.10	A strong health service in school is an essential part of a good child health service.
5.19	Left to themselves, resources simply do not flow where health care needs are greatest.
5.20	A way must be found for children's rights to be more clearly defined and for their needs to be made regularly known.
7.25	All those providing primary health care for children should see themselves as part of a wider comprehensive pattern of services for children.
7.27	Within community nursing there should be a distinct group of nurses with combined preventive and curative nursing responsibility for children.
7.35	In each health district there should be a special handicap team

178   HEALTH AND SOCIAL SERVICES

	... (which) would work from a child development centre and would provide a special diagnostic assessment and treatment service for handicapped children and advice and support for their parents.
7.36	There should be a single supporting child psychiatric service that would embrace the functions of the present child guidance services and the hospital-based child psychiatric services.
9.31	We are convinced that home visiting has an indispensable and increasing place in the future child health services.
10.37	There is an increasing desire to include the handicapped child within the normal school as far as possible and to provide his special education as part of his individual curriculum.
12.10	The community is too often thought of as what happens outside the hospital: for us the hospital is one important activity in a community health service.
12.20	The district hospital services for acutely ill children should be centralized in one department, in one part of the main hospital, accommodating all children and providing paediatric and specialist services.
12.51	A multiplicity of small hospitals caring for children will lead to continuing inefficiency and waste of our present fragmented system of child care.
18.16	Integration means leaving behind false divisions between clinical and social paediatrics, treatment and prevention, hospital and community.

Doctors in the British Child Health Service

General practitioners
The general practitioner is the doctor of first contact in most instances of illness or injury, although in emergency or when the doctor is unavailable, a child may be taken directly to the accident and emergency department of a hospital. The general practitioner also frequently gives general advice on child health and may participate in screening, immunization and other organized programmes of preventive paediatrics. Such duties are not universally undertaken, however, for not all practitioners have the interest or time to acquire the necessary skills or to put them into practice. Where a group of general practitioners practise from a health centre, one or more of their number may take a special interest in child health, while remaining a general practitioner inasmuch as he continues to care for patients of all ages. He may run special clinics for screening and other paediatric purposes, help to maintain the standard of paediatric practice in the group as a whole, and act as a link between the health centre and the child health services in general. The Court Report (1976) recommended that this concept should become more formalized in terms of both responsibility and training and that such 'general practitioner paediatricians' might amount to as many as

40 per cent of all general practitioners. Whether this is a desirable development is a matter of opinion: some believe that it is a satisfactory compromise between the American paediatric practitioner and the traditional British general practitioner, while others consider that it has the disadvantages of both with none of the advantages. Government policy in Britain tends to favour the emergence of group practices with a variety of 'special interests' among the general practitioners concerned, but has not accepted the more formal Court recommendation. There is a contrary view that the development of general practitioners with special interests would diminish the status of general practice as the only true generality in medicine and would result in the metamorphosis of a group practice into an aggregate of specialists. This anxiety was unintentionally fostered by the Court Committee when it introduced the label GPP, though be it noted that the Committee itself rejected any suggestion that the GPP would cease to practice family medicine or his colleagues to practise paediatrics.

Paediatricians

Any doctor who practises wholly among children may reasonably be called a paediatrician. He may work mainly or entirely in preventive paediatrics or mainly or entirely in therapeutic paediatrics. He may practise general paediatrics across the whole spectrum of child health and disease: alternatively, he may channel his interest towards a particular specialty—a system specialty such as cardiology or a wider field such as educational medicine or nutrition—and practise as a general paediatrician with a special interest or entirely as a paediatric specialist. Whatever the pattern of his practice may be, if it is devoted to children, he is by definition a paediatrician.

Consultant paediatricians. In the United Kingdom, the title consultant implies that the paediatrician has undertaken an approved pattern of postgraduate training, has passed examinations or fulfilled such other criteria as are prescribed, and has been appointed to a consultant post in the Health Service in open competition with others. Accreditation as a paediatric specialist may become obligatory in the future before application for a consultant post but such formal recognition is not yet mandatory in the United Kingdom. A consultant paediatrician may be qualified to practise general paediatrics at the level of skill expected of a consultant or may be a consultant paediatrician in a designated specialty, such as educational medicine or paediatric nephrology, when a very high level of competence will be required in the special field but not necessarily in all other aspects of paediatrics. With greater specialization in paediatrics, these distinctions become increasingly important and imply that the title 'consultant paediatrician' should always be qualified to indicate the range of competence: where competence is right across the board, the title 'consultant general paediatrician' is appropriate.

The consultant paediatrician should not be considered as synonymous with the hospital paediatrician as has tended to be the case in the past. It is true that many general paediatricians work largely, or sometimes entirely, in hospital, and that paediatric system specialists spend most of their working time in hospital units. However the majority of consultant paediatricians have commitments both in and out of hospital, the emphasis depending on their particular interest and responsibilities. Thus a consultant may be responsible for in-patient and out-patient care of children in one or more hospitals, may hold clinics in health centres or assessment centres, may have commitments to special schools, and may act in a consultative capacity to various community services and to general practitioners in domiciliary practice. The consultant paediatrician with a special interest in educational medicine may spend the largest part of his time in schools and school clinics and have little or no commitment to hospital work: the academic paediatrician in the university medical school may spend a portion of his time in patient care and a larger part in teaching, research and university administration. What all have in common is that they are paediatricians, they have been rigorously trained to a high professional standard, and they have been appointed to their posts in competition with their peers and with the approval of paediatricians already established as consultants.

Child health practitioners ('clinical medical officers'). In a child health service there is a large amount of clinical work which requires paediatric expertise beyond that of the average general practitioner and yet does not necessitate the full breadth and depth of training of the consultant. Such work includes examination of newborn infants, developmental diagnosis, and some aspects of child health clinic work and school health work (see Chs 10 and 15). While the general practitioner with special interest in paediatrics could and sometimes does undertake this work, it is unlikely that there will ever be sufficient interested general practitioners to assume total responsibility for it. Moreover, it is arguable that some at least of the work will be carried out more efficiently by a doctor wholly committed to paediatrics than by a general practitioner who must necessarily maintain competence in all fields of medicine. There is, therefore, a need for a considerable number of paediatricians trained in these aspects of paediatrics, but not necessarily fulfilling all the requirements for appointment as consultants. While such doctors are paediatricians in that they practise medicine wholly among children, a distinctive title to recognize their particular level of expertise and responsibilities is desirable. The title 'area paediatrician' was proposed in Scotland (Scottish Home and Health Department, 1973), but does carry with it the connotation of a geographical responsibility: 'child health practitioner' was suggested by the Court Committee (1976) and may find favour, although there is a risk of confusion with health professionals in other countries who function in a different way. For the time being, these doctors are referred to as 'clinical medical officers', a title which indicates their former service with the local authorities. Whatever title eventually achieves general acceptance, the nature of the work and the responsibilities and limitations of these appointments are evident and will become more precisely defined as time goes on. The doctors concerned will sometimes work in schools and child health clinics, and sometimes in general practitioner health centres. Appropriate programmes of postgraduate medical education for these doctors are being developed but there is an urgent need to establish for them a clear career structure and an assured place as clinicians in the child health service (Royal Colleges of Physicians and British Paediatric Association, 1979; Faculty of Community Medicine, 1980).

The administration and organization of services, especially in large and complex urban areas, may necessitate a gradation of responsibilities within the generality of clinical medical officers, so that some are designated 'senior'. The National Health Service has always been opposed to a hierarchical structure, maintaining that *any* clinical responsibility implies complete independence. Nevertheless, what seemed right for a comparatively simple therapeutic service is not necessarily appropriate for the complex organization needed to provide a pattern of total care for infants and children of all ages. The educational system alone is sufficiently varied to require a matching school health service which will ensure proper liaison between all concerned and an acceptable level of advice to the school authorities.

Other clinical specialists
Many of the special health needs of children are met by a large number of consultants, only a small proportion of whom are practising wholly among children. In some centres there are paediatric surgeons, although most children's surgery is in the hands of general surgeons with varying degrees of interest and skill. The larger children's medical centres sometimes have paediatric otolaryngologists, paediatric orthopaedic surgeons, and so on, but they are few in number and the great majority of consultants in these specialties deal with patients of all ages, though some may concentrate more on children than others.

Child psychiatrists work more closely with paediatricians than most other specialists, but the nature of family psychiatry is such that most child psychiatrists concern themselves with the treatment of parents and other members of the family as well as with the child, and so are technically not 'paediatric' in that they do not confine their practice to children, although it is child-centred.

When a child has a disorder which is rare, obscure or difficult to treat, the appropriate paediatric specialist is generally the best person to provide the special diagnostic and therapeutic skill required. Thus a complex neurological disease is likely to need the attention of a paediatric neurologist and so on. Where such specialists are not available—and their small numbers and specialist skill necessitate their concentration in a few large centres—the next best thing is combined care by a consultant paediatrician and an adult physician specializing in the appropriate system specialty. Such a symbiotic working relationship can be very effective, for the one provides the paediatric knowledge and experience and the other the specialized skill. Complementary care of this kind will only work satisfactorily if each consultant respects the other, neither becomes possessive, and they work together in harmony with the general practitioner who understands the professional relationship.

This principle of mutual trust and respect and practical co-operation is increasingly applied to the care of children with chronic disabilities, where optimum care can only be achieved by a multidisciplinary team including family doctor, paediatric and other medical specialists, workers from education, social work, and psychology, and therapists of different kinds (see p. 251).

Specialists in community medicine
A complete child health service on a national scale requires competent organization and administration, a good records system, data analysis, evaluation of services, and consultative and advisory machinery. It also needs expertise in

epidemiology, community health, health education, and related aspects of health care. If the word 'clinical' is used to imply concern with individual patients, then the medical expertise required for the activities outlined above is 'non-clinical' though it is obviously very relevant to, and indeed necessary for, the effective application of clinical skills.

A feature of the unified health service in the United Kingdom is the central position of the specialist in community medicine, who originated from the twin streams of hospital medical administrators and public health doctors, but is more than either of these. As training programmes for specialists in community medicine become more clearly defined, they will certainly include the acquisition of skills in integrating medical work and in epidemiological methods together with other experience which may vary according to the special interest of the individual.

The existence of a specialty of community medicine implies an expertise of its own which should be applicable to any part of the health service. In the English child health service, however, it is considered that the specialist in community medicine must have had a significant amount of training and experience in clinical paediatrics in order to understand its problems. It follows from this concept that there must be specialists in community medicine (child health) who, once trained, will remain within the child health service and will not normally move to other branches of the health service, and that specialists in community medicine from other branches will not be readily acceptable in the child health service. In Scotland, on the other hand, it is recognized that a skilled specialist in community medicine may move from one part of the service to another, bringing to each his expertise in community medicine, without necessarily having special knowledge or experience of the medical specialty or service concerned. Indeed, special knowledge of the particular specialty may sometimes be a positive disadvantage, for it may tempt the specialist in community medicine to go beyond his sphere and make policy decisions which are properly those of the clinicians.

Time will no doubt tell which is the preferable way, but meanwhile the administrative and epidemiological expertise in the child health service is provided in England by specialists in community medicine (child health) and in Scotland by undifferentiated specialists in community medicine. What is clear in both countries is that the specialist in community medicine does not have responsibility for individual patients and is therefore by definition not a clinician. At the inception of the integrated service, it was necessary for doctors in the health departments of local authorities to opt either for community medicine posts or for clinical work: while this distinction is quite clear, it is not understood or not accepted by everyone and some confusion of identity and responsibility still persists.

REFERENCES

Bamford F N, Mitchell R G 1976 Child health and paediatrics in the USSR. Developmental Medicine and Child Neurology 18: 320–327
Bhatia J R 1973 Health planning for children. Indian Pediatrics 10: 393–395

Brim O G 1975 Macro-structural influences on child development and the need for childhood social indicators. American Journal of Orthopsychiatry 45: 516–524

Butrov V N 1974 The education of medical personnel in the USSR. American Journal of Public Health 64: 149–154

Cunningham N 1978 The Under Fives Clinic—what difference does it make? Journal of Tropical Pediatrics and Environmental Child Health 24: 239–334

Court S D M (chairman) 1976 Fit for the future: Report of the Committee on Child Health Services. HMSO, London

Elliott K (ed) 1979 Auxiliaries in primary health care: an annotated bibliography. Intermediate Technology Publications, London

Faculty of Community Medicine 1980 Clinical medical officers in the child health service. British Medical Journal 280: 385–386

Forfar J O 1973 Child health services, today and tomorrow. Community Health 4: 261–267

Forfar J O 1979 Effectiveness and cost in the paediatric service. Scottish Medical Journal 24: 233–239

Ghai O P 1973 Health planning for children. Indian Pediatrics 10: 1–4

Henderson J 1978 A crusade for children. People 5: 23–26

Hyde G 1974 The Soviet Health Service. Lawrence & Wishart, London

Kempe C H (chairman) 1979 The future of pediatric education: Report by the Task Force on Pediatric Education. American Academy of Pediatrics, Evanston, Illinois

Kerr L E 1975 The poverty of affluence. American Journal of Public Health 65: 17–20

Madeley R J, Latham A 1979 Management aspects of high risk strategies in child health. Community Medicine 1: 36–39

Mellander O 1973 Nutrition and health care in preschool children: report from China. Environmental Child Health 19: 253–257

Mitchell R G 1976 Child Health Services in the United Kingdom—present and future. In: Wallace H M (ed) Health care of mothers and children in national health services: implications for the United States. Ballinger, Cambridge, Mass.

Mitchell R G 1977 Health services for children: the Donald Paterson Memorial Lecture. In: Robinson G C (ed) Re-designing the child care encounter. University of British Columbia, Vancouver

Morley D 1978 Priorities in manpower for child health services: a view from England. Bulletin of the International Paediatric Association 2: 35–37

Paxman J M, Shattock F M, Fendall N R E 1979 The use of paramedicals for primary health in the commonwealth. Commonwealth Secretariat, London

Petersson P O 1978 Aspects on the European and especially Swedish MCH services. Journal of Tropical Pediatrics and Environmental Child Health 24: 65–69

Royal Colleges of Physicians and British Paediatric Association 1979 Clinical medical officers in the child health service: Report of the Joint Paediatric Committee. British Medical Journal 2: 1563–1565

Rudolph A M 1974 Child health in the People's Republic of China. In: Schulman I (ed) Advances in pediatrics. Year Book Medical Publishers, Inc., Chicago, vol 21

Ryan M 1978 The organization of Soviet medical care. Blackwell & Robertson, Oxford

Schorr L B 1978 Social policy issues in improving child health services: a child advocate's view. Pediatrics 62: 370–376

Scottish Home and Health Department 1973 Towards an integrated child health service. HMSO, Edinburgh

Scottish Home and Health Department 1974a Reorganization and the School Health Service: Report of a Sub-committee of the Consultative Committee of Medical Officers of Health. SHHD, Edinburgh

Scottish Home and Health Department 1974b The Child Health Services: a systematic planning approach. Report by a joint team from the SHHD and the WHO. SHHD, Edinburgh

Senewiratne B 1975 Emigration of doctors: a problem for the developing and the developed countries. British Medical Journal i: 618–620

Silver H K 1971 The school nurse-practitioner program. Journal of the American Medical Association 216: 1332–1334

Silver H K, Ford L C, Day L R 1968 The pediatric nurse-practitioner program. Journal of the American Medical Association 204: 298–302

Silver H K, Ott J E 1973 The child health associate. Pediatrics 51: 1–7

Wallace H M 1971 Children and youth projects and related comprehensive health care programs. Clinical Pediatrics 10: 487–494

West R R, Lowe C R 1976 Regional variations in need for and provision and use of child health services in England and Wales. British Medical Journal 2: 843–846
World Health Organization 1978a Risk approach for maternal and child health care. WHO Offset Publications No 39. WHO, Geneva
World Health Organization 1978b Alma-Ata 1978: primary health care. A Joint WHO/UNICEF report. WHO, Geneva
World Health Organization 1979 The International Year of the Child and WHO. WHO Chronicle 33: 3–6
Wynn M, Wynn A 1974a The protection of maternity and infancy. Council for Children's Welfare, London
Wynn M, Wynn A 1974b The right of every child to health care. Council for Children's Welfare, London

Preventive aspects of child health practice

Introduction

For many health workers it continues to be a strange idea, or at most a low priority, to pay careful clinical attention to apparently healthy children. Western medical practice is traditionally curative in its emphasis and medical teaching has until recently been dominated by hospitals. It is becoming more than merely fashionable, however, to question health care priorities and active measures to prevent ill health will in future be necessary on economic as well as humanitarian grounds. The Report of the Committee on Child Health Services (Court, 1976) has pointed to a lack of weight on the preventive side of the balance as one of the basic shortcomings of present child health services and, although the distinctions between 'prevention' and 'cure' need to be minimized from the consumer's viewpoint, the relatively neglected preventive aspects of clinical practice require the separate consideration which is the purpose of this chapter.

Achieving continuity of health care for children implies abandoning arbitrary distinctions such as those between 'child health' and 'school health', and establishing more effective links between perinatal, pre-school and school health services and with facilities for handicapped children. Provision of effective services for families with children in the 0 to five years age group presents special problems, however, because between the 'captive populations' of neonates (nearly all babies now being delivered in hospital) and children attending school compulsorily at five it is exceptionally difficult to bring services to bear where they are most needed, during a period of great potential vulnerability.

Health care is one contribution to a multidisciplinary concern for the well-being of children. The overlap with educational services is obvious and especially relevant to nursery education and early educational intervention with handicapped children. Psychologists have made an extensive contribution in research and practice to the monitoring of developmental progress in young children. More effective co-operation with social services in numerous respects is urgent. It behoves the medical profession not to assume that it is automatically the pivot of professional concern for children and parents in a multidisciplinary context: although this is often the case, no divine right of doctors operates in this respect. Health personnel have much to learn as well as much to offer in these areas of co-operation.

The deliberate restriction of this discussion to clinical considerations is not intended in any way to belittle the contribution made to the health and well-being of children by other measures in the fields of community medicine and public health.

Preventive child health practice

The need for preventive services
With the notable exception of infectious disease prophylaxis (Office of Health Economics, 1964), no objective evidence is available as to the contribution of personal preventive services to the improved well-being of children in the United Kingdom, although they have undoubtedly had a considerable effect in various ways. The past performance of fragmented and impoverished health services is in any case not necessarily a helpful guide to the potential of adequately financed preventive services in the future. Furthermore, difficulties in measuring some aspects of care (e.g. the alleviation of distress, or the maintenance of well-being) in no way diminish their importance to the individuals concerned. The patterns of mortality and morbidity among children today, the nature and extent of health problems in the community and their relationship to education and ultimate social well-being, and the desirability of avoiding costly curative medical care and social remediation, all point to the need for a deliberate emphasis upon preventive medical oversight of children and their families, in close co-operation with other professions concerned with children in the community. A preventive dimension to health care is particularly relevant to the following problems and requirements:

1. There is continuing avoidable mortality and morbidity among children in the community; causes include (a) accidents, on roads *and in homes*; (b) cot deaths; (c) non-accidental injury; (d) infectious disease.
2. There are socio-economic gradients, to the constant disadvantage of the less privileged, in most parameters of health (Davie et al, 1972; Office of Health Economics, 1962). The reasons are undoubtedly complex and far from entirely 'medical' but contributory factors are:

   a. Differences in child-rearing attitudes and practices (Newson & Newson, 1965).

   b. Differences in effective use of available health services. Paradoxically, those whose need of help is greatest often have most difficulty in obtaining it. The emphasis upon patient-initiated contact in primary health care has tended to place inarticulate, socially ineffective parents at a disadvantage, although their higher morbidity rates and continuing health and educational disadvantage are now clearly documented (Davie et al, 1972; Wedge & Prosser, 1973; Field, 1974; Wilson & Herbert, 1975).

   c. Differences in distribution of health (and other) services. An 'inverse care law' operates (Hart, 1971), whereby those areas with the greatest need have fewest resources available to them. Inner urban areas are an obvious example, and there are wider regional variations showing the same inverse ratio between socio-economic need and health provision.

3. The environments in which some children spend much of their time lack adequate stimulation, particularly so far as play opportunities, emotional

warmth and security, and language stimulation are concerned. This problem has been related (but is certainly not confined) to certain cultural groups (Pollak, 1972), and is also serious in the context of child-minding (Jackson, 1974).

4. All children and parents are particularly vulnerable during a child's earliest years, the child during a period of rapid and complex development, the parents because they are under real and imagined pressure—from modern society and through the mass media—to guide their children's development. Realistic, informed and self-critical medical support and intervention could be of great potential benefit to families during this period, especially because most parents are highly motivated to promote their children's health, and welcome good advisory facilities.

5. The early recognition of potentially handicapping disorders, established as the basis of ongoing support of the handicapped child and his family, necessitates the serial monitoring of the development of all children, so that early signs of deviation from accepted normal developmental patterns can be investigated in detail.

6. Effective medical supervision of older healthy and handicapped children during their school years depends upon the input of relevant recorded information concerning each child's progress in the pre-school period.

The nature of clinical preventive practice
Prevention may be:
 1. primary—action taken to prevent a problem occurring;
 2. secondary—early detection of abnormality or deviation from normal;
 3. tertiary—action to contain and minimize an established abnormal condition.

Effective preventive child health practice must include discrete and purposeful medical intervention of all three types on a broad, well-informed, developmentally orientated foundation of training and knowledge.

Tertiary prevention involves the care of children with established handicaps and is not discussed further here, except to emphasize the obvious need for the closest possible dovetailing of primary child health care in general with services to meet the special needs of handicapped children.

Successful primary prevention is an end in itself. Secondary prevention, however, is only a first step in a sequence of events, otherwise this approach cannot be justified. The implications for services are obvious: recognition of disorder and subsequent assessment of the child's deficiencies and assets must be much more closely linked with remediation than at present is commonly the case.

The aim, admirable in itself, of integrating prevention and cure into a single type of health care should not be allowed to obscure essential differences between the two approaches. The well-known patient-initiated contact of traditional curative medicine is replaced in preventive practice by a doctor–'patient' relationship with the following characteristics:

1. The 'patient' (parent) does not present himself (or the child) to the doctor with symptoms. A preventive service has a responsibility to the whole population concerned: if it is a personal (clinical) preventive service, it is offered to

each individual who is encouraged to use it and who, if he does so, should derive benefit from it. The service itself, and the curative and supportive services backing it up, must therefore be adequate. Sufficient time for unhurried two-way communication is essential.

2. Health personnel involved in such contacts face the problem of offering advice which has not been directly solicited by the recipient.

3. Unsolicited advice about the health of children, developmental examinations, and the search for early signs of disorder involve the doctor in a continuing professional relationship in which it is frequently impossible to avoid subjecting parents to stress; moreover, such stress cannot always be immediately resolved, especially when 'diagnosis by increasing suspicion' (Ingram, 1969) is involved. The sensitive handling of parents and children must be foremost among the preventive clinician's skills.

The importance of 'non-disease'—symptomatology in the absence of an underlying disease or abnormal state—has received attention in the context of adult medicine (Hart, 1973). 'Non-disease' is often doctor-aggravated, and preventive child health could readily provide fertile soil for the proliferation of 'developmental non-disease', much of it iatrogenic, in the minds of parents concerning their children. Avoidance of such proliferation depends on careful structuring of the services and the exercise of appropriate professional skills.

The scope of clinical preventive practice
The roles of primary medical care services have been defined (Ministry of Health. 1971) as follows:

1. The diagnosis and management in or near the home of undifferentiated illness in a defined population of individuals or families to whom the general practitioner is directly accessible and for whom he accepts a continuing responsibility.

2. The prevention of disease and the maintenance of health both physical and mental including the detection of the earliest departure from normal in the individuals and families of this population.

The first role has been performed by the general practitioner service, but the second, with notable exceptions particularly in the field of 'developmental screening' (Hooper & Alexander 1971; Starte, 1971, 1974; Bain 1974), on the whole has not been fulfilled by general practitioners, despite the intended impetus of the Sheldon Report (Ministry of Health, 1967) in this direction.

Local authority health departments, which provided a qualitatively variable preventive service for children, no longer exist, but the need remains for services which are relevant to local community requirements and which contribute this preventive and health-promoting dimension to primary child health care.

To avoid confusion over terminology, and to help make further discussion both precise and comprehensive, the concept of 'health surveillance' is put forward here both to describe preventive practice and to indicate how it dovetails with other aspects of primary care.

Health surveillance is defined as:

'The unsolicited serial professional observation of the health and development of the child and of the well-being of the family as a whole' (DHSS, 1972).

To be fully effective, it must include the following components:

1. Oversight of growth and development, and early recognition and initial investigation of children showing significant deviation from accepted norms.

2. An advisory service for parents and children which covers health, normal development and common deviations therefrom, and important social and environmental hazards. This service must be readily available and adapted in scope and venue to meet any particular needs of those who may use it.

3. Intervention of all types as appropriate, as an integral part of the services. Drugs and medicines should be fully prescribable by all doctors clinically involved. Intervention also includes advice (with follow-up to check whether any advice given was taken and whether it was effective, with appropriate feedback), direct referral for more specialist help, and involvement of other personal supportive services.

4. A programme of effective infectious disease prophylaxis.

Present practice and future needs

Child health clinics

Attention paid to the Sheldon report (Ministry of Health, 1967) and plans to implement its recommendations have tended to overlook the sub-committee's limited terms of reference which, particularly in the 1970s context of health service reorganization and integration, were an inadequate basis in themselves for a preventive dimension in primary health care. A clinic service, however friendly and efficient, will never reach all children: clinics are a valuable supplement to, but can never replace, domiciliary visiting, and families most in need of advice and support are usually among those who never darken a clinic door.

There is remarkably little up-to-date information about who attends clinics and why, and research into the reasons for non-attendance would be particularly valuable. Bax & Hart (1976) have shown that high attendance rates can be achieved by dedicated clinic staff, at least in the short term. In general, mothers will come if they derive benefit from coming. At present many attend much less frequently once first babies become toddlers, even with subsequent infants.

An effective clinic service can be provided in many settings, such as purpose-built premises, health centres, general practitioners' surgeries and church halls. The setting should, above all, be appropriate to its function. Design and decor should be child-orientated. Rooms should be sufficiently large, well ventilated and illuminated. The atmosphere should be cheerful, informal and lacking in 'clinical' overtones so far as possible. The areas used for clinical assessments should be adequately sound-insulated and large enough for assessment of vision and hearing: at least part of the floor should be carpeted. Appropriate 'nursery-size' furniture is essential for small children: the children need to be comfortable and it helps the adults concerned to make contact at the children's level, in every sense.

Domiciliary visiting
Surveillance in the home has an indispensable place in child health services. The health visitor's role as a 'health' worker and her access to the child at home give her unique and invaluable opportunities to observe children in their natural environment. Domiciliary health visiting is relatively expensive in time, but one visit often yields much more relevant information than several visits by some members of the family to clinic or surgery. In the general practice context, the tendency towards fewer home visits by doctors makes this contribution to the primary health care team's understanding of the family even more important. Home visits by health visitors and doctors are vital for contact with the disadvantaged 'non-attending' family.

Advice to parents—the need for research
It is not surprising that health education campaigns which have been undertaken in this country have not been conspicuously successful in the past in view of the minuscule proportion of the annual health budget which is allocated to finance both the campaigns themselves and the research into attitudes upon which they should be based.

Parents in general are highly motivated to help their children, and the advertising industry already has a wealth of knowledge about how people's behaviour can be changed, some at least of which should be applicable without ethical offence to help persuade parents to adopt health-promoting child-rearing practices. What is lacking at present is a sound research basis for such campaigns. Much more needs to be known about *how* parents bring up their children, and *why* they adopt the attitudes they now have to child health and development. Studies already carried out (Newson & Newson, 1965, 1968) both provide information and also emphasize how much more we need to know.

Advice given to parents about their children needs to be sound, authoritative and scientifically based. It is salutary to reflect that, in the past, advisory services such as 'the welfare' have been abundant sources of conflicting, non-substantiated advice to mothers (e.g. on infant feeding), and that many children have thrived in spite, rather than because, of the counsel of such 'experts'.

'Developmental paediatrics'
Paediatrics is the 'medicine of dependent and developing persons' (Court & Jackson, 1972). The whole new dimension of observation and clinical evaluation of children's developmental skills, pioneered in the United States by Gesell and in Britain by Illingworth and Sheridan, is relevant to all aspects of child health, but is properly a dominant component of community child health practice.

Normal child development, usually subdivided for convenience into the fields of gross motor, fine motor (eye–hand co-ordination), hearing and language, and social skills, has now been described qualitatively in great detail, and normal patterns of development, as well as common variations of the normal, are well documented. In addition, special attention has been paid to techniques for assessing hearing and language and vision, because of the overriding importance of normal sensory input through the channels of hearing and vision to development as a whole. Manuals relating knowledge of normal development to clinical practice are readily available (e.g. Illingworth, 1962, 1975, 1977; Sheridan, 1973; 1975; Egan et al, 1969). All emphasize the importance of the developmental and medical history, although Hart et al (1978) have reappraised critically some aspects of the conventional developmental history. The *clinical skills* required to make an accurate assessment of a child's development are stressed, as are the need for experience and care in interpreting the significance of apparent deviations from 'normal' (this is also of crucial importance in the context of what is said, *and what is not said*, to parents), and the need for serial evaluations, both to check on certain aspects at the optimum age (e.g. hearing at eight to nine months), and to monitor individual skills and their interrelationships as the pattern of development unfolds with time.

The practical problem of meeting the need for repeated checks within the limitations imposed by manpower and other resource restrictions is bound to cause controversy, and has yet to be settled with a wide measure of agreement. A programme which is integrated into the broader concept of health surveillance is suggested at the end of this chapter.

Early recognition of handicapping disorders
This is established as a sound basis for the management of handicapping disorders in childhood (Rogers, 1971; Lancet, 1975). It is not, however, the only, or even the most important, reason for seeking an effective health surveillance programme for children, nor is it the sole purpose of close attention to children's physical and mental development. *Nothing could be worse for the promotion of health than to surround professional interest in children with the aura of hunting for hidden handicaps.* Doctors in particular need to be aware that the traditional morbidity bias of their medical education can easily colour their contact with children and parents unless care is taken to manifest a positive attitude to children's health.

Much more needs to be done to establish 'recognition—assessment—remediation' as a closely knit sequence of attitudes and events in all cases where potential handicap is suspected or established. Enthusiasm for identifying affected children has forged well ahead of the provision of adequate remediation and practical help for the families concerned.

The problems involved in recognizing handicapping disorders at a sufficiently early stage for effective habilitation to be achieved vary according to the age at which the disorder itself or its effects upon the child's development become evident. At risk of over-simplifying the situation, four broad overlapping groups may be distinguished:

1. In a considerable proportion of cases of severe disability, early recognition is a relatively small problem and is likely to be achieved in hospital, the condition either being manifest at or soon after birth, or becoming apparent during very early life. Obvious examples are congenital malformations, such as spina bifida or severe multiple abnormalities associated with microcephaly, and very marked delay in early motor development.

2. Neuromotor disorders, cases of mental handicap without obvious physical stigmata, and defects of vision and hearing comprise the important group of

conditions which present later, often by delaying or distorting normal development. These 'developmental disorders' are those for which primary care health services must seek to provide presymptomatic recognition through effective health surveillance.

3. A third rather ill-defined group comprises children who have problems which often emerge later in the pre-school period, who may be disadvantaged in peer group activities and later in their schooling. Examples are children whose slowness in maturation in one or more aspects of development is outside wide normal limits; poorly co-ordinated children and those with signs of minimal cerebral dysfunction; and children with disorders of language development. More research is needed, with particular reference to the relationship of such problems to later 'learning difficulties', to determine whether even earlier recognition would be feasible and helpful.

4. Surveys of the results of developmental screening in general practice (Hooper & Alexander, 1971; Starte, 1971, 1974; Bain, 1974) reveal a fourth group of children, variously described as showing 'developmental delay' or 'significant developmental delay' or having 'minor developmental defects', all of whom were subsequently found to be normal. This confirms the frequent clinical impression that the development of many children may temporarily lag behind the 'normal' pattern in one or more respects—common examples are gross motor and language development—but that, in terms of reaching the maturity of the immediate pre-school years within the very wide range of normal abilities of three- and four-year-olds, these developmental laggards 'get there in the end' and are entirely normal children. Important issues (also discussed under 'screening', below) are raised, such as the irrelevance and inaccuracy for these children of many of the milestone norms upon which 'developmental screening' programmes are based, and the dangers of attempting pass/fail scoring against this background of wide ranges of normality (Starte, 1974, has mitigated the latter difficulty by devising a short scale of responses to each test item). The 'non-disease' dangers implicit in managing this group are also obvious (see p. 188).

Where primary prevention of handicap is still not practicable, secondary prevention, presymptomatic diagnosis, by primary health care services must be the aim. Parents themselves, however, are often the first to notice that all is not well with their child (Sheridan, 1962, 1969; Bain, 1974), and health services *must* provide them with opportunities to obtain advice without delay.

Screening
Holt (1974) has provided a comprehensive review of screening in childhood, and in many fields the potential and limitations of the screening approach are reasonably clear. So far as 'developmental screening' is concerned, however, the present situation is confused: even if it is regarded as 'the simple determination of developmental status' (Scottish Home and Health Department, 1973), in practice it is often far from easy and tends to be most difficult in those cases where it is most important. Medical screening itself can be a complex and sophisticated concept, and the term may imply some or all of the following features:

1. Application to the whole of a defined, apparently healthy population to detect the minority who are possible sufferers from the condition being sought, at a presymptomatic stage.
2. Administration on a single occasion (to minimize cost and non-cooperation).
3. Simplicity of administration.
4. Objective pass/fail interpretation of the response.
5. Use of relatively unskilled personnel, who need to be trained in the test procedure but do not need training in the underlying discipline.
6. Use of quantitative measures in evaluation, for example sensitivity (minimizing false negatives), specificity (minimizing false positives), repeatability, and interobserver reliability.

The first of these is the best known and is the basis of developmental examinations being referred to as 'screening', but there are obvious problems in attempting to apply any of the other features to child development.

The second criterion does not apply because, in general, attention to development must be serial to be meaningful.

The most serious difficulties surrounding 'developmental screening' relate to the search for a simple procedure with pass/fail scoring, for the use of other than highly skilled personnel. In the words of Illingworth (1977): 'He who thinks that a sensible developmental screening can be made on purely objective findings on the basis of some psychologist's test reveals a regrettable lack of understanding of the complexities of human development' and, one must add, of the complexities of psychological test structure and standardization. Part of the confusion does seem to relate to misunderstandings about the *different* and *complementary* roles of clinical assessment and psychometric testing, ironically at a time when some psychologists in this field are moving away from norm-referenced testing, i.e. comparison of an individual with norms derived from the performance of other individuals on the same test (Evans & Sparrow, 1975).

Pass/fail scoring is inappropriate without standardization based upon detailed knowledge of ranges of normal, and investigation of four commonly used developmental milestones (Neligan & Prudham 1969a 1969b) reveals how inaccurate and misleading most schemes for 'screening' on a pass/fail basis would be. The 3rd to 97th percentile ranges for the milestones investigated, quoted to the nearest half month and relating to girls (slightly different ranges applying to boys) are:

Sitting (1 minute)	$4\frac{1}{2}$ to $9\frac{1}{2}$ months
Walking (10 steps)	$9\frac{1}{2}$ to $18\frac{1}{2}$ months
Words (3 or 4)	$8\frac{1}{2}$ to 20 months
Sentences (3 or 4 words)	16 to 36 months

The clinician concerns himself not only with the abilities of a child of a certain age, but with determining (as accurately as is feasible) when a skill was first achieved, the maturity with which it is now performed, whether there are any unusual features about its accomplishment, and how it relates to other aspects of the child's development. All these nuances are lost in a pass/fail evaluation.

The use of ancillary workers for 'developmental screening' is a matter which needs the greatest care. It must be clearly understood that clinical skills, based upon understanding of and training in child development, are being deployed; that appropriate training (i.e. not just in a test procedure but in underlying principles) must be given; and that supervision and support by clinical doctors must be adequate to maintain high standards of practice. Furthermore, attention to 'screening' with a view to detection of disorder *must* be given against the backcloth of health surveillance, with its wider implications of promoting health in the social context of the individual family.

The Denver Developmental Screening Test (Frankenberg & Dodds, 1967) represents the most thorough attempt so far to devise a test for 'screening' development in a stricter sense of the term. The care taken to overcome many of the difficulties discussed above is impressive (Frankenberg et al, 1971a; Frankenberg et al, 1971b). It is nevertheless less simple than it might appear on first acquaintance, and its widespread use in the United Kingdom would require careful attention to standardization of test items (Bryant et al, 1974).

In the Cardiff study of the DDST (Bryant et al, 1973), health visitors carried out test procedures, but it was suggested that the results should be scrutinized by a doctor trained in developmental paediatrics. If universally applied, this approach to 'screening' would have two undesirable effects: doctors would be required to give opinions on the development of children with whom they had not themselves been clinically involved, and the value of the health visitor's interaction with parent and child would be greatly reduced by deferring comments and advice about development to another place, person and time.

The subtleties of early human development are such, and the problems of deciding developmental status in the all-important 'difficult' and 'borderline' cases at any age are so great, that it still remains an open question whether the clearcut distinction, so desirable in theory, between 'screening' and 'assessment' of development can be made a practical reality.

Screening tests of vision and hearing, such as the Stycar tests (Sheridan, 1973) and the hearing tests associated with Manchester, illustrate many of the problems which have been discussed. They are relatively simple techniques, designed for application on a population basis for early detection of disorders such as severe hearing loss or impaired visual acuity, which can have a seriously adverse effect upon development but which are often particularly amenable to *early* treatment and ongoing supervision.

The tests concerned are, however, clinical procedures par excellence and require to be administered and interpreted with great skill in quiet, non-distracting surroundings. Health visitors are frequently deployed for this purpose, particularly for tests of hearing, and there is no doubt that, where training, ongoing supervision and facilities for testing are of sufficiently high standard, satisfactory results can be achieved. Such conditions, however, often do not apply: training and supervision may be inadequate for sufficient skill to be acquired and maintained, and most homes and many clinics are too noisy and distracting. The skills required in this field continue to be almost universally underrated. This has led to a situation where current efforts to 'screen' babies for hearing loss are probably not only contributing little if anything to detecting cases of deafness, but may even have a delaying influence because of the misleading sense of security given by 'false negative' results at nine months. Other problems relating to the tests themselves and to service delivery and acceptance have been discussed by Boothman & Orr (1978). There is urgent need to evaluate an alternative whole population approach, such as a carefully structured questionnaire combined with the overall developmental vigilance of well-trained health visitors.

The child 'at risk'

Risk registers were devised in an attempt to chart a valid short cut through the enormous task of whole population surveillance to early recognition of children with potential handicaps; they were widely used, but have been abandoned in their original form.

The exercise was, however, useful in several respects. At the outset it encouraged interest in the problem of hidden handicap and its later effects upon the children and families concerned. Its failure reinforced the growing apprehension that, for many medical and social reasons, whole population health surveillance was unavoidable in spite of tremendous problems in terms of manpower and resources.

The most important lesson learnt from the failure of risk registers has been that two related but distinct concepts were involved (Rogers 1971; DHSS, 1972):

1. *The concept of the child 'at risk':* some children are considered to be at increased risk of subsequent handicap because of genetic endowment or adverse environmental influences during fetal, perinatal, neonatal or post-neonatal development.

Disentangled from risk *registers* (see below), this concept is valuable within the limits of current knowledge about the natural history of developmental disorders. Accurate relevant data should be available in the medical records of every child, so that any 'at risk' factors can be taken into account during developmental examinations. In this way, too, due weight can be given to combinations of factors (Alberman & Goldstein, 1970).

2. *The risk register concept:* this mistakenly assumed that a small group of infants, suitably selected (those with relevant 'at risk' factors in their history), would include most of those who would subsequently develop handicapping conditions.

The idea was based upon invalid assumptions about the distribution of both 'at risk' factors and handicapping disorders in the child population (Rogers, 1968). For most children included on risk registers, the risk of subsequent handicap was little if any higher than that for non-selected children, only a minority of the selected children being at appreciably increased or 'high' risk. This led to unduly large numbers of children being selected for registers, and an unacceptably low yield in that many cases of handicap (up to 50 per cent with some registers) were not among selected children, thus defeating the object of the rather complicated exercise.

It may be worth giving extra attention to the small group of highly vulnerable children mentioned above, provided that this occurs within the framework of surveillance services for all children (because most handicaps occur outside such a group) and that sufficiently precise and flexible selection procedures can be devised.

Davie et al (1972), using data from the National Child Development Study, showed that a few criteria could be used to identify a small group (13.2 per cent of the 1958 cohort) among whom 25.3 per cent of subsequent cases of 'severe physical or mental, or multiple handicap' occurred. Such criteria could form the basis of selection for additional surveillance, taking local facilities and channels of communication into account: indeed the use of this approach in future, including the type of extra attention bestowed on selected children, should be related to the overall effectiveness of local surveillance services in achieving early recognition of handicaps (Alberman & Goldstein, 1970; Davie et al, 1972).

Professional roles

Health visitors and primary care doctors are the key professional groups in preventive child health care and the Court Report's blueprint must be regarded as the desirable pattern for the future, even though the detailed recommendations for 'child health visitors' and 'general practitioner paediatricians' as such are unlikely to be implemented.

The health visitor. The contribution of health visiting to past improvements in child health is probably underestimated. The potential of such a service, making use of the health visitor's unique blend of medical and social skills, her image as a preventive health worker, and her unrivalled opportunities for access to children in their home environment, has never been achieved or even approached because of past professional isolation and inadequate staffing to allow effective work in depth.

The traditional child health role of the health visitor has been modified during the past decade by the effects of attachment to general practice which, though generally welcomed as a contribution to integrating health services, has created problems. So relevant are health visiting skills to the needs of all age groups in the community (particularly the elderly), that health visitors now have a cradle-to-grave commitment which, in the absence of an expansion of the service, has reduced the time available for attention to young children. Domiciliary visiting in particular has suffered. Most serious of all has been the loss of a geographical area commitment to families, since general practice is now unique among health, education and social services in not being organized on a uniform geographical basis. The families most in need are those most likely to fall through the resultant large holes in the preventive net.

For health surveillance to be effective, the health visiting service must be responsible for establishing contact between all families with children and the preventive health services. To achieve this it will be necessary:

1. To increase health visitor time available to children, so that case loads can be reduced to allow more effective work, including time-consuming involvement with disadvantaged families.

2. To establish a working relationship with child health doctors in which the ability of health visitors to undertake skilled clinical work (following appropriate training and under close supervision) is fully accepted.

3. To revise health visitor training courses to meet these requirements.

4. To accept a return to geographical deployment of health visitors in all areas other than those where efficient group practices make whole population coverage by practice-attached health visitors feasible.

The primary care doctor. The essential qualification for child health practice must in future be appropriate and adequate training. The doctor so equipped must have time for unhurried clinical work and the opportunity to maintain his skills and experience, both of normal development and behaviour and of the commoner handicapping disorders of childhood (which are each numerically relatively uncommon), by being responsible for a child population of adequate size and appropriate age structure.

It would be ideal for most aspects of health surveillance to be the family doctor's responsibility, and some appropriate training is being included in vocational training schemes for general practitioners. It would, however, be essential to encourage a greater degree of specialization or 'special interest' in child health than is common at present if the conditions of professional time and adequate ongoing paediatric experience which are inherent in the 'general practitioner paediatrician' concept are to be met in the context of group general practice in the United Kingdom.

The preventive attitudes and skills of former local authority clinical doctors are crucial for the maintenance of services, at least until longer-term planning can take effect. There will probably be a permanent role for the Scottish 'area paediatrician' (Scottish Home and Health Department, 1973) and his English and Welsh counterpart, to the extent that efficient group general practice cannot be established, for example in remote rural or inner urban areas (see p. 180).

To meet community health needs, undergraduate education in child health needs to shift its centre of gravity from the hospital environment, which by its very nature is least appropriate for teaching preventive medicine, to the wider community. A thorough grounding in child health and development and the commonest deviations therefrom (primary health care problems) should be the basis of undergraduate paediatric teaching, the care of the ill child in the hospital bed being largely the postgraduate concern of those aiming at a career in specialist paediatrics.

The role of parents

There is a danger that improved services and greater professional competence could lead parents to feel elbowed aside, rather than supported, in caring for their children. The pre-eminence of the parental role demands more than lip service from health professionals for many reasons, among them the following:

1. Parents know their own child better than anyone else. Some parents are completely unrealistic about their children's capabilities, but most are not and some are astute if untutored observers. The doctor's observations of the child are fragmentary in contrast, though they have a depth based upon training and

experience, and the doctor is able to compare very broadly with normality and common deviations therefrom. A synthesis of the parental and medical viewpoints, if it could be achieved, would provide invaluable insights: this is the rationale of various attempts to devise a new type of record to which parents (under appropriate supervision) and health personnel contribute, to build up a picture which is less norm-referenced than conventional records and emphasizes the individual child's relative strengths and weaknesses (Evans & Sparrow, 1975). Such an approach, at present being actively explored so far as handicapped children are concerned, might have great potential in surveillance of healthy children.

2. Doctors tend to exaggerate parental shortcomings in observing children, and to ignore their own. Many young children, for example, show up poorly in a test situation in the unfamiliar environment of a clinic, yet this disadvantage to the child is often underrated or ignored and clinic personnel are likely to discount (politely) the mother's insistence that tests failed in the clinic are within the child's competence in his home surroundings.

3. The danger of unsolicited professional interest in children provoking parental anxiety has been a recurring theme of this chapter. Skilful involvement of some parents in assessment procedures (such as the new approach to records mentioned above), and overt acknowledgement by health personnel of the parent's status as an expert on her/his own child, could do much to avoid or minimize such distress.

4. Many handicapping disorders would be identified earlier if parents were confident of an informed and interested response from their doctor. In spite of lip service paid to Sheridan's insistence that a mother's concern about her child should *never* be ignored (Sheridan, 1962, 1969), the experiences of parents with young handicapped children in some areas suggest a continuing dismal situation, even allowing for retrospective inaccuracy and the projection of grief and bitterness on the medical services. Many such parents continue to report great difficulty in evoking a helpful response when they sought advice and support from doctors and others concerning their early anxieties about their children.

5. Whenever remediation, of whatever kind, is necessary, parents are the most important people involved in helping their child. This applies to every family situation, from infant feeding to management of the severely handicapped child at home.

Co-operation with social services

Effective partnership between health authorities and social service departments, essential for tackling many community health and social problems, has not easily been achieved in the past decade, and liaison could be greatly improved in many parts of the country. Staff shortages and myopic professional self-interest on both sides have not helped. Two points deserving special mention are:

1. The need to rationalize the interface between the work of social workers and that of health visitors who, in attachment to general practice, have tended to have their considerable social work skills exploited.

2. The need for close co-operation in identifying and contacting families requiring intensive support, including health surveillance.

Records

Good records do not by themselves constitute good practice, but they do much to encourage it. The converse is also true, and the present chaotic state of child health records has probably contributed to the poor services received by some families.

It is tempting to look to computers for salvation in this respect, but the universal computer age in medical records has yet to dawn and many records will have to continue to be made and stored using conventional methods.

A single health record for each child is, similarly, an attractive but impracticable idea. The design of child health records should nevertheless be standardized on a national scale, to encourage uniformity of practice and also to facilitate transfer of surveillance data and responsibility when families move from one health district to another. The record card for use during the 0 to five years period should be designed with continuity with fetal health and with school health needs in mind, even if a separate school health record is necessary for administrative reasons.

The design of record should be flexible enough to allow for variations in need and in detailed approach. A difficult and importance balance has to be struck between too much printed detail which could encourage a 'tick-the-shopping-list' attitude on the one hand, and a blank page with no headings or reminders of relevant information on the other. This is particularly important while so many problems surrounding the concept of 'developmental screening' remain unresolved. No health visitor or doctor should be required to record any information the medical or developmental significance of which they do not understand. The 'health surveillance' section of the record should include space for the following:

1. relevant family, antenatal, natal and neonatal data ('at risk' factors);
2. adequate social information about the family;
3. recordings of height, weight and head circumference compared with percentile norms;
4. notes of intervention and its outcome;
5. an adequate record of developmental progress.

Immunization

Infectious disease prophylaxis is made available in the United Kingdom through primary health care services, according to a schedule of procedures laid down and monitored by the Joint Committee on Vaccination and Immunization of the Departments of Health. The objectives of immunization against infectious diseases are two-fold:

1. To protect the child from specific infectious diseases by provoking and maintaining a state of active immunity.
2. To influence the overall prevalence of the disease in the community and to break the cycles of epidemics which are characteristic of non-immune populations, by maintaining a constant high level of immunity among children.

At present immunization procedures against tetanus, diphtheria, pertussis and poliomyelitis are recommended for and made available to young children. BCG vaccination against tuberculosis is usually offered to older schoolchildren who have a negative skin (Heaf or Mantoux) reaction, and rubella vaccine is offered to girls at pre-adolescence. Vaccination against smallpox has been discontinued as a routine procedure in infants. Pertussis prophylaxis is under close review following concern about major reactions to the vaccine with permanent sequelae (see also p. 227).

The impact of immunization procedures upon mortality and morbidity has been immense, even allowing for the facts that some causative organisms appear to have declined in virulence, and that the advent of effective chemotherapy made a (relatively small) contribution (Office of Health Economics, 1964). Indeed, the very success of immunization programmes has created problems in maintaining the present generally satisfactory situation, because a whole generation of parents and doctors has never seen the effects of unchecked epidemic disease upon children, and there is understandable concern about the possibility of serious side-effects to the prophylactic agent being more common than the disease itself. The doctor, in his advisory role to parents, may find a conflict between his responsibilities to the individual child and those to the community of children at large. Current concern about pertussis vaccine illustrates this dilemma. Sufficient parents, understandably scared by the apparent risk of neurological sequelae, have refused the vaccine on their children's behalf to result in a situation where levels of immunity have fallen far enough to allow epidemic pertussis to re-occur, greatly increasing the risk of mortality and morbidity from the disease, especially in very young babies.

There are no simple answers to these problems, but the health departments and clinical doctors both have a responsibility to discharge:

1. The health departments should keep clinical doctors informed of the up-to-date epidemiological and immunological situation. Because these are complex fields, relevant research and other data need to be abstracted and interpreted for the clinician, so that the practical implications are made clearer. A regular bulletin devoted to infectious disease control and circulated free to doctors might be a practical approach worth considering.

2. Clinicians have a responsibility to keep themselves informed of the contemporary situation. They should thoroughly understand the 'official' policy, and be prepared to have their own divergent views on any issues where, on the evidence available, there are reasonable grounds for differences of opinion. In advising parents they should be prepared, if necessary or helpful in individual circumstances, to give both their own and the 'official' point of view, explaining how and why they have reached their own standpoint. Examples of possible divergencies from official policy could relate to the problem of pertussis and to reservations about the relatively high incidence of reactions to measles vaccine.

All parents' queries and doubts about any aspects of immunization should be treated with respect, and they have a right to know about possible side-effects before deciding about their child's involvement in the programme.

The schedule for giving triple antigen (diphtheria, tetanus, pertussis) and oral polio vaccine does not fit into a rational schedule of health surveillance, and there are sound reasons for separating surveillance encounters, which must be made pleasurable for the child, from the more or less uncomfortable process of receiving injections. The disadvantages of requiring mothers to make extra visits for immunization procedures, however, have been minimized in those areas where local immunization records have been computerized. The computer can be programmed to send appointments, follow up non-attenders with reminders, and reduce the clerical work involved in keeping records to a minimum: this service can be made available to family doctors in their own surgeries or health centres. Increased administrative efficiency leads to reduced delays for mothers at immunization sessions, so that the inconvenience of extra visits is minimal, non-attendance is reduced and acceptance rates correspondingly increased.

Although clinical responsibility for all immunization procedures must be accepted by a doctor, it is common practice for the sessions to be conducted by a nurse. However, the doctor in training for community child health will do well to give himself plenty of direct experience in all aspects of conducting a session, since it provides a different but often very informative opportunity to observe the interaction between mother and child.

One of the most important components of the immunization procedure is to elicit a medical history of the family and child which is sufficient to reveal any valid contraindications to the procedure, with which all personnel concerned must be familiar and up to date.

An approach to health surveillance

This section outlines an approach to health surveillance which takes into account the comments already made, and would be adaptable to local needs. The basic aims are to reach all children, and to offer most help where help is most needed.

Surveillance has been defined (p. 189) as essentially unsolicited, but the services concerned must be readily accessible to parents with 'acute' problems (e.g. a screaming baby), so that appropriate help can be provided and the situation prevented from escalating. Ready accessibility implies some 'open door' access to clinic personnel (in addition to an appointments system) and health visitors who have time to visit homes sufficiently frequently to become known and approachable while on their 'beat'.

The scheme involves:

The health visitor as the key figure who establishes and maintains contact with the family of every child within her responsibility, the health visiting service collectively being responsible for reaching all children. Health visitors participate in the surveillance programmes (see below), and work closely with child health doctors by whom they are directly supervised in their clinical role.

The child health doctor who has the necessary training, skills, facilities and *time* for medical and developmental examinations of all children referred to him by health visitors, as well as for his routine involvement in the surveillance programmes.

Specialist medical and other supporting (social and educational) services which are not routinely involved but are readily available as necessary.

The scheme as a whole must have the professional capability to deal promptly and appropriately with any query or concern from whatever source about the health or development of any child, arising from the surveillance programme.

It is suggested that there should be:
1. A basic surveillance programme for all children.
2. Additional surveillance to meet the special needs of:
   a. many families from time to time;
   b. developmentally vulnerable ('high risk') children;
   c. 'non-utilizers' of health services.

The basic programme (see Schedule p. 204)
This is suggested as a minimum programme for every child. It should be flexible, and is intended to allow checks on important parameters of growth, health and development and to anticipate the most likely needs for support and advice in the family context.

The first and sixth encounters are integral parts of perinatal and 'school' health respectively, thus building continuity of health care into the programme.

The complexities of child development are such that any practicable scheme has to be a compromise with inherent disadvantages. High standards of clinical practice and regular professional contact, with facilities for prompt further assessment, are the best safeguards against missed opportunities for early preventive intervention.

Additional surveillance
1. All families are liable to stress and need extra support from time to time. There may be ongoing strain, such as a handicapped family member, or an acute 'crisis' caused by such events as death or illness, or parental disharmony or desertion. The ability of a family to cope is influenced by many factors such as family structure and size, the strength of family bonds, socio-economic circumstances, housing, and health (particularly of the mother). The modern health visitor is trained to apportion her time according to her assessment of need, and to encourage use of supportive facilities.

2. A group of children may be identified as being developmentally vulnerable (at 'high risk' of subsequent handicap). Problems of selection criteria, and the need for the final decision to be a flexible one, have been discussed above (p. 195), and practical details need to be worked out locally.

Appropriate supervision of this group is a combined hospital and community paediatric responsibility (Rogers, 1971) and needs to be carefully organized, co-ordinating the hospital and community contributions with special care being taken to avoid wasteful duplication of effort. Health visitors can be directly involved in the additional surveillance and can also assist by encouraging extra attendances for assessment by the child health doctor.

3. A major commitment of time and personnel will be required to extend surveillance to those children least likely to receive it without such extra effort. These are 'non-attenders' at facilities such as child health clinics, and probably include a disproportionate number of children with medical, behavioural, emotional and complex social problems.

The difficulties of bringing preventive services to bear upon what is an ill-defined and heterogenous section of the population include:

a. *identification* of the families concerned: many are, or should be, known to social service departments;

b. *making effective contact*.

The extent of the difficulties in these two respects varies according to the circumstances. Families in need of this kind of support are likely to come within one or more of the following broad groups (although it does not follow that all families so described are necessarily to be regarded as needing special help).

1. *Socially disadvantaged and 'problem' families*. These, unless they are also 'mobile' (see below), are usually known to health and social services, and already absorb much time and resources. Research into the needs of this group suggests that, although they are readily identified and contacted, the practical advice given may be less relevant to the realities of 'grinding poverty', and therefore less effective, than health personnel dealing otherwise with relative affluence may imagine (Wilson & Herbert, 1975).

2. *The 'mobile' population*. In some inner urban areas the families who move frequently with constant chronic accommodation problems comprise a substantial minority of the population. Characteristically they seldom register with general practitioners, often using hospital casualty departments in lieu of primary health care services, and the problems of both identifying and contacting them has been made more difficult by the loss to health visitors of their exclusive home visiting responsibilities within a defined area, consequent upon the policy of attachment to general practice. It is in such areas that there is a particularly strong case for retaining geographical deployment of health visitors.

3. *Children who lack adequate stimulation* for normal social and language development, or who are emotionally deprived, including some with working mothers and many who are 'child minded', children in local authority day nurseries, and those who attend state or private nursery schools for other than 'educational' reasons.

Extension of preventive surveillance to children in nursery facilities run or supervised by local authorities would be relatively simple administratively, although there are problems of communication with the mothers at work. More difficult problems are associated with registered child-minding, the diffuse nature of the service making effective oversight difficult for under-staffed social service departments. Most serious of all are the problems associated with unregistered child-minding. It is difficult both to identify and contact these children and their families, yet their need of health surveillance and intervention is certainly great (Jackson, 1974).

4. *Children in care*. This group are vulnerable because of the circumstances which have taken them out of their family setting, and because there are great practical problems in providing alternative care of adequate quality on a long-term basis for all who need it. The Home Office regulations which required frequent statutory medical examinations (the rationale of which was, on the whole, to prevent abuse, monitor nutrition and ensure 'freedom from infection') have been relaxed. They should be replaced by examinations carried out by

child health doctors with preventive and developmental training, and this should be regarded as a special aspect of community child health surveillance.

5. *Children in long-stay hospitals.* There are good reasons for giving serious consideration to the extension of at least some aspects of community-based health surveillance to these children, whose great need is now documented (Oswin, 1975, 1978). Although most have handicapping conditions, they are often not predominantly in need of medical and nursing care, and both the nursing care attitudes of the staff concerned and the serious staff shortages in such hospitals are liable to be detrimental to the children's emotional and social needs. Furthermore, isolation of these institutions from the community in all respects is a serious problem which co-operative involvement of community-based personnel could help to overcome.

Conclusions

The 1974 reorganization of the health services should have eliminated the divisive tripartite anomalies of the 1948 structure and the Court Report should have provided fresh impetus and long-term objectives for the child health services. The emerging reality, however, is different: there continue to be divisions and there is still no satisfactory training or career structure for those trying to maintain preventive services. None of the important recommendations of the Court Committee have been implemented, other than the setting up of a Joint Committee for Children. Furthermore, schemes devised to make the best of the present situation, such as that described by Trefor Jones (1979), also underline (probably unwittingly) that nothing which falls far short of the 'general practitioner paediatrician' concept in comprehensiveness will give family doctors the central role in prevention which it was hoped they would wish to claim.

Should there be no further progress towards implementing at least some of the Court proposals, this would indeed be a dismal outcome to a decade of opportunities for change which are unlikely to occur again. Ignorance of need can no longer be an excuse and the gap between what we know and what we do should nag the conscience of every health professional concerned with children. It is above all difficult to conceive of a future pattern of child health services relevant to children's needs which is not built on a firm foundation of preventive practice.

Schedule of suggested basic surveillance programme

	Age (approx)	Personnel	Location	Main objectives
1.	At birth	Doctor (paediatrician)	Hospital maternity unit	Recognition of defects. Reassurance of mother. Start of ongoing medical record (including carry-over of relevant obstetric data, etc.).

Comments. Mothers require positive reassurance (i.e. more than mere absence of adverse comment) about the normality of their infants.

Age (approx)	Personnel	Location	Main objectives

Problems in carrying out this examination associated with policies of early discharge from maternity units include the time factor, and the onset later than 48 or 72 hours after birth of certain cardiac and other physical signs.

2. 6 weeks	Doctor	Clinic	Introduction to clinic—premises and facilities. Support for young mothers (glamour of motherhood wearing thin; fatigue; depression; isolation; potential relationship problems in family).
	For 'non-attenders' Health visitor	Home	

Comments. Full medical follow-up by a doctor of the neonatal examination is very desirable. Nevertheless, there is otherwise a relatively low emphasis upon detection of disabilities at this stage. The opportunity is taken to *listen*, encourage and advise.

3. 7 to 8 months	Health visitor	Clinic or home	Review of health and development. Attention to hearing and vision.

Comments. Close supervision and support of the health visitor by a doctor are essential, so that all queries can be investigated in more detail.

Timing is important; 6 months is too early for hearing tests and relatively unrewarding for motor development: from 9 months hearing tests are difficult and many babies are shy of strangers.

4. 18 months	Health visitor	Clinic or home	Hearing and early language development. Mobility. Social development.

Comments. Close supervision and support of the health visitor by a doctor are essential, so that all queries can be investigated in more detail.

5. 3 years	Doctor	Clinic	Opportunity to discuss development: e.g. behaviour (tantrums, jealousy if new baby arrives), toilet training, language development. Vision testing (e.g. Stycar). Cover test for squint.

Age (approx)	Personnel	Location	Main objectives

Comments. Rather early for reliable vision tests (Stycar) on some children. Often not easy (and not necessarily desirable) to carry out 'traditional' clinical examination at this age. May be linked to nursery school education where relevant.

6. $4\frac{1}{2}$ to 5 years	Doctor	Clinic	Pre-school summing up of early development. Link with school health service: early warning to teachers of potential or established difficulties, e.g. speech, behaviour affecting well-being at school. Vision testing: cover test for squint.

Comments. Information made available from this encounter should be the basis of a selective (i.e. non-routine) approach to ongoing health supervision of individual children in school.

REFERENCES

Alberman E D, Goldstein H 1970 The 'at risk' register: a statistical evaluation. British Journal of Preventive and Social Medicine 24: 129–135

Bain D J G 1974 The results of developmental screening in general practice. Health Bulletin 32: 189–193

Bax M, Hart H 1976 The health needs of pre-school children. Archives of Disease in Childhood 51: 848–852

Boothman R, Orr N 1978 Value of screening for deafness in the first year of life. Archives of Disease in Childhood 53: 570–573

Bryant G M, Davies K J, Newcombe R G 1974 The Denver Development Screening Test. Achievement of test items in the first year of life by Denver and Cardiff infants. Developmental Medicine and Child Neurology 16: 475–484

Bryant G M, Davies K J, Richards F M, Voorhees S 1973 A preliminary study of the use of the Denver Developmental Screening Test in a health department. Developmental Medicine and Child Neurology 15: 33–40

Court S D M (chairman) 1976 Fit for the future: Report of the Committee on Child Health Services. HMSO, London

Court S D M, Jackson A 1972 Paediatrics in the seventies. Oxford University Press, London

Davie R, Butler N R, Goldstein H 1972 From birth to seven. Longmans and National Children's Bureau, London

Department of Health and Social Security 1972 Report of the Working Group on Risk Registers. Unpublished

Egan D F, Illingworth R S, Mac Keith R C 1969 Developmental screening 0–5 years. Clinics in Developmental Medicine No. 30. Spastics Society and Heinemann, London

Evans R, Sparrow M 1975 Trends in the assessment of early childhood development. Child Care, Health and Development 1: 127–132

Field F 1974 Unequal Britain. A report on the cycle of inequality. Arrow Books, London
Frankenburg W K, Dodds J B 1967 The Denver Developmental Screening Test. Journal of Pediatrics 71: 181–191
Frankenburg W K, Goldstein A D, Camp B W 1971a The revised Denver Developmental Screening Test: its accuracy as a screening instrument. Journal of Pediatrics 79: 988–995
Frankenburg W K, Camp B W, Van Natta P A, Demersseman J A 1971b Reliability and stability of the Denver Developmental Screening Test. Child Development 42: 1315–1325
Hart F D 1973 The importance of 'non-disease'. Practitioner 211: 193–196
Hart H, Bax M, Jenkins S 1978 The value of the developmental history. Developmental Medicine and Child Neurology 20: 442–452
Hart J T 1971 The inverse care law Lancet i: 405–412
Holt K S 1974 Screening for disease: infancy and childhood. Lancet ii: 1057–1060
Hooper P D, Alexander E L 1971 Developmental assessment in general practice. Practitioner 207: 371–376
Illingworth R S 1962 An introduction to developmental assessment in the first year. Little Club Clinics No. 3. National Spastics' Society, London
Illingworth R S 1975 The development of the infant and young child, normal and abnormal, 6th edn. Churchill Livingstone, Edinburgh
Illingworth R S 1977 Basic Developmental Screening 0–2 years, 2nd edn. Blackwell, Oxford
Ingram T T S 1969 The new approach to early diagnosis of handicaps in childhood. Developmental Medicine and Child Neurology 11: 279–290
Jackson S 1974 The educational implications of unsatisfactory childminding. Childminding Research Unit. Unpublished paper
Lancet 1975 Developmental screening (editorial). Lancet i: 784–785
Ministry of Health 1967 Child Welfare Centres: Report of the Sub-Committee of the Standing Medical Advisory Committee (The Sheldon Report). HMSO, London
Ministry of Health 1971 The organisation of group practice. HMSO, London
Neligan G A, Prudham D 1969a Norms for four standard developmental milestones by sex, social class and place in the family. Developmental Medicine and Child Neurology 11: 413–422
Neligan G A, Prudham D 1969b Potential value of four early developmental milestones in screening children for increased risk of later retardation. Developmental Medicine and Child Neurology 11: 423–431
Newson J, Newson E 1965 Patterns of infant care in an urban community. Penguin, Harmondsworth
Newson J, Newson E 1968 Four years old in an urban community. Allen & Unwin, London
Office of Health Economics 1962 The lives of our children: a study in childhood mortality. Office of Health Economics, London
Office of Health Economics 1964 Infants at risk: an historical and international comparison. Office of Health Economics, London
Oswin M 1975 Handicapped children and the 'hospital scandal reports'. Child Care, Health and Development 1: 71–75
Oswin M 1978 Children living in long-stay hospitals. Spastics International Medical Publications and Heinemann, London
Pollak M 1972 Today's three-year-olds in London. Spastics International Medical Publications and Heinemann, London
Rogers M G H 1968 Risk registers and the early detection of handicaps. Developmental Medicine and Child Neurology 10: 651–661
Rogers M G H 1971 The early recognition of handicapping disorders in childhood. Developmental Medicine and Child Neurology 13: 88–101
Scottish Home and Health Department 1973 Towards an integrated child health service. HMSO, Edinburgh
Sheridan M D 1962 Infants at risk of handicapping conditions. Monthly Bulletin of the Ministry of Health and Public Health Laboratory Service 21: 238–244
Sheridan M D 1969 Definitions relating to developmental paediatrics. Health Trends 1 (no. 2): 4–7
Sheridan M D 1973 Children's developmental progress from birth to five years: the Stycar sequences. National Foundation for Educational Research, Slough
Sheridan M D 1975 The developmental progress of infants and young children. Report on Public Health and Medical Subjects, No. 102 3rd edn. HMSO, London
Starte G D 1971 'Child's play', or paediatric developmental screening in general practice. Practitioner 209:84–89
Starte G D 1974 Developmental assessment of the young child in general practice. Practitioner 213: 823–828

Trefor Jones R H 1979 Integration of hospital and community child health services. Health Trends 11: 10–13

Wedge P, Prosser H 1973 Born to fail? Arrow Books and National Children's Bureau, London

Wilson H, Herbert G W 1975 Parents and children in the inner city. Routledge & Kegan Paul, London

Primary paediatric care

The care of children, both preventive and therapeutic, is an important part of general practice. The continuing involvement with a family, often over many years, that is a feature of practice, and the mutual respect and trust that are usually evident, frequently have their origins in the doctor's involvement with the young child. Paediatric care, however, begins with the first antenatal visit that the mother makes: in addition to ensuring that the pregnancy remains normal and results in a healthy mother and infant, the general practitioner has a responsibility to prepare his patient for her role as a mother and through education to help her to ensure that her child, when born, remains healthy. The preventive aspects of child care in general practice should start, therefore, in the prenatal period and, together with the management of episodic illness, should continue until the child leaves school. The adult's reaction to health and illness is, to a large extent, conditioned by his experiences and training during childhood and the standard of paediatric care that is offered by the family doctor has an importance that extends beyond simply the maintenance of good organic health.

The organization of general practice

The general practitioner has been described as 'a doctor who provides personal, primary and continuing care to individuals and families'. Over the last 20 years general practice has been in a state of increasing change and the family doctor of today differs from his predecessor in almost all aspects of his work—its organization, its workload and even its philosophy. One of the constant features, and one which should be retained, is that contained in the above quotation. One of the more significant changes has been the growing move away from the single-handed practice towards the formation of group practices. In 1951 in England and Wales, 43 per cent of practitioners worked alone and 19 per cent in groups of three or more doctors: in 1974 these figures had changed to 18 per cent and 61 per cent respectively. Paralleling this change has been the development of health centres and the attachment of community nurses and health visitors to form the basis of a practice team.

The health centre
A health centre is simply a purpose-built building designed to serve a predetermined population and staffed by general practitioners and community nursing

staff organized into one or more practice teams. It is now the policy of central government to continue and expand the health centre building programme and it must be anticipated that by the end of 1980 the majority of the urban population of this country will receive their first-line medical and nursing care from such centres. It should not be assumed, however, that a purpose-built centre is a prerequisite for good general practice. There have been steady improvements in the premises, staffing and equipment of many group practices so that they are, to all intents and purposes, providing the same standard of care that is the potential of the health centre. In general practice, as in all other branches of medicine, the final denominators of the quality of service are the interest, experience and motivation of the individual doctor or nurse.

Nursing staff
Since 1964 there has been a steady increase in the number of community nurses and health visitors who have been attached to specific general practices rather than, as hitherto, to patients living in a defined geographical area. A survey of all general practices in England in 1974 (Reedy et al, 1976) showed that 68 per cent had one or more attached home nurses. Such attachments existed in 92 per cent of health centre practices and in 68 per cent of non-health-centre group practices. 51 per cent of single-handed practitioners had an attached nurse as compared with 81 per cent of all practices with four or more principals. Problems of recruitment and staffing, together with the real fact that the work of these nurses is likely to be more efficient if they are responsible for a circumscribed area rather than for the scattered patients of individual practitioners, have hindered this development. The advantages to doctor and nurse, and more importantly to the patient, of a team rather than an individual approach to health care outweigh any disadvantages, and the policy of the attachment of nursing staff to general practice is likely to be steadily implemented. The attachment of health visitors to general practice began earlier than did that of home or district nurses. By 1973, 79 per cent of all health visitors in England were attached and this figure is continuing to rise.

The health visitor is a registered general nurse who has completed a further training course of 12 months. The theoretical aspects of the course include an understanding of the normal growth and development of children, the psychosocial factors that are important to the welfare of a family, the recognition and management of behavioural problems in young children, adolescents and families, and the opportunities for and techniques of health education. The syllabus also includes teaching in sociology and psychiatry, communicable diseases, and the care of the elderly. The health visitor is trained, therefore, principally for the preventive and supportive role. She has a responsibility for the health and welfare of the pre-school child through developmental screening and immunization clinics and by visiting families of young children at home; for children with physical or mental handicap; and during the antenatal period to prepare the mother for the care of her child. Mention has been made of the importance in general practice of both the preventive and therapeutic aspects of child care. The general practitioner who from choice or geography is single-handed and whose contact with his district nurse or health visitor is both infrequent and by telephone, is unfortunately less able to offer a comprehensive child care service. The health visitor has a growing range of responsibilities additional to her primary concern with the pre-school child. Increasingly she is involved in preventive programmes for adults of middle age and in supportive visiting of the elderly. It is unlikely however that her involvement with patients other than the pre-school child amounts to more than perhaps 10 per cent of her total workload.

Training for practice
One further development in general practice requires mention. Since 1968 a period of vocational training has been considered desirable for all doctors before entering general practice as a principal and this will become a statutory requirement after 1981. The existing schemes of vocational training consist of two years in a variety of hospital specialties and one year in general practice as a trainee assistant.

In almost all areas the year spent as a trainee in general practice is an apprenticeship, in which the trainee steadily expands his range of work and responsibility. The amount of formal training that he receives varies from one practice to another and is mainly dependent on the motivation and abilities of the practice doctors. In many areas day release programmes, which attempt to fill gaps that are evident in the schedule of training, are organized throughout the training year in practice. The dangers of a relatively unstructured training course are that the supervision of the young doctor may be inadequate and that more stress may be placed on the service than on the training aspects of his course. In the paediatric component of practice work an unstructured method of training can mean that the young doctor may only see those patients and problems that, by chance, come his way: there may then be areas of paediatric care and illness in the practice, particularly handicapping conditions, of which the trainee doctor has had no practical experience at the end of his training year.

The hospital posts involved represent partly those in which a sufficient number of junior staffing positions are available and partly those specialties thought to be appropriate for general practice. Paediatric medicine is included in the majority of such schemes and the vocational training that is thus given to the general practitioner is likely to be further improved in the future by a more specific and structured period of training in general practice in the paediatric component of practice work.

Child care
The changes in general practice that have been mentioned have perhaps more potential for child care than for other aspects of clinical work. General practice covers such a wide spectrum of medicine that no doctor can fail to have a particular interest or expertise in one area or another. In group practice the added interest and knowledge of the doctor is available to his colleagues both as a form of continuing education and as an informal second opinion. When this interest is reinforced by adequate specialist education during the period of vocational training, the range of preventive and clinical skills that the general practitioner can then offer is potentially much greater than has previously been possible. The Report of the Court Committee (1976) included the recommendations that

general practice and health visiting should include semi-specialists in child care: the 'general practitioner paediatrician' and the 'child health visitor'. The CHV would specialize in and be restricted to work with children, while the GPP, for a proportion of his working week, would be involved in 'specialist' paediatric care for selected children from his own and his partner's lists. These proposals of the Court Committee have met with considerable opposition both from general practice and from health visiting. Practitioners fear that the adoption of these recommendations would so dilute the generalist aspect of practice as to open the door to the polyclinic approach. What has been accepted, however, is the need for an upgrading of the overall standards of paediatric training and of the care given to the child population by general practitioners. The pattern of the future is likely to be that the young doctor, after a comprehensive period of vocational training, will join a group practice where the surgery accommodation and equipment, together with the attachment to the practice of community nurses and health visitors, will allow a high standard of child care to be offered. Not all doctors will be so fortunate: there will always be those who have to work on their own, and for them training in the paediatric aspects of general practice, both vocational and continuing, must be carefully planned and freely available.

Workload in general practice
In Britain the 'average' general practitioner has 2500 patients registered with him, of whom 500 will be children below the age of 15. Variations in this figure will naturally occur and are most marked in the new towns, as in Livingston, West Lothian, where 16.7 per cent of the population are under school age and 40 per cent are under 15 years of age. Between 25 and 30 per cent of the doctor's work is with children: those below school age have approximately six to eight consultations per patient per year, while there is a reduction in the annual consultation rate for schoolchildren to three or four per patient.

Other factors influence the consultation rates for children apart from the age distribution of the practice. In general terms, consultation rates for all patients are higher in practices which have a smaller patient list, in urban as opposed to rural areas, and where the practice population is biased towards social classes IV and V. Consultation rates for children tend to follow the overall pattern for the practice population, reflecting these parameters and the method and pattern of work of the individual doctor.

Home visits
Over the last 10 years there has been a steady reduction in the numbers of home visits, a trend encouraged by general practitioners and influenced by factors such as the availability of public transport, car ownership, and the flexibility or otherwise of appointment systems. The average ratio of consultations to home visits for all patients is 4:1, but the reduction in the number of visits is less marked in respect of children: the difficulties that a young mother may have in bringing a sick child to the surgery is a frequent and often justifiable reason for the doctor to make a home call. The author's workload figures for a new town practice in which 40 per cent of the population were under 15 years are

Table 11.1 Paediatric workload in general practice: percentage of patients and annual number of doctor contacts

Age groups (years)	0	Consultations per year 1–5	6–10	10+
0–4	13.2	65.0	14.7	7.1
5–14	17.9	64.5	11.2	6.4

given in Table 11.1. The seasonal variations in consulting rates for children in the same practice are shown in Figure 11.1, a variation which is present but less marked in the adult population.

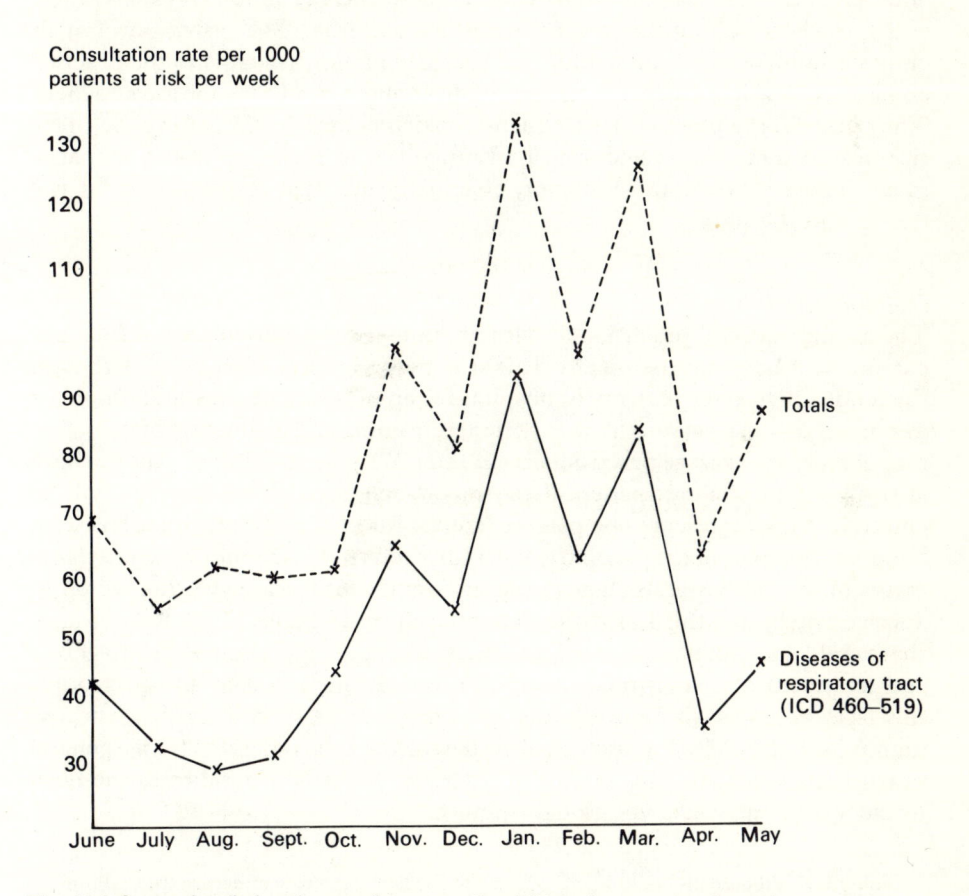

Fig. 11.1 Seasonal variations in consulting rates for children in one general practice

Observer variation
Consultation and visit rates such as have been quoted are derived from the workload studies of many practices. The individual doctor can also influence the apparent workload for certain groups of patients, such as the young and the elderly, and for different disease categories. This 'observer variation' is most noticeable in the differences reported in the incidence of psychiatric illness: the

doctor who is sympathetic to and has an affinity for a specialty will tend to attract a higher number of such patients than will his partners and may thus report a higher real or apparent incidence of illness within his area of interest. This observer error should be kept in mind in relation to other parameters such as morbidity patterns, handicap registers, and referral rates to hospital or other agencies.

Special clinics
In addition to sickness consultations and home visits, many practices offer additional services such as 'well-baby' clinics, chronic illness review clinics, and special consulting sessions set aside for children. The provision of such clinics is influenced by the staffing and accommodation available to the practice and is more feasible when a community nurse and a health visitor are attached. The nurses in the practice are frequently instrumental in stimulating the practice to start these clinics and are closely involved in their day-to-day management. These services are, however, essentially the dual responsibility of the doctor and the nurse.

Hospital referrals
The average general practitioner, with an annual consultation rate of four per patient, will have approximately 10 000 patient contacts each year. Although the tendency to refer patients to hospital for an out-patient consultation or for in-patient care can vary with the experience, training and inclination of the referring doctor, the average practitioner will refer 375 patients (15 per cent of those at risk) to a hospital out-patient department each year, of whom seven will be children. This represents one patient referral for every 357 consultations with children. A survey of the paediatric morbidity referred to the out-patient departments of several hospitals showed that no significant disease was discovered in approximately one third of those patients referred (Table 11.2). Reassurance that a child does not have a significant illness can be as important as the diagnosis and treatment of a confirmed disease. Although important in all age groups, this facet of a specialist consultation is perhaps more so in childhood and the high figure of NAD ('no abnormality detected') referrals reflects the general practitioner's need for this service. This figure perhaps also indicates the need for adequate paediatric vocational training.

Table 11.2 Proportions of conditions referred to paediatric out-patient departments. (From Forsyth & Logan, 1968)

Morbidity	% of paediatric referrals
No significant disease (NAD)	31
Congenital abnormalities	11
Genito-urinary disorders	9
Respiratory disease	8
CNS disorders	8
Alimentary disease	6
Cardiovascular system (including congenital heart disease)	6
Allergic illnesses	5

Morbidity patterns

A diagrammatic representation of health and disease would show five main levels (Fig. 11.2). The position of the dividing line between the pre-symptomatic and symptomatic phases in this diagram alters with different age groups in the population. In paediatric care the pre-symptomatic stage is usually small and the threshold level at which professional advice is sought shows that there is a reduced tendency for illness to be self- or mother-treated than is the case with adult patients.

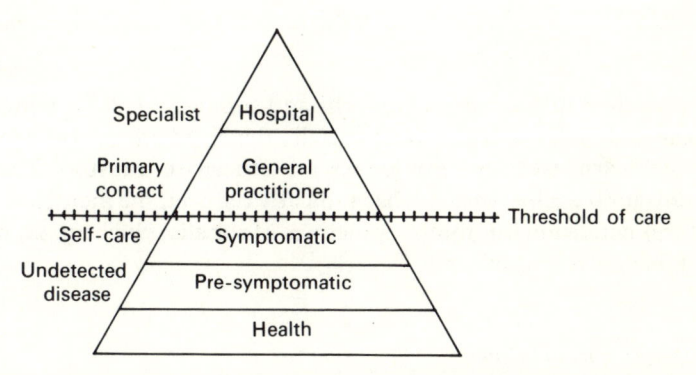

Fig. 11.2 Diagrammatic representation of levels of care available. (From RCGP 1973 Present state and future needs of general practice. Reports from General Practice XIII)

The factors which stimulate a patient to seek medical help are many and varied, and are particularly important in childhood illness. The mother's perception of health and illness, her confidence in her own abilities as a mother, her knowledge of the normal growth and development of a child, her experience of previous illness in the family, and a multitude of familial and social factors all influence her decision. A relatively high consultation rate for the pre-school child is the result and the factors that have been mentioned are at least as important in understanding the morbidity patterns in childhood as is the differing susceptibility of the child to infection. It is also worth noting that many of the factors which influence a mother to seek medical help for her child are potentially amenable to change through both formal and informal health education.

Acute illness

Table 11.3 shows the patterns of childhood morbidity seen by the general practitioner working in a group practice which has 3500 children under the age of 15 years.

Almost half of the episodes of illness (47 per cent) are caused by respiratory and infective and parasitic conditions, and the majority of these are upper respiratory and intestinal infections. Apart from mental disorders, between one third and one half of all consultations in the practice in each of these disease groups relate to children. Illness in childhood is prone to seasonal variations (Fig. 11.1). Respiratory disease, accounting for about one third of all episodes of illness, increases significantly in the winter months and is a major cause of the higher consultation rate in this season. Diarrhoea, usually viral or chemical,

Table 11.3 Patterns of childhood morbidity. (From Barber & Boddy, 1975)

Disease groups	% of total child consultations	% of consultations (all ages) child patients
Respiratory system	32	47
Infective and parasitic disease	15	55
CNS and sense organs	12	44
Symptoms and ill-defined conditions	10	31
Skin diseases	9	36
Accident, poisoning and violence	5	25
Mental disorders	4	11

is more prevalent in the summer months and sonne-dysentery, which is a common cause of diarrhoea in the more socially deprived areas, also becomes more common in warm weather. Epidemics are otherwise unusual. The campaign of immunization against measles has radically reduced the incidence and prevalence of this condition but minor epidemics of rubella, chickenpox, mumps and infective hepatitis still occur.

Handicap and chronic illness

Handicap is difficult to define and the estimations that have been made of the numbers of children in this category vary with the criteria used. One method of assessing handicap is to relate the numbers and types of handicapping conditions to the resources of staff and equipment that are necessary for patient management. Conditions such as enuresis, asthma or behavioural disorder seldom require skills that are outwith those of the general practitioner and the health visitor: approximately 6 per cent of children in the practice will be in this group. More serious or complex disability, such as spina bifida, which requires considerable and varied resources and the skills of many specialties, is present in about 3 per cent of children. Handicap and chronic illness of all kinds involve the practice team in therapeutic, preventive, and supportive care and a handicap register is an important, if not essential, administrative tool in general practice. Table 11.4 shows the handicap and disability statistics in the pre-school population of a practice of 9122 patients.

Table 11.4 Handicap and disability statistics of a general practice. (From Bain, 1974)

Number of pre-school children (0–4 years)	1524
Number on handicap register:	
behavioural disorders	28
asthma	24
CNS disorders	9
musculo-skeletal defects	6
metabolic disorders	5
mental subnormality	4
sensory defects	4
cardiovascular disorders	2
Total	82 = 5.4%

Congenital abnormalities
In the average practice congenital abnormalities are rare and relatively insignificant in terms of total morbidity and workload (Table 11.5). However, the few such patients in the practice have a considerable and continuing involvement with all members of the team and the supportive responsibilities to the patient and the family are an important and time-consuming aspect of their care.

Table 11.5 Numbers of children with congenital abnormalities: 'average' practice of 2500 patients. (From RCGP, 1973)

Congenital disorders	Expected number of patients
Congenital heart disease	1 new one every 5 years
Pyloric stenosis	1 new one every 7 years
Talipes	1 new one every 7 years
Spina bifida	1 new one every 7 years
Mongolism	1 new one every 10 years
Anencephaly	1 new one every 10 years
Cleft palate	1 new one every 20 years
Congenital dislocation of the hip	1 new one every 20 years

Practice organization for child care

The promotion of health
Many general practitioners are moving away from a system of offering care only 'on demand'. The administrative improvements that have taken place in group practices, together with the increasing application of team care, mean that a planned approach is more practical and can bring greater benefits. Preventive medicine and health education play a large part in community paediatric care and should be specifically allowed for: the organization of the child care service is therefore an important part of the practice administration.

Ill health and disability are prevented or minimized principally through a combination of developmental screening and 'well-baby' clinics. The promotion of health, as opposed to the detection of illness, ought to occur at each and every patient contact through informal advice and discussion. Formal health education is mainly the responsibility of the health visitor and is built into her contacts with the pregnant mother at the antenatal clinic and at relaxation, motherhood and parenthood classes. This important facet of the work of the health visitor continues during her periodic visits to the family in the pre-school years of the child's life.

Acute illness
The arrangements that are made for the care of the sick child vary from practice to practice. At the least they involve home visiting when requested and the provision of consulting time within the practice's regular surgery sessions. More sophisticated arrangements include consulting sessions set aside for children, chronic disease and handicap review clinics, time set aside for a more leisurely and in-depth assessment of complicated illness, either physical or psychosocial, an accident and emergency service, and case discussions with other members of the team.

Illness patterns in children are affected by seasonal variations and this factor becomes more important as the proportion of children in the practice population rises above the national average of 20 per cent. Much of this increased workload is due to respiratory illness which is normally less complicated than in the adult and requires less consulting time. A 'sick child' consulting session, held in the early afternoon, can ensure that children are seen at a more convenient time of the day, enables the health visitor to be involved in both the presenting illness and its after-care, and leaves the traditional evening surgery free for adult patients. Even more benefit can be obtained if the health visitor holds her own consulting session in parallel with that of the doctor and can see patients referred to her or who elect to see her as their first contact.

Chronic illness

The assessment of the progress of chronic illness or handicap cannot be adequately completed during a normal, busy consulting session. In general the prospective care of the child needs to be carefully planned, with consideration being given to psychological, social and rehabilitation factors as well as to the organic aspect of the disease. Inevitably this will involve the community nursing sister and health visitor but the social worker, the physiotherapist, the specialist in paediatric medicine, the educationalist and others may need to be involved. The relatively small number of children in a practice who have chronic disease or handicap (25 to 30 per general practitioner) means that these review clinics, at each of which four to six children would be seen, need only be held once every four weeks. The administrative arrangements include an adequate postal appointment system, in addition to ensuring that all the disciplines involved in the care of the patient are represented when this is necessary. Chronic disease review clinics may be organized for each doctor in the practice or the responsibility for the clinic can be given to one doctor who has a particular interest and knowledge of this work. If this latter arrangement is made, it is important that each patient is fully discussed with the patient's own doctor who retains the responsibility for the day-by-day management of the child. His partner, by mutual consent, acts in an advisory capacity. There are several advantages to this system. The doctor involved in the clinic gains a continuing experience in the assessment and management of handicapping conditions and it is easier and more fruitful if disciplines and specialists outwith the immediate practice team relate to one doctor in the practice rather than to several members of a group.

Emergencies

The accident and emergency aspects of paediatric care refer to trauma and physical accident and the emergency out-of-hours service for the practice population. Illness emergency is normally adequately managed through the usual consulting arrangements.

A casualty service is only practical when the practice has attached nursing staff and when, as in a health centre, there is an adequately equipped and staffed treatment room. The majority of the conditions seen will be traumatic—bruising and lacerations, sprains and fractures—but the equipment provided in the treatment room should include drugs necessary for the treatment of medical emergencies such as status asthmaticus or status epilepticus. The treatment room should also contain oxygen equipment, a neonatal airway and mucus aspirator and an emergency obstetric bag. Most of the patients seen in the treatment room can be cared for in part, if not in whole, by an experienced nursing sister: the full potential of this service can only be achieved if the treatment room is continually staffed and the patients can be seen, and when necessary treatment started, in the absence of the doctor. The doctor is responsible for the provision and maintenance of equipment, for the training and supervision of the nursing staff, and with his nursing colleagues for decisions relating to the responsibilities of the nurses involved in the treatment room.

Illness which starts or becomes more severe during the night is always more frightening and distressful than if it had occurred during daylight hours. Illness in children is further compounded by the anxieties it arouses in the parents: the emergency night visit to a child is concerned with relief of these tensions as well as with the emergency therapeutic measures that may be necessary. For these reasons, the emergency care of children is best achieved if it is organized from and among the practice doctors. There is evidence to show that the referral rate to hospital for children is increased if the night emergency cover is provided by doctors unknown to the patient and untrained in general practice. It is impracticable for each doctor to give continuing 24-hour care to his patients: in a group practice all the doctors will be known by name, if not by face, to the patients and the night care of the practice and particularly of the child population is best achieved by a rota system amongst the practice doctors. Following the emergency call the continuing care of the patient is handed back to the child's own family doctor.

Conferences
Practice meetings and case conferences are a common feature of group practice work. Arrangements for these vary with individual wishes but it is preferable for these meetings to take place at regular and predetermined times rather than to be left to chance. There is little need to discuss the normal patterns of episodic illness in children save during times when epidemics prevail, but patients with handicap or chronic disease, or cases of serious psychosocial illness, can be discussed with all involved so that the skills of each member of the team can be optimally utilized. Such case conferences can be arranged following the monthly chronic disease review clinic: again, this must be planned in advance.

Management of minor illness
The doctor's response to a consultation affects the patient's future behaviour and his interpretation of the 'sick role'. When the patient is a young child, the doctor, through his philosophy and approach in the surgery, can influence the future pattern of demand by the patient and by other members of the family.

A breakdown of total practice morbidity shows that, in approximate figures, 64 per cent of all consultations are for minor self-limiting conditions, 15 per cent are for serious illness and 21 per cent for chronic disease. The pattern of child morbidity seen in practice is that between 85 and 90 per cent of all consultations are for minor illness with chronic and serious illnesses constituting the remainder. The importance to the doctor of the large volume of minor illness rests more in his approach to these consultations than in his therapeutic objectives, however important they may be at the time.

Many consultations are prompted by the presence of a symptom such as pain which is causing distress or discomfort to the child and the treatment of the illness with prescribed drugs is mainly concerned with the relief of such symptoms. In some cases, notably in upper respiratory tract infections, antibiotics are used in a prophylactic sense rather than as a specific treatment for an established pathogen. The majority of cases of acute otitis media are likely to resolve spontaneously without treatment, but it could be considered unethical to fail to use all available measures to reduce the child's discomfort. The absence of acute mastoiditis in present-day practice is to some extent related to the habit of prescribing an antibiotic as a routine treatment for otitis media. This example illustrates a philosophy that is a realistic and justifiable approach to antibiotic prescribing for children in general practice: the differing conditions of practice mean that the prescribing rules learned in medical school are not always justified in the management of illness in the community. The large volume of acute respiratory tract illness in childhood means that antibiotics constitute a major part of the general practitioner's pattern of prescribing.

Drug prescribing is, however, a two-edged weapon and its adverse effects can be seen in the too-ready use of the prescription for all chilhood illnesses. In the absence of specific and distressing symptoms, consultations can be prompted by the mother's inability or unwillingness to assume responsibilities for her child's illness or by some fears of illness resulting from past experience. The delegation of this responsibility to the doctor when there does not seem to be a justifiable illness present can result in an increased workload and in feelings of annoyance and irritation. The doctor's use of prescribed drugs in such a situation simply reinforces the mother's belief that her child's consultation has been justified and she will repeat this pattern of behaviour on each and every occasion that her children are ill.

The doctor's response to this aspect of his work is easier to describe than it is to achieve. The practice can make policy decisions relating to the prescribing habits to be followed by all: this is as necessary for such drugs as cough syrups and diarrhoea mixtures as it is for antibiotics and sedatives. Such an approach will tend to prevent patients shopping-around, and patients can be more reassured if all partners in a practice have a consistent pattern of prescribing. Restrictions in drug prescribing for minor illness mean that the therapeutic effect of the consultation must be exploited to the full and adequate time must be available in which to explain the significance and probable outcome of the illness. This is best achieved in the special 'sick child' consulting session, when the patient can be referred to the health visitor if necessary for more specific advice.

Minor illness in children can also be used by an adult as a 'ticket' with which to approach the doctor and high consulting rates among the children of an individual family are often an indication of psychosocial stress. Such frequent attenders are usually only identified if there are good medical records; the family can then be referred to the health visitor for more detailed assessment and continued support and advice. Similar policies can be adopted for home visits to children and in many instances the community nurse or health visitor can usefully be asked to supervise the illness and the way in which the mother copes with her sick child.

To respond to consultations for minor illness in children simply with drug prescriptions only perpetuates a high level of indiscriminate demand, influencing the way in which a future generation will use the health service. In addition to the therapeutic objectives, the approach to minor childhood illness in general practice is aimed at giving the mother an understanding of the 'normal' illnesses of young children and the techniques of nursing care at home, and the ability to seek help from doctors and nurses at the optimum time and for the most appropriate reasons. One of the difficulties of general practice medicine is the recognition of the few cases of potentially serious or life-threatening disease amongst the mass of more trivial illness seen in the day-to-day work. This can only be achieved if the doctor retains a high level of suspicion, if his techniques of history-taking and examination are sound, and if he subjects his work to a continuous process of audit and analysis.

The management of chronic illness

Chronic illness in childhood demands the highest standards of medical care: the child's full potential in life is threatened, the future effects of even small errors of judgement can be profound, and the final outcome of treatment and the way in which the child is managed can have significant effects on the family unit. While the care of the child will usually involve many individuals and disciplines, the general practitioner, by virtue of his continuing responsibility for the child and the family, has a central and important role to play. The majority of cases of chronic disease or handicap are first detected, if not diagnosed, in general practice and the specialist in paediatric medicine is usually the first of the other disciplines to be involved. This in itself can present a potential hazard if a pattern becomes established that the specialist has the total responsibility for the management of the disease or handicap, working in isolation from the general practitioner who is still involved with the patient in the ordinary illnesses of childhood. Care that is optimum can only be achieved if there is a close working partnership between all disciplines involved with the patient and if the skills of each are thus appropriately used.

While most group practices have attached nursing staff, many of the larger health centres have the additional resources of a dietician and a physiotherapist, X-ray and ECG equipment, and consulting rooms for visiting hospital specialists. Most of the facilities and disciplines needed for the care of chronic disease and handicap are thus present in the centre, which can be the locus from which the continuing care is given. Much of the benefit that can result from the health centre-based specialist's review clinic will be lost unless the general practitioner or health visitor is also present at the clinic and unless the specialist is involved in a 'case conference' with the other disciplines involved with the patient. The number of patients in each practice who would require to be reviewed indefinitely is small (approximately 15 patients or 3 per cent of the child population) and a health centre serving 20 000 patients would have a continuing workload of about 120 children. This figure would represent a monthly clinic of 10 patients if each child required one annual review and the clinics can be arranged as far as is possible so that the patients seen at any one are those from one of the practices. This arrangement makes it more feasible for members of each practice team to attend the specialist clinic and to be involved in the review consultation.

In addition to his responsibilities for part of the care of a child with chronic disease, the general practitioner is involved in the management of intercurrent illnesses and with the health visitor in the supportive care that many such families require. These families frequently show anxieties and tensions which are reflected in higher consultation rates for the other siblings, and particularly for the mother. Many of these anxieties centre around questions of schooling, recreational activities, and later employment. Behavioural disorders are more common in children with handicap, particularly during puberty and adolescence. The care of a handicapped child involves the anticipation of crises, be they organic, psychological or social, and many of the difficulties faced by such children can be avoided by action taken through foresight. This involves liaison with schoolteachers, educational psychologists and, if the choice of future employment is limited by the handicap, with the disablement resettlement service. The management of chronic disease and handicap in childhood is concerned with maximizing the patient's potential to enable him to have as full as possible a life, with the care of the whole person in his environment.

Preventive paediatric care

To a limited extent preventive medicine is practised at each consultation or home visit when the opportunity is taken to make the contact educative and advisory, as well as therapeutic. Additionally, an increasing number of practices have organized more formal clinics for preventive medicine: the well-baby, preschool developmental screening, and immunization clinics.

The 'well-baby' clinic is almost a misnomer. This clinic is usually organized and run by a health visitor and gives the mother of a young child the opportunity to consult the health visitor in an informal way with any worries or difficulties which she may have about her child's development. The clinic also allows the health visitor to keep a continuing check on the child's developmental progress although in a less precise way than is possible when a separate developmental screening clinic is held. If a more objective and structured programme of developmental screening is attempted, it is better if the two aspects of screening and 'minor ailments' are kept separate. The 'well-baby' clinic then becomes in effect an open access consulting session at which the health visitor can give advice about problems brought to her and can use the clinic as an important opportunity for health education. There is likely to be some degree of overlap between the 'well-baby' clinic and the 'sick child' consulting session, and a doctor should be available in the surgery or health centre during the time that the clinic is held so that the health visitor can turn to him when necessary for further advice.

Pre-school developmental screening
It is not yet clear whether the results of a pre-school developmental screening programme in general practice justify the time and resources that are involved. Developmental screening is an emotive subject and many practitioners feel that it is a service which they ought to provide despite the lack of objective proof of its value (see also Ch. 10).

It is important to differentiate between screening and assessment, as the two activities require different levels of training, knowledge and skills. It has been shown that screening can be competently done by the interested general practitioner or health visitor, and any such programme must be constructed in such a way that it is appropriate to the doctor or nurse who is motivated but has not had additional specific experience or training. The assessment of the nature and severity of abnormalities of development, on the other hand, is generally outwith the ability of the general practitioner and health visitor. Two levels are therefore necessary for a developmental screening programme: first, the screening clinic organized in and by the practice, from which those children who are detected as having a possible developmental abnormality are referred for a 'Second Tier' assessment; and second, the hospital paediatric unit or the child development centre, where this assessment is made. In the larger health centres the assessment aspects of the programme can be organized by one of the practitioners, if he has had adequate training and experience in this work, or by a child health doctor attached to the centre on a part-time basis for this duty.

Most screening programmes are based on the work of Egan et al (1969), who recommend that there should be seven examinations in the first five years of life—at six weeks, six months, 10 months, 18 months, two years, three years and four and a half years. Each examination comprises a set of developmental tests appropriate to the age of the child and measurements of height or length, weight and skull circumference. The number of physical examinations varies from one scheme to another but must include at least two, at six weeks and at four and a half years.

Developmental screening is thought to be worthwhile because it promotes the optimal development of each child and the early identification of handicapping conditions, thus allowing remedial measures to be introduced at an early stage.

Aims of screening
A developmental screening programme is seen by many solely as a method of detecting neurodevelopmental disability and, as the number of children so affected is small, such a programme may not seem to be justified by the number of abnormalities detected. In one year, Bain (1974) reported that 96 children out of a total of 1204 (7.9 per cent) were considered to show some facet of abnormal development and subsequent assessment of these children revealed only six cases of continuing significant handicap (0.5 per cent of all children examined). Similar figures have been given by other workers in this field. The value therefore of a screening programme which involves the doctor or health visitor in the routine of one clinic each week of two to three hours, which is

associated with a high default rate and which identifies only a small number of handicapped children, does not appear to be compatible with the workload and resources of general practice. To regard identification of neurodevelopmental defect as the sole aim of the programme is, however, to take too narrow a view of its potential. Developmental disability can be described in four levels of severity. The first level includes conditions such as spina bifida and other severe and easily recognized abnormalities which are usually discovered at or immediately after birth. The second level includes less severe and obvious conditions, for example, spasticity, which generally become obvious during the first year of life and which can thus be detected in a practice-based developmental screening clinic. Minor degrees of speech and hearing loss are typical of disabilities at level three. These conditions may only be detected through some formal developmental screening clinic and may not become obvious until the child is two years of age or older. The fourth level—and the least severe and obvious level—includes children who suffer delay in one or more areas of development as a result of emotional deprivation or lack of opportunity. This level of handicap is only identifiable through a developmental screening clinic and developmental delay may occur at any time during the pre-school years. The importance of delay rests in the concept that the longer a child is prevented—for whatever reason—from developing some new skill, the less will be the eventual achievement. The child's potential in that skill is thus permanently lessened. Disabilities at level one are usually detected in hospital and those at level two may be first identified by the child's parents. Disabilities at levels three and four, however, can only be discovered if there is a formal developmental screening clinic in the community. Other benefits are less easy to measure but may be summed up by saying that such a programme demonstrates to patients that the general practitioner has an interest in health as well as disease; affords a valuable opportunity for health education; is on the whole popular with patients; and has been shown to be accompanied by a fall in the sickness consultation rate in those children who have attended.

Almost without exception, all community-based developmental screening systems have important drawbacks. They are rigid in that they rely on children appearing at a particular age for which specific tests have been designed and are applied. Difficulties can thus be experienced in interpreting the results of say the six-month examination if the child attends at an age of four or seven months. Rigidity is also seen in the failure of most screening procedures to allow for the normal variations in age at which different abilities and skills are achieved. The second drawback is that the systems rely heavily on a subjective opinion as to the normality or otherwise of the child's developmental status. The third drawback is that only normal and abnormal development can be competently determined: there is no way in which developmental delay, which can be the precursor of abnormal development, can be detected.

The author's view is that a developmental screening programme should be offered in general practice and should be part of the work of a practice team. While it is certain that, ideally, all children should be included in a comprehensive screening programme, practical difficulties have emerged from almost all the schemes that have been reported from general practice.

Attendance. One of the most fundamental problems has been that of attendance. Bain (1974) has reported a default rate of 28.8 per cent at the six-week examination stage, rising to 37.8 per cent at the three-year examination, and the author's figures show an increase in default rate from 14.6 per cent at the six-week examination stage to 39.9 per cent at the 18-month examination. Clearly default rates of this magnitude seriously reduce the value of the screening programme, particularly since those who default are frequently those to whom the programme has potentially most to offer. Default rates can be minimized if the health visitor visits such patients at home and either persuades the mother to re-attend with her child or completes the screening examination in the home. This remedy depends on the health visitor having the necessary time to visit all defaulters, and on the form of examination being sufficiently flexible for it to be used in the home and at ages which do not correspond strictly to those detailed above. The author's figures show that the health visitor who is attached to a practice of 3500 patients examines approximately five children at each weekly clinic and has an average default rate of 5.4 per cent, whereas comparable figures for the health visitor attached to a practice of 9700 patients are 20 children at each clinic and an average default rate of 15 per cent. The lesson is obvious: the programme is likely to be progressively more impracticable as the practice population increases above a figure of 3000 for each health visitor.

Decision making. Most screening programmes rely on the doctor or health visitor making a global and subjective decision as to whether a child's developmental progress is considered normal or abnormal. Such an approach is realistic since one that is more precise and determined would tend to change the programme from one of screening to one of assessment. Subjective decisions, however, are affected by variations in the standards applied, and screening programmes which rely on this method of decision making are of limited value. More needs to be done on the design of a programme so that it can be more easily integrated into the realities of practice work and the 'second generation' scheme recently developed in Glasgow may go some way towards this end.

This new system is based on percentile-like charts for the four main areas of development—gross motor; vision and fine motor; speech and language; and social adaptation—in addition to specified schedules for physical examination, and percentile height, weight and head-circumference charts (Fig. 11.3). A minimum of four attendances are recommended at six weeks, between seven and ten months, and at two and four years. Three physical examinations—at six weeks, two and four years—are also recommended. This minimum schedule can of course be expanded as necessary, since there are developmental tests appropriate to the following ages: six weeks, three, six, nine, 12, 18 and 24 months, three and four years.

In each of the four main areas of development there is a pair of tests for each three-month stage in the first year of life, each six-month stage in the second year, and annually thereafter. The advantages of this system are impressive. The ages at which developmental testing can be applied are unlimited and the system does not therefore depend on a child attending precisely at the predetermined ages. The decision on the need for assessment is made more objective

226 HEALTH AND SOCIAL SERVICES

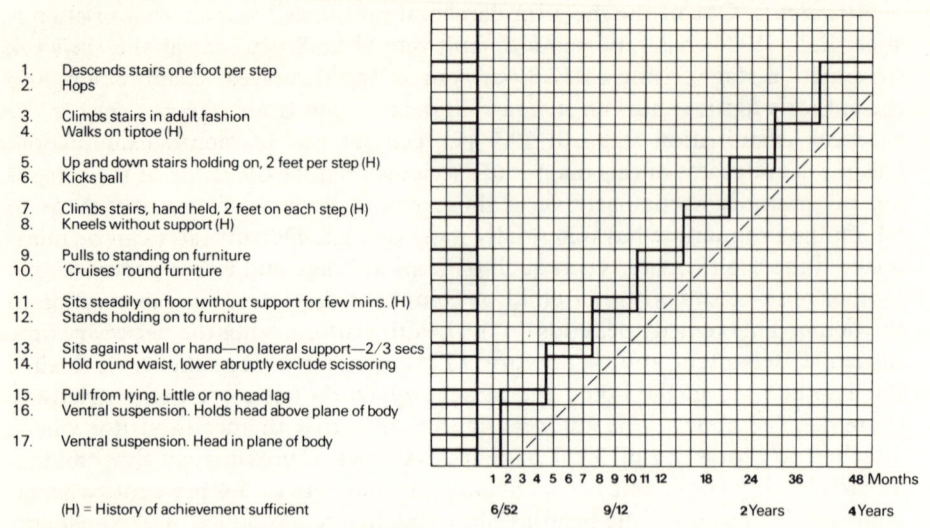

1. Descends stairs one foot per step
2. Hops

3. Climbs stairs in adult fashion
4. Walks on tiptoe (H)

5. Up and down stairs holding on, 2 feet per step (H)
6. Kicks ball

7. Climbs stairs, hand held, 2 feet on each step (H)
8. Kneels without support (H)

9. Pulls to standing on furniture
10. 'Cruises' round furniture

11. Sits steadily on floor without support for few mins. (H)
12. Stands holding on to furniture

13. Sits against wall or hand—no lateral support—2/3 secs
14. Hold round waist, lower abruptly exclude scissoring

15. Pull from lying. Little or no head lag
16. Ventral suspension. Holds head above plane of body

17. Ventral suspension. Head in plane of body

(H) = History of achievement sufficient

Fig. 11.3 Chart for gross motor development

in that a child is considered to have abnormal development if he shows a delay of more than three months in the first year of life, or six months in the second. The display of a child's progress in a visual form means that faltering development can also be spotted. This is an important facility in that deprivation, which potentially at least is remediable, can thus be detected through a falling-off in the child's developmental ability.

The Woodside System has to date (1979) been adopted as the standard Child Health Record in four Scottish Health Board areas representing approximately one third of the population. It is likely therefore that this important facility will progressively be included in the service that the general practitioner can offer to his patients.

Immunization

For many years a composite schedule of immunization has been available for all children. The responsibility is taken either by the general practitioner or by the clinical medical officer of the community child health service (previously of the Local Health Authority). BCG is no longer routinely given to the newborn child but, with rubella vaccination, is offered to senior school entrants by the School Health Service. Immunization against smallpox is no longer recommended except when a child is moving to an area where the disease is endemic.

The standard immunization programme begins when a child is three months of age and a suitable schedule is as follows

    3 months   1st triple antigen (diphtheria, pertussis, tetanus)
                           1st oral poliomyelitis
    5 months   2nd triple antigen
                           2nd oral poliomyelitis

9 months	3rd triple antigen
	3rd oral poliomyelitis
15 months	measles
4½ years	triple antigen and poliomyelitis boosters.

A reliable call-forward system is essential if this service is offered in general practice, and computer systems are available in some parts of the country which relieve the practice secretaries of this duty. It is important that accurate records are kept of the child's immune status. This information is usually also given to the mother of the child with the details of immunizations completed, entered on one of the many record cards available from drug manufacturers. The immunizations are best arranged at intervals of two or four weeks in the form of regular clinics depending on the number of children in the practice. The clinic is usually run by the practice nursing staff but it is preferable if a doctor is also available in the surgery or health centre at the time the clinic is held. It is not usually practical to combine immunization with either a 'well-baby' or a developmental screening clinic: crying children do not form the most appropriate background against which to test a child's development. Similarly, immunization cannot be combined with sick child consultation. Children who are unwell when immunization is due should be recalled to the next clinic.

Recent controversy over the safety or otherwise of pertussis vaccination has led to a greater awareness of factors that would make immunization unwise. A history of cerebral irritation at birth or of convulsive seizures during infancy are absolute contraindications, and children who have a history of meningitis should, in the view of some doctors, not be offered pertussis immunization. Systemic reactions to immunization are relatively rare. Local reactions are more common and need only local treatment and reassurance. Children with a known history of allergy or drug sensitivity are more liable to suffer systemic reaction and advice should be sought from a paediatrician before such children are immunized. A similar rule should hold for children who are debilitated by illness or who have a known chronic disease.

Health education

Few general practitioners have much interest in formal health education and even fewer have had experience or training in the techniques of the subject. The doctor's contribution, as has been mentioned, tends to be opportunist and informal and is usually confined to consultations and home visits. This small but important involvement in health education is, however, subject to several constraints. Some doctors are just not interested in this aspect of work and believe that their duty is to prescribe treatment: most find that the time required is so critical that an advisory and educative consultation is seldom feasible in the context of a busy consulting session. One should not be too critical of the apparent lack of interest shown in health education. The traditions of the profession are towards therapeutic medicine and the training of doctors from their earliest student days has been towards a belief that the doctor's job is to diagnose illness and to use an expanding therapeutic armoury of treatments for his patient.

The health visitor, in her training and inclination, represents the opposite standpoint, and one of the advantages of the team approach in general practice is found in the blending of the different skills of health visitor and doctor. Although programmes of preventive medicine and education are slowly being introduced for adult patients—in 'well-woman' clinics, family planning clinics and schemes of screening for conditions such as hypertension—their potential is probably greatest in childhood. It is the usual practice for the antenatal care of a patient to be shared between the general practitioner and the hospital clinic and a common scheme is for the patient to have an early visit to the hospital booking clinic and to be seen by her own doctor thereafter until the 36th week, after which she attends the hospital on alternate weeks. In recent years it has become standard practice for the general practitioner to have a separate antenatal clinic rather than to include this work during his normal consulting hours. This allows a better standard of antenatal care to be given and enables the health visitor to contribute in an educative and advisory capacity throughout the pregnancy, establishing an understanding and rapport with the patient which leads naturally into her care of the young child.

While the doctor's main interest is in ensuring that the pregnancy is progressing normally, the health visitor is concerned with such factors as diet, exercise, hygiene and clothing, and advising on the layette and bedding required for the baby. In many practices the health visitor organizes more formal classes in relaxation, mothercraft and parenthood, at which such topics as childbirth, the postnatal period, the feeding of infants and young children, and the normal growth and development of the child are discussed. This contact is particularly important for the welfare of the unmarried mother and her child. By visiting the patient at home the health visitor can ensure that the arrangements that have been made for the new baby are suitable, and more importantly can strengthen her relationship with the family. During pregnancy, and particularly in a first pregnancy, the young mother is most receptive to advice and health education and the contacts that the health visitor has with her can be used to include discussions on the 'normal' illnesses of the young child, the recognition of stages of illness and recovery and practical details of the nursing care of the sick child at home. The latter information used to be handed down from mother to daughter and when families were large the older children were accustomed to looking after younger brothers and sisters. In recent years the reduction in the size of families, the loosening of family ties and the mobility of the population mean that an increasing number of mothers lack any real knowledge of the care of the young child. This aspect of the health visitor's work is correspondingly of increasing importance.

The contact with the mother continues throughout the pre-school life of the child. The health visitor is not primarily concerned with traditional nursing duties and moreover, because of her statutory duty to visit and supervise the child's development, she has access to patients who for many reasons may not be well known to the doctor. She is thus able to identify tensions and problems in the family which can be reflected in child abuse, in high consultation rates or in behavioural disturbances, and more importantly she may be able to initiate action before a crisis point is reached. In this respect her continuing supportive involvement with the handicapped child is of particular value.

Much of the benefit of the health visitor's work is lost unless there is close and continuing contact with other disciplines involved with the child, and particularly with the general practitioner. This is not to say that communication can only occur if the health visitor is attached to and working from a specific practice. A contact that is always by telephone and between people who do not know each other as individuals is always less than it can be when the doctor and health visitor work together as a team. The information that the doctor has concerning the pattern of illness in the family, and the health visitor's knowledge about the health and inter-personal relationships within the family, are complementary and the general practitioner who works in isolation from his nursing colleagues is less able to achieve a comprehensive child health service for his practice.

The beneficial contacts that the practice team has with the young child are inevitably reduced when school-age is reached. In many families the mother takes on full or part-time employment at this stage and fall-off in parental control can nullify much of the health visitor's work in the first four years of the child's life. Poor habits of health and hygiene can become established during later childhood which may continue into adulthood and can influence the welfare of the next generation. The care of the older child is therefore an important but somewhat neglected part of the practice responsibility.

The care of the school child is shared between the general practitioner, who is mainly responsible for the management of episodic illness, and the School Health Service which organizes periodic medical examinations for all schoolchildren and has a responsibility for handicapped children and those in special schools. In some instances the practice health visitor is involved in school medical examinations but it is more usual for the School Health Service to be organized by a separate team of doctors and nurses. The disadvantages which can result if the care of the individual child is the responsibility of different disciplines working in isolation from each other are commonly seen in the School Health Service as it is organized at present. Except in rural areas this is difficult to remedy: one of the more valuable aspects of the service is that there is a good working relationship between the medical and nursing staff and the schoolteachers whose knowledge of the child, and in particular the child's behaviour and aptitude, is thus available to those responsible for the medical examinations. There have been moves to transfer the responsibility for some aspects of the School Health Service to the general practitioner and his health visitor but the practical difficulties of arranging that each child is examined in the school by his own doctor seem to be almost insuperable. In many respects it is preferable not to alter the present system but to insist on an adequate exchange of information between the School Health Service and the general practitioner.

Formal health education, including sex education, is becoming an increasingly important and recognized part of the school curriculum. Until recently this subject has tended to be organized on an 'ad hoc' basis confined mainly to senior pupils, and to be the responsibility of a teacher with an interest in the subject but with no special experience or training. Questions such as the extent and content of sex education and the degree to which this subject should be the responsibility of the school as opposed to the parents, have hindered the development of a more formal programme. If it is to make a useful contribution to the school curriculum, health education should constitute a well-prepared programme which is taught at all stages from primary to senior secondary school, by teachers who have received some training in the subject to supplement their interest, and with the help of the many professional audio-visual aids that are available. In recent years there has been some progress towards this end and the work that has been done in Scotland by Forth Valley Health Board to initiate a certificate course in health education for schoolteachers deserves special praise. It seems logical that as this trend continues, the general practitioner and health visitor should become more involved in programmes of health education in schools—in the continuation of what was first started at the antenatal clinic.

Relationship with other disciplines

Throughout this chapter many references have been made to the benefit of the 'team' approach to the care of children in the community.

The change in philosophy which this represents is one of the most significant that has occurred in general practice and is central to many of the other changes that have taken place, such as the attachment of community nursing staff and the development of the health centre. Initially the team was thought of strictly in community terms but this view has been widened and the team can include every discipline which is concerned with the care of the patient in the community, regardless of whether or not the discipline usually works in general practice.

It has been increasingly realized over the last 10 years that the most effective management of an illness is that which is concerned with the whole person as an individual and as a member of a family unit in the community. From this has stemmed the philosophy that ill health is seldom if ever simple and that organic disease is always compounded by social and psychological factors, the relative size and importance of each factor varying from patient to patient and from one disease to another. Similarly, the care of a patient in the community does not simply consist of the treatment of the disease process: it extends from primary prevention through early diagnosis to rehabilitation and the eventual re-establishment of a state of health. A traditional and narrower view of illness was that it constituted simply a disease process and the training of a doctor reflected this view. It was a natural consequence therefore that the general practitioner was expected to give total, personal and continuing domiciliary care to his patients, to be a Jack-of-all-trades, and to respond to every patient contact with a standard formula of history, examination, diagnosis and treatment. When it is accepted that ill health is made up of physical, psychological and social factors, and when the responsibility is extended to include prevention, rehabilitation and the maintenance of a state of health, it is clear that a doctor is only partially able to fill this commitment. The realization that, in the care of the ill patient, the doctor has a restricted role to play and in some cases his contribution, as compared with that of other disciplines, may be of only limited value to the patient, is one that some general practitioners have found difficult to accept. It involves an appreciation of personal limitations as well as skills, a knowledge of the attitudes and abilities of other professions, and a willingness to delegate to others some of the responsibilities previously assumed to belong to the doctor. Some of the other disciplines involved, such as social workers, educational and clinical psychologists, and even health visitors, have a method of working and of assessing priorities which may appear unusual to a doctor who, by virtue of his specialized training, may have had no previous experience of the range of skills others can offer (Barber & Kratz, 1980).

Despite these difficulties and the threat to his position that such delegation can entail, the concept of team care has been welcomed, and indeed further developed, by many general practitioners who see in it a method by which the care that is given to the patient can be improved. The integration in 1974 of the hitherto tripartite health service has given further stimulus to the concept that the community has a single medical service, part of which is sited in the community and part in the hospital, and that the optimum use of the varying skills of individual members can only be achieved through team work. Team work itself can only become established when attitudes, sincerely held by the different disciplines but bred by isolation, are modified and it is the isolation of one profession from another that holds the key. The general practitioner whose contacts with the community nursing service, the social work department and the hospital specialist are by telephone or letter will have a limited knowledge of the skills of others and will thus be more inclined to soldier on alone or may lose contact with his patient through a formal referral to another discipline. If all those working in the community do so from the same group practice or health centre, know and respect each other as individuals, and meet together to consider the care of specific patients, wasteful and duplicated effort can be avoided and the appropriate skills of other professions can be used for the benefit of the patient.

The hospital specialist has much to offer the community team and his involvement in a health centre clinic has a potential which so far has not been fully appreciated. The periodic review of the patient with chronic disease or handicap can become more meaningful, and for the specialist less time-consuming, if it is organized as a case conference in which the specialist, the general practitioner, the health visitor, and others are involved. At such a conference, decisions about the policy to be followed for the ongoing care of the patient can be made by all those concerned and the contribution of the specialist is of the greatest importance.

Much of what has been said applies to all ages of patients but is of particular relevance to children with chronic disease and handicap. The need for a team approach to the care of these patients is self-evident, but the importance of preventive medicine and of health education in the care of all children is such that without this approach the community child health service is a pale shadow of its full potential.

REFERENCES

Bain D J G 1974 The results of developmental screening in general practice. Health Bulletin (Edinburgh) 32: 189–193

Barber J H, Boddy F A 1975 General practice medicine. Churchill Livingstone, Edinburgh

Barber J H, Kratz Charlotte R 1980 Towards team care. Churchill Livingstone, Edinburgh

Court S D M (chairman) 1976 Fit for the future: Report of the Committee on Child Health Services. HMSO London
Egan D, Illingworth R S, Mac Keith R C 1969 Developmental screening 0–5 years. Clinics in Developmental Medicine, No. 30. Spastics International Medical Publications Heinemann, London
Forsyth G, Logan R F 1968 Gateway or dividing line? Oxford University Press, London
Reedy B L E C, Philip P R, Newell D J 1976 Nurses and nursing in primary medical care in England. British Medical Journal ii: 1304–1306.
RCGP 1973 Present state and future needs of general practice. Reports from General Practice, No. 16 3rd edn. Royal College of General Practitioners London

Hospital services for children

Introduction
Paediatrics in the United Kingdom has changed profoundly during the 35 years since the Second World War. The distribution of disease among children in hospital in 1980 is dramatically different from the pattern of 1950. The introduction of new drugs and the refinement of surgical techniques have brought many previously untreatable conditions within the scope of correction and cure. These developments have been matched by remarkable advances in diagnostic precision which have in turn called for huge increases in technical and laboratory resources. Changes of this kind across the whole field of childhood disease have required and continue to require corresponding changes in the buildings, staffing and operation of children's hospitals.

Along with these far-reaching developments in relation to organic disease of childhood, there has been an equally or more important advance in the understanding of the development needs of children. The serious consequences of separating a young child from his mother and family have been identified and evaluated by numerous workers, notably Spence (1947) Robertson (1958) and Bowlby (1960), and the importance of a mother being with her infant or toddler during his admission to hospital is increasingly recognized. The close relationship now clearly established between factors in a child's home and immediate environment and defects of growth and development, as well as some forms of organic disease, has highlighted the need for close collaboration between health and social services in and outside hospital.

Advances in knowledge, techniques and understanding are unfortunately made very much more easily and rapidly than the adaptation of buildings and the generation of the specialized skills and other resources needed to implement them. Progress with implementation is inevitably uneven, so that the pattern of hospital services for children is a slowly changing patchwork. The description which follows must be read with this in mind. It is neither an exact account of the services in any one region, nor a blueprint for what the service might be, but rather a varying compromise between the two, between the realities of the present and reasonable aspirations for the future.

The role of the hospital
There is no doubt that in the past the hospital has been regarded by many as the heart of the health service, with the teaching hospital the ace among the

hearts. It remains true that scientific knowledge of disease and medical research are concentrated in the teaching centres and academically the teaching hospital is inevitably central. But in a health service the assumption of a privileged status for the hospital is inappropriate. It is intelligible only if society measures achievement primarily in terms of expertise in medical science, if the viewpoint is disease-oriented rather than health-oriented, and this is not the viewpoint of contemporary paediatrics. The health services for children must be judged by their success in enabling all children to achieve their innate potential for physical, intellectual, emotional and social development. The child grows up in the context of his family, neighbourhood and school. These are the primary guardians of his health and well-being and are guided and supported in this task by the primary health care team and other community health services. The role of the hospital is one of support for these services and through and with them of the family. Understood in this way the achievement of the hospital in relation to the health of the community it serves can still be measured by its success in curing disease, but a truer measure will include the contribution it is making to the more effective operation of the community services of which it is inevitably an integral part.

Within this general understanding of role, the specific functions of the hospital can be defined as:

1. The diagnosis and treatment of major illness.
2. The evaluation and management or guidance regarding management of continuing or chronic illness or disability.
3. The diagnosis and treatment of mental and behavioural disturbance.
4. The provision of short-term care for children whose homes are found to be unsafe or seriously inadequate for their needs.
5. The provision of long-term care where the needs in terms of nursing and medical supervision are beyond the resources of the community health and social services.

In numerical terms the hospital services for children are concerned chiefly with the first and second of these functions. The third is a smaller but very necessary service with an important educational responsibility to impart its insights and skills to others working with children. The fourth represents a small but peculiarly difficult and demanding responsibility. The fifth is a major service requiring specialized hospital provision.

Organization

Children's hospital services in England and Wales are organized by regions and in Scotland by areas. The basic unit is a children's department which is normally located in a district general hospital. The department is in the charge of one or more consultant paediatricians (Neligan & Webb, 1968) and is competent to handle most of the illnesses and health problems occurring in the population of the district which are beyond the capability of the primary health care team. However, its competence is not complete and a significant proportion of disorders requiring knowledge and technical resources beyond its capacities are cared for at the regional centre, in association with the university teaching department.

The district general hospital
The facilities available to children's departments in district general hospitals vary widely. Some are occupying well designed purpose-built units: others are still using old buildings adapted to their new functions with varying degrees of success. However, the requirements of such departments are now very well understood. The Platt Committee (1959) established sound guidelines, and more recent reports by the Department of Health and Social Security (1971a) and the British Paediatric Association (1974) have given authoritative, well argued, detailed recommendations for their design and operation. The broad requirements are facilities for handling accidents and emergencies, for an out-patient consultant service, for the comprehensive assessment of children suffering from physical and/or mental handicap, and for the diagnosis and treatment of acute medical, surgical and psychiatric conditions with separate provision for children suffering from chronic physical illness or handicap. There is no need here for a detailed account of all these physical facilities, but some features of design recommended by the DHSS and the BPA deserve mention because of the important principles they embody.

Accidents and emergencies are normally cared for initially in the adult accident room (AR). Separate waiting areas for children, with direct access to examination and treatment rooms and easy access to the children's ward, should be available. The ideal of a 24-hour children's AR in the charge of a consultant paediatrician is practicable only in children's hospitals in large centres of population.

Out-patient facilities should be separate from the adult out-patients' department, so that the waiting area can be a playroom. Consulting rooms need to be large enough to accommodate several members of a family, to allow a toddler to continue playing during a consultation, and to allow medical students, student nurses, health visitor, social worker, or visiting doctor to be present without undue intrusion on the personal quality of the consultation.

The assessment centre requires generous provision of space for examinations by the different disciplines which may be involved in comprehensive evaluation (see p. 252). The centre is most conveniently located in close proximity to the out-patient department, with opportunity for sharing facilities.

The size of the in-patient section will vary with the particular needs of the district. The DHSS suggests as a rough guide 0.5 beds per 1000 total population as adequate provision for acute medical, surgical and psychiatric conditions, for assessment of children with mental and/or physical handicaps, and for the long-stay care of all handicapped children requiring it. This figure excludes regional specialties, but includes 0.13 beds per 1000 for the mentally handicapped, estimated on the assumption that local authority domiciliary, residential and other services are reasonably developed.

These figures are bound to be subject to revision from time to time. Nursing staff shortages and deficit budgets will encourage hard-pressed administrators to examine bed-occupancy figures in their search for legitimate economies.

Children's wards are always vulnerable to this sort of scrutiny. Because so much of childhood disease is acute, requiring immediate hospital admission, fluctuations in occupancy rates are inevitable, and peak bed requirements as occur during the winter epidemics of lower respiratory tract infections need to be taken into account in the formulation of these norms.

Ward units should be no larger than 24 beds in the interests of nursing efficiency. Six of the beds should be in single rooms: these should be large enough and suitably equipped for a variety of uses, including a child requiring isolation and high dependency care; two small infants; one adolescent; a child accompanied by a parent; or a resident parent. Two additional rooms for parents should be provided with each unit of 24 beds and these should be large enough to accommodate a sibling. While such provision should ensure that the need of vulnerable infants and toddlers for their mother's presence is met, the mothers themselves have additional needs. Meadow (1969) studied a group of mothers in hospital with their children and found that boredom was their dominant experience. A sitting-room, television and access to simple cooking facilities are the least that should be available for parents throughout the day. Space and play facilities for toddlers and older children and provision for a teacher to conduct classes for all school-age children well enough to participate are also essential.

Although most of the infectious diseases of childhood can be nursed with suitable precautions in single rooms on general children's wards, occasional cases requiring more stringent isolation are best cared for in the separate infectious disease unit of the hospital. This in the interests of economy may be designed for both children and adults. Although a consultant in communicable disease may be in charge of the unit, children who are admitted should remain the responsibility of the paediatrician.

One other facility forming part of the children's department in district general hospitals providing a maternity service is the special care baby unit (SCBU) for those newborn infants needing more specialized medical and nursing care than is available on routine lying-in wards. An Expert Group on Special Care for Babies (DHSS, 1971b) has recommended that in such units there should be six cots per 1000 deliveries in a ward specially conditioned with a stable environmental temperature, with an appropriate range of incubators, ventilators and monitoring equipment, with appropriate laboratory back-up, and with its own specially trained nursing staff and suitable medical cover. Apart from these technical requirements, a development of general interest has been the recognition of the importance of early bonding in the formation of normal mother–baby relationships (Brimblecombe et al, 1978). Promoting this is, of course, primarily a matter of policy: a mother may be encouraged to enjoy her baby or refused access to him irrespective of the design of the unit. However, a BPA Working Party (1974) recommends that in a 20-cot unit there should be four bed-sitting rooms for mothers of babies receiving high dependency care to enable them to stay nearby and thus have maximum opportunity for personal contact.

The exacting requirements for SCBUs recommended by the Expert Group (DHSS, 1971b) can clearly be met only in larger units serving populations of

200 000 or more. In many smaller maternity units, the standards are not being and cannot be achieved. And yet even these standards fail to meet the needs of babies requiring surgery, or artificial respiratory support for periods of longer than a few hours, or intravenous nutrition. Such highly specialized services, which constitute 'intensive care', have been shown to reduce mortality among immature and ill neonates and also to reduce the sequelae of neonatal illness. The benefits of intensive care, which is now available in most regional centres, should be accessible to all through transfer of selected at-risk mothers before delivery, or by means of a suitably equipped and staffed flying-squad service to transport babies born in peripheral units to the regional centre with optimal supervision and technical support during the journey.

In addition to these important principles of design are a number of complementary functional principles also stressed by the Platt Committee (1959). These are that children who require to be in hospital should always be in children's wards, that the nurses in charge of such wards should be children's trained, that mothers, particularly of children between the ages of six months and four to five years, should be able and be encouraged to stay overnight in hospital with their children and that visiting on children's wards should be unrestricted. Although all these principles enjoy increasingly general acceptance, their implementation remains very far from general. The Court Committee (1976), after stating baldly that 'there are still many aspects of hospital care where the special needs of children are not recognized', cites some examples—that in many accident rooms, special arrangements are not available for the children seen there, even though children comprise one quarter to one third of all AR patients; that of 654 hospitals in England and Wales surveyed in 1973, only two out of three could provide overnight accommodation for a parent of at least one child and only about half had unrestricted visiting; and that of nursing sisters in charge of wards of departments where children are nursed, only 57 per cent were Registered Sick Children's Nurses (RSCN).

The regional children's department
The regional children's department is organized in association with the university department of child health. It provides a hospital service analogous to that of a district department for the local population, but in addition provides certain specialized services for the region. The extent to which a given specialty service is fully regional varies with the uniqueness of its resources. These are partly a matter of technical knowledge and skills, partly of equipment. In practice, cardiology and cardiac surgery, neurology and neurosurgery, paediatric surgery (especially for the newborn) and plastic surgery provide comprehensive regional services. Child psychiatry is also organized as a regional service but few units are as yet in a position to meet regional needs in full. Other branches of medicine now developing as special paediatric interests include nephrology, gastroenterology, haematology, immunology, endocrinology and oncology, and these also may offer a regional or sub-regional service.

There is no doubt that the grouping of all these services in a single children's hospital or in a concentration of children's beds in one general hospital has great advantages (BPA and BAPS Memorandum, 1971). Such concentration facilitates consultation between specialists, the efficient distribution and use of trained children's nurses and balance in the training experience of doctors and nurses. By allowing a flexible use of beds between different specialties, a smaller total number of beds can suffice than when specialist services are located in different hospitals. The laboratories, radiology and other supporting services required for a single children's department or hospital of this size need to be on a scale which justifies and makes possible specialization in the paediatric aspects of these disciplines, and the development of techniques and facilities specially adapted to the needs of children. A large children's unit also favours the development of an integrated academic department and thereby contributes indirectly to the quality of undergraduate and postgraduate teaching and of research. Regional centres therefore aim to achieve the maximum feasible concentration of children's beds in one location. However, the technical requirements of some specialized services may have to be given precedence over these more general considerations. This applies to neurosurgery and cardiac surgery where all patients, children and adults, need to be close to the concentration of equipment and skills and therefore in one hospital. Where sheer numbers preclude the location of all specialties in a single hospital, some dispersion of children's beds may have to be accepted.

The service

The essential features of the service provided by hospitals are most simply described through hospital statistics. A general picture of the operation can be presented by the use of broad diagnostic categories, with an indication of the specialist services involved and a grouping of patients according to whether they are drawn from the local or regional population. The experience in 1974 of the hospitals of the Newcastle Area Health Authority (Teaching) as a regional centre and of Durham as a district hospital in the same region has been analysed. Information about in-patients is relatively complete and accessible and is presented in Table 12.1.

The data relate to children aged 16 years or less, discharged during 1974 from the Newcastle and Durham hospitals. The figures do not include children in psychiatric units or hospitals for long-term handicap, but are otherwise complete. Cases have been grouped into 20 broad diagnostic categories; two of these, congenital malformations and trauma, have been broken down further into the subgroups which are normally admitted under different services.

The absolute numbers for each diagnostic category give some indication of the distribution of disease requiring admission to hospital. It is worth noting that in the regional centre, eye and ear conditions, congenital malformations, and trauma together comprise 45.5 per cent of all admissions, correction of squint being the main eye condition, various infections of the middle ear the main ear condition, and fractures, burns and accidental poisoning making up more than half of the trauma group. Of all these, only accidental poisonings come normally under the direct care of a paediatrician. The congenital malformations are all cared for by regional specialties: spina bifida by neurosurgery, orthopaedics, urology and paediatrics jointly; heart lesions by cardiology and

Table 12.1 Total discharges aged 16 years or less for 1974 from Newcastle AHA(T) Hospitals and Durham Hospitals, showing percentages from outside 'local' areas and arranged by diagnostic groups

Diagnostic groups	International Classification of Disease Codes	Newcastle AHA(T) Hospital Total	Per cent from 'other areas'	Durham Hospital Group Total	Per cent from 'other areas'
Infective and parasitic	000–139	263	23	74	12
Neoplasms, benign and malignant	140–239	319	64	21	14
Endocrine	240–258	114	37	26	12
Nutritional deficiencies and metabolic	260–279	144	38	20	35
Blood	280–289	164	34	32	6
Mental	290–315	116	34	23	4
Nervous system	320–358	276	46	20	—
Sense organs, eye and ear	360–389	1923	43	131	10
Circulatory system	390–459	66	59	10	—
Respiratory system	460–579	1869	34	141	8
Digestive system	520–577	1212	26	163	7
Genito-urinary	580–629	469	44	130	7
Pregnancy and puerperium	630–678	103	14	36	6
Skin and subcutaneous tissue	680–709	401	42	105	28
Musculo-skeletal	710–722	253	26	49	12
Congenital malformations	740–759	2015	57	63	6
a. spina bifida	741	157	65		
b. heart	746	236	72		
c. cleft lip and palate	749	109	72		
d. digestive tract and genital organs	750–752	575	53.5		
Perinatal	760–779	47	57	41	7
Symptoms	780–796	1095	24	284	10
Trauma	800–998	2187	25	516	16
a. fractures	800–829	532	30		
b. burns	940–949	194	24		
c. poisoning	960–989	280	16		
Other conditions		379	80	29	14
Total		13 415	38	1914	12

cardiac surgery; cleft lips and palates by plastic surgery; and malformations of the digestive and urinary tracts by paediatric surgery.

An analysis of the 13 415 discharges from Newcastle hospitals by the clinical services responsible for their care is given in Table 12.2. This table again emphasizes the large proportion of children in hospital who are cared for primarily

Table 12.2 Distribution of Newcastle AHA(T) children's discharges (1974) by clinical services

Service	No. of children	Per cent
Paediatrics	6320	47
General surgery	533	4
Ear, nose and throat	2489	18
Ophthalmology	1196	9
Orthopaedics	915	7
Plastic surgery	949	7
Other	1013	8
Total	13 415	100

by services other than medical paediatrics. The proportion is in fact higher than the table suggests because children with cardiac and neurological problems are included in the paediatric service although they are in fact cared for by cardiologists and neurologists jointly with paediatricians. In the same way some surgical, orthopaedic, haematological, or psychiatric cases are a joint responsibility with paediatricians and might therefore be assigned to these services.

This apparent confusion may be something of a nightmare to the statistician, but in fact implies an arrangement of clinical responsibilities which can be very much in the interests of patients. Under this arrangement children are admitted to a ward where the paediatric house officer and registrar are in immediate charge. If, as an example, the problem proves to be surgical, the surgical service is called and from then on the child can enjoy the benefit of joint paediatric and surgical care with consultants of both services available if needed. The arrangement facilities the sharing of skill and insights between specialties and the possible hazard that responsibility for immediate care and final decisions may be assumed by neither service is avoided if there is complete understanding between all concerned—doctors, nurses and the child's family—regarding which house officer and registrar are immediately responsible and which consultant is in ultimate charge. The statistician's requirements can be catered for by an agreed convention in the records department and consistency in its application.

It may be considered instructive to relate these in-patient statistics to the populations served. The district population served by Durham is 166 000. For all but two categories of disease where the service arrangements are atypical, 86 per cent or more of cases are drawn from this district population. For the regional centre the position is very different. It is providing both a general service for the commoner conditions occurring in the local population, and specialized services for the region. The general service is utilized by a wider population than that of the AHA(T), and some allowance has been made for this in Table 12.1 by adding several of the adjacent localities to the AHA(T) population. Even with this adjustment, the service provided by Newcastle is significantly more regional for all categories of disease than that provided by Durham, and for certain specialties like plastic surgery (72 per cent) and cardiology (72 per cent) a substantial majority of the cases treated is drawn from 'other areas'. The total population of the northern region in the 1971 census was 3 142 036, of which 28 per cent were aged 16 years or less. A regional study of strictly paediatric patient flow in 1973 suggested that the population served by Newcastle hospitals was 862 000; a recent broad analysis indicated that 24 per cent of all paediatric admissions in the region were to the Newcastle group of hospitals, which gives an equivalent population of about 746 000 (McNay, 1975). Clearly these populations are being served to a very variable extent by different specialties. This variation effectively limits the usefulness of hospital experience in any determination of disease incidence.

Child psychiatry
Child psychiatric services in Britain are still developing, with substantial needs as yet unmet. Only a minority of district children's departments have a consult-

ant child psychiatrist; in these departments patients requiring admission to hospital are admitted to the paediatric wards. Only in regional centres is there likely to be a fully established in-patient child psychiatric service. This service calls for a concentration of highly developed skills in a relatively large staff of psychiatrists, psychologists, psychiatric social workers, psychiatric nurses and teachers to provide care for a relatively small number of particularly difficult and demanding children. The Nuffield Child Psychiatry Unit in Newcastle, with 25 day-patient and in-patient beds, admitted 26 new day-patients and 42 new in-patients during the year 1974. These children were drawn from the region as a whole and represented a selection of the most severely disturbed. A significant number of less seriously disturbed children were cared for jointly with paediatricians in general children's wards. By contrast, in its out-patient service, the Unit treated 693 new patients in 1974, with a total of new and old out-patient attendances of 5706.

Out-patients

The huge volume of disease defined by the in-patient data is the main focus of concern of out-patient and accident room services. Reliable data for out-patients are not readily available, and generalizations must suffice to convey the picture. For most surgical services, the content of out-patient clinics must correspond very closely to their in-patient material. However, in general paediatric out-patients and to a lesser extent in specialist medical services like cardiology and neurology the spectrum of clinical problems is significantly different from the cases in the wards. There is a very much higher proportion of children with symptoms requiring the exclusion of organic disease, or an evaluation of the psychogenic, family or social factors which may be contributing to the problem. In a consecutive series of 549 new out-patients seen over a 22-month period by one consultant paediatrician in Durham, 151 cases came clearly into this category, and many of the remainder undoubtedly had significant psychosocial components (Stansfeld, 1975). Steiner (1975) made a meticulous analysis of 211 consecutive out-patients seen in a general paediatric clinic over a two-year period for additional social, family, emotional or educational problems requiring specific attention in management. He identified more than one problem of this sort in 55 (26 per cent) of the patients.

Developmental assessment centres

Developmental assessment centres function largely on a day-attendance basis, children requiring in-patient investigation being admitted to one of the general children's wards. The service provided by a regional centre can be illustrated by the experience of the Newcastle Child Development Centre in 1974. One hundred and ninety-two new cases were seen during the year, 51 per cent from Newcastle and Northumberland reflecting the local service, and 49 per cent from other areas in the region. They ranged in age from less than one year (7 per cent) to over 10 years (12 per cent); diagnostic categories of handicap are shown in Table 12.3. Fifty per cent of cases were referred to the centre by paediatricians, 14 per cent by local authority doctors and 22 per cent by general practitioners. As in psychiatry, the service offered is expensive because assessments may involve all skills represented on the staff and extend over many months:

nevertheless it is an extremely valuable service, helping to ensure in the only way possible that children with learning problems or physical disabilities are correctly placed in the normal or special school in which they can most certainly realize their true developmental potential.

Table 12.3 Diagnostic categories of handicap seen at Newcastle Child Development Centre (1974)

Diagnosis	Percentage ($n=192$)
Physical	17
Visual	6
Hearing	6
Neurological	29
Language	56
Intellectual	54
Total	100 (many multiple)

Communication

Earlier in this chapter the role of the hospital services as one of support for the primary care team was stressed. This role is clearly played in part through the treatment actually given to children and the advice given to their parents, but it is also dependent in part on the communication that takes place between those working in the hospital and those in contact with the child and his family outside. The normal form of communication is a letter. In an emergency, or for an early out-patient appointment, the family doctor may telephone, but usually a letter explains the problem to the consultant who gives his opinion and advice in a written reply. When a child is discharged home from the ward, it is usual for the parents to be given a short letter for their family doctor which includes information of immediate practical importance. This is later followed by a fuller letter, possibly accompanied by a case summary. This traditional pattern of communication between family doctor, consultant and hospital ward staff is well established and in general well maintained. It proved satisfactory when the family doctor had sole charge of the child at home but this is no longer the case. Today, the health visitor attached to the practice, a second health visitor in the child health centre which an infant or pre-school child may be attending, a school doctor in the case of older children, and occasionally a social worker from the Social Services Department or representatives of other agencies may all be in contact with the family. In these circumstances a traditional letter to the family doctor with a copy to the Specialist in Community Medicine (Child Health) may be very inadequate communication. Steiner (1975) in his study of Newcastle experience in this regard found that even where educational, family or social problems had been recognized in addition to the primary medical problem, direct communication about these between the hospital and community services concerned was often lacking. Although Steiner's survey was undertaken as recently as 1972–4, it was at that time something of a pioneering venture by a paediatrician in the relatively unexplored interface between hospital and community services.

Since then, this interface has been more thoroughly studied, nationally by the Child Health Services Committees, and locally by specialists in community medicine, paediatricians with a community interest, and child health care planning teams. The Court Committee's various recommendations for integrating services for children and making them more child-centred would certainly have simplified lines of communication, and might have been expected to lead to better communication between those with common or overlapping responsibilities. However, the Committee's specific proposals have not been accepted. There is therefore as yet no central directive for a rationalization of services and improvements in communication must continue to depend on local initiatives.

While the Court Committee's specific proposals may have been rejected, their general appraisal of child health and child health services has gained wide acceptance. The Report has stimulated wide discussion which has undoubtedly created a greater interest in exploring ways of achieving more effective collaboration between hospital paediatric departments, clinical medical officers and general practitioners. One development has been the creation of appointments which span traditional boundaries of responsibility. Such bridging posts may be held by a consultant paediatrician who takes on defined responsibilities in the community services, or by a specialist in community medicine or clinical medical officer who carries responsibilities within a department of paediatrics or a hospital. In addition, training posts which offer both hospital and community paediatric experience are being developed. These may be at senior house officer level in the form of a one-year rotation with six months in hospital and six months in community services, as recommended by the Council for Postgraduate Medical Education (1979), or at registrar or senior registrar level when appointments include sessions in both hospital and community.

Such joint appointments and the discussions that have led to them are resulting in better mutual understanding and in turn in the freer use of telephone and letter. Communication between disciplines is also being improved by liaison appointments, as for example by a health visitor who attends ward rounds or out-patient clinics in hospital and then undertakes to communicate about selected children with colleagues in the referring practices. The 1973 reorganization of the social services changed the status of the hospital social worker (HSW) from a hospital to an area social services department employee. There can now be no doubt that this accountability to the area department has helped the HSW to identify with area social workers: at the same time, wherever the HSW remains based primarily in the hospital, there is no indication that identification with the hospital team has been in any way compromised. Communication between health and social services departments has unquestionably improved and reorganization may well have contributed to this.

However, other factors are also contributing to this freer communication. The steps that have been taken by all AHAs to deal more effectively with non-accidental injury and child abuse include the formation of policy and case review committees on which the different professions concerned with children are represented. In committees such as these and in the context of case conferences, paediatricians, family doctors, psychiatrists, health visitors, social workers and the police are learning to understand each other's problems and responsibilities and to work together. From this understanding new patterns of communication are already beginning to flow. The deficiencies in communication which Steiner was able to identify may now be the exception, and direct communication by telephone, by personal contact or by letter between hospital and community services may become increasingly the norm. Certainly it is in this way above all others that the hospital services will fulfil their role in contributing to the more effective operation of community services, and justify their claim to be integral to them.

While this need for improved communication between hospital and all those concerned in the care of an individual child or family cannot be questioned, there is an equally clear need for discrimination in this regard. The confidential nature of much of the information in hospital case records must limit the extent to which these can be made freely available. Many consultants in the past have interpreted their responsibility in this regard as limiting their communication about patients to a personal letter to the family doctor. However, the care of patients is increasingly a joint responsibility of multidisciplinary teams and conventions regarding confidentiality are bound to change. It is proving impossible to define rigid guidelines. With the need for legal safeguards on the one hand and for trust and goodwill on the other, this whole question of confidentiality is bound to remain a subject for continuing debate. A sensitive regard for the interests of the child and family and a thoughtfully responsible handling of the information imparted in trust is all that is possible.

The future

The hope entertained when the National Health Service was inaugurated that improved health care would lead to diminished requirements for hospital services has not so far been borne out in practice. Although many of the diseases of children caused by infection have been almost or completely eradicated, other diseases have come within the scope of effective therapy. Often the therapy, as in relation to congenital malformations and leukaemia, has imposed very heavy demands on hospitals. Changes of this sort in the shape of the hospital service will certainly continue, so that predictions of future need are difficult. The fall in the birth-rate and the general improvement in child care must lead to a reduction in the absolute numbers of certain disorders so that a measure of contraction of some services may be possible in the future. But there is a continuing irreducible quantum of childhood disease which will remain the primary responsibility of the elaborate complex of disciplines making up the present hospital services for children. The need to sustain and improve on the present high level of this service is obvious.

At the same time there is an obvious need to draw on this hospital-based expertise more effectively in relation to primary health care. In so far as the level of primary care can be improved, so the objective to which all must be committed, of caring for children as far as possible at home and in their community, will be realized. The educational and training role of hospital departments needs to be developed further. This is true of all branches of paediatrics but especially true of the more recently developed disciplines of child psychiatry and the developmental assessment of severe or complex handicap. The small numbers of children these disciplines handle restrict their opportunities for education through shared responsibility, though such opportunities as arise are generally well exploited. This imposes on them a responsibility for formal training courses open to all the concerned professions and this should and does form a very substantial part of their work. The even newer discipline of community paediatrics carries a still heavier responsibility in this regard. The exact form of this discipline is only now beginning to emerge, but its scope for creative liaison with general practice on the one hand and community health services on the other and thus for further improving the health and care of children must be unrivalled.

REFERENCES

Bowlby J 1960 Separation anxiety; a critical review of the literature. Journal of Child Psychology and Psychiatry 1: 251–269

Brimblecombe F S W, Richards M P M, Roberton N R C 1978 Separation and special care baby units. Clinics in Developmental Medicine No 68. Spastics International Medical Publications and Heinemann, London

British Paediatric Association and the British Association of Paediatric Surgeons 1971 Memorandum on the desirable size of major children's centres serving larger regions or conurbations

British Paediatric Association Working Party Report 1974 Planning of hospital children's departments. British Paediatric Association, London

Council for Postgraduate Medical Education 1979 Report on Training of Clinical Medical Officers. CPGME, London

Court S D M (chairman) 1976 Fit for the future: Report of the Committee on Child Health Services. HMSO, London

Department of Health and Social Security 1971a Hospital facilities for children. HM (71)22. HMSO, London

Department of Health and Social Security 1971b Report of the Expert Group on Special Care for Babies. Reports on Public Health and Medical Subjects No. 127. HMSO, London

McNay R A 1975 Personal communication

Meadow S R 1969 The captive mother. Archives of Disease in Childhood 44: 362–367

Neligan G A, Webb B 1968 The work of consultant paediatricians employed by regional hospital boards. British Paediatric Association, London

'The Platt Committee' 1959 Report of the Committee on the Welfare of Children in Hospital. HMSO, London

Robertson J 1958 Young children in hospital. Tavistock Publications, London

Spence J C 1947 The care of children in hospitals. British Medical Journal, i: 125–130

Stansfeld J M 1975 Personal communication

Steiner H 1975 Paediatrics in hospital and community in Newcastle upon Tyne. In: Bridging in health. Published for the Nuffield Provincial Hospitals Trust. Oxford University Press, London

13

Werner H. Schutt

Handicapped children

Individuals in society are considered 'normal' when they are able to participate in a wide range of human endeavour on equal terms with others, without requiring special consideration or undue help. Most people acquire competence in the basic skills needed for daily living and, with increasing maturation, become independent and able to contribute to the common good, whether in the setting of the family or of the wider community. A few are prevented from acquiring this natural versatility because of a defect resulting in a disability. Human diversity and the complex structure of modern society often create alternatives which allow the affected person to compensate and so ensure his independence and his ability to contribute. The disability leads to handicap when it retards, distorts or adversely affects normal development and adjustment to life (Younghusband et al, 1970). Compensation is therefore an all-important phenomenon which requires sufficient flexibility on the part of individual and community to alter attitudes and life-styles so that harmonious co-existence is possible. For this to be a reality, awareness of the problems, sensitive community organization and appropriate training are essential prerequisites.

Handicap has far-reaching consequences for the lives of affected individuals and those around them, and can result in economic hardship and social isolation. These effects may be cumulative and make an already difficult situation intolerable. A disability causing handicap is invariably restrictive, curtails experience and seriously interferes with the process of adaptation. Nowhere is this more obvious than in children, who are inhibited from getting to know the world they live in with all its pleasures and pitfalls. Intellectual and emotional stunting is a common consequence which further reduces the child's ability to participate fully in the life of his community.

Incidence
The incidence of handicapping conditions varies from one community to another according to genetic background, geographic location and cultural sophistication, as well as the medical services available. Repeated estimates of incidence make it possible to recognize changes in frequency from one year to the next and from one age group to another, and allow analysis of the reasons for such changes. Studies of this kind can lead ultimately to prevention. Data on incidence are also essential for effective planning of special medical, educational and social services. Table 13.1 lists all major handicapping conditions

detected in Bristol City in 1967. Children with learning difficulties without any obvious neurological or other disability form the largest group, followed by those with a specific nervous system defect and then by children with congenital malformations of the heart. The table clearly illustrates the continuing medical dilemma of recognizing some conditions by their specific structural defects without stating the degree of handicap, and others solely by the presence of a functional deficit. Both approaches are important but have different applications. For the purposes of clinical management and personal adaptation, recognition of the degree of functional loss is of particular relevance. For example, to the deaf individual it matters little whether his handicap is due to congenital rubella infection or inherited as a genetic disorder; it is crucial to determine whether his loss of hearing is mild, moderate or severe, and whether he has selective high or low frequency deafness. These functional issues will determine the appropriate provision, as well as the ultimate competence of the handicapped individual in society. On the other hand, aetiological considerations remain important for prognostication and prevention.

Table 13.1 Point prevalence of disabling conditions among 2456 children in Bristol

Condition	Number of children with each diagnostic label	Rate per 1000 Bristol children
1. *Central nervous system disorders*		
Cerebral palsy	262	2.8
Convulsive disorders	382	4.1
Spina bifida	36	0.4
Hydrocephalus	36	0.4
Microcephaly	38	0.4
Other CNS defects	29	0.3
2. *Visual disorders*		
Cataracts	19	0.2
Other visual defects	100	1.1
3. *Hearing disorders*		
Perceptive hearing loss	214	2.3
Conductive hearing loss	112	1.2
Other hearing loss	20	0.2
4. *Respiratory disorders*		
Asthma	116	1.2
Chronic respiratory infections	26	0.3
Other respiratory disorders	10	0.1
5. *Cardiovascular disorders*		
Surgically repaired heart lesions	73	0.8
Ventricular septal defects	24	0.3
Atrial septal defects	13	0.1
Fallot's tetralogy	37	0.4
Other congenital heart lesions	186	2.0
Acquired heart disorders	19	0.2
6. *Intellectual disorders*		
Down's syndrome	103	1.1
Other severely subnormal (SSN)	281	3.0
Other educationally subnormal (ESN)	489	5.2

Detection and screening

Disability may be detected at any time from birth to school age, and screening procedures are now well established in the services for the newborn, the child health clinics and the school health service. Their importance cannot be denied but the most effective way of organizing screening has been the subject of much debate, centred around the respective roles and responsibilities of the primary care team, the specialist in child health and the paediatrician. These may be expected to vary from one part of the country to the next, depending on the characteristics of the population served as well as the expertise available, and details are less important than ensuring that professional standards are high and that communication between different parts of the service is good (see Ch. 9). Special training of medical, educational and social work staff, both before and after professional qualification, is essential. Early detection encourages more effective planning of help; particular attention should be paid to the less privileged sections of the community, where incidence may be higher and recognition tardy. Awareness amongst both the professions and the public is increased by open discussion in the news media and by the activities of voluntary bodies with a specific interest in the handicapped.

There are distinct age-dependent ways in which disabilities are ascertained. Severe congenital malformations usually become obvious in the neonatal period, whilst milder variants are detected later. The presence of a structural defect does not by itself determine the degree of handicap and it is only as development proceeds that the functional deficit becomes obvious. Congenital defects of the eye may be evident at birth but blindness is generally detected later when the child fails to follow the mother with his eyes and begins to adopt alternative methods of exploration. The degree of visual impairment is clearly graded and mild variants will only declare themselves when age-appropriate vision testing reveals a defect for near or distant vision. Deafness can present early as non-responsiveness to sound, or later with defective acquisition of speech. The diverse ways in which behaviour develops demonstrate the wide spectrum of handicap, ranging from the child whose responses to people and his environment are moderately or profoundly delayed to the one who makes steady progress, though his behaviour remains less mature than is accepted for the age-related norm. Again, severe retardation is detectable early, whilst mild intellectual underfunctioning is manifest as learning difficulty which will often only come to light when the demands of the school show that the child is unable to maintain the pace of the majority. It is worth restating that the cause of both mild and severe disability may be the same and that an aetiological classification may indicate prognosis and methods of prevention but does not define the degree of handicap. The organization of the educational system into services for children with motor handicaps, for those with severe visual impairment and partial sight and for the deaf and partially hearing, emphasizes the overriding need for functional grading within that system. Clearly, medical models and disease classifications have only limited application in this context. Tuberose sclerosis affords a good example. This condition has a dominant mode of inheritance and may show with skin manifestations only; as epilepsy in an otherwise normal child; or as profound mental handicap with hypsarrhythmia. Each of the affected individuals requires an educational approach suited to his developmental status rather than to the diagnostic category.

It becomes clear that the surveillance of the child population must be a continuous process covering all children, but one that pays particular attention to a defined group which is known to have a greater incidence of disability and is considered to be 'at risk'. This group includes children who have had a variety of perinatal problems, children with a family history of genetic or acquired disease and children in adverse social circumstances (see Ch. 10).

Referral

Parents, and sometimes the wider family, are daily involved in the critical appraisal of their children and, where a defect has not been obvious in the neonatal period, they will usually be the first to draw attention to a deviation from normal. Discussion of parental fears may first start with the health visitor who in turn will alert the family doctor. His advice will depend on the particular findings but must be based on sound knowledge of normal development. The action to be taken may be relatively simple and may involve referral to one or two specialists only, for example the confirmation of deafness by the audiologist and the subsequent involvement of the teacher for the deaf. An interested family practitioner can at times achieve the necessary co-ordination himself but, as these children do not occur frequently in any one general practice, he will not usually have the experience to deal with all aspects effectively. In most cases the fact that the disabilities are multiple and that each may have a profound effect on learning makes referral to a developmental assessment centre advisable.

Multiple disabilities

Disabilities rarely occur in isolation and the detection of one should focus attention on the likelihood of associated disorders which are often less obvious but may nevertheless affect the prospect of habilitation in the open community. Appreciation of the natural history of the disorder will determine what features need special consideration and what form further investigation should take. Again, early detection results in effective remedial planning. This is well exemplified in hydrocephalus and spina bifida, where the problems encountered demonstrate the importance of screening and a co-ordinated multiprofessional approach. Initial detection occurs at birth and, after estimating the probable prognosis, selection for aggressive treatment is made. Immediate closure of the spinal defect and control of the hydrocephalus are the concern of the neurosurgical team: present-day techniques do not guarantee reliable control of intracranial pressure, so long-term follow-up is essential. Paralysis of the lower limbs may be accompanied by developing contractures and secondary deformities which require careful orthopaedic supervision. Urological malformations and recurrent pyelonephritis are common and some children develop epilepsy. Many have visual defect and the occasional child with spina bifida is deaf. These children often show maturational problems and have learning difficulties in school. Disturbed behaviour is not uncommon.

The initial diagnosis of spina bifida thus alerts the medical team to the possibility of associated disorders and the need to exclude or treat them. Planning must proceed sequentially and in a way that causes least disruption to the life of the family. Other conditions have different associations. Cleft palate, for example, is particularly likely to be accompanied by feeding difficulties, recurrent chest infections, deafness and dental malocclusion: affected children not infrequently have problems with cognitive development and need supervision in the toddler years and beyond. Each condition has its own features and associations which need attention from a wide range of specialists. Whilst it may be possible to simplify the process of diagnosis and assessment, no one clinic is likely to combine enough professional expertise to meet all eventualities.

The needs of handicapped children and their families

The children

Most needs of handicapped children do not differ significantly from those of their normal peers. They are best met within the framework of a stable and caring family that understands and has come to terms with the situation and is able to make appropriate adjustments. Other more specific requirements are dictated by the nature of the disability and the developmental level the child has reached. Young children may need extra help with feeding or special encouragement to recognize and become familiar with parents, brothers and sisters, and the domestic environment. Those with motor problems will require aids to assist sitting, standing and walking; the visually impaired may need glasses and the deaf hearing aids. All will benefit from the skilled application of training and teaching methods specifically designed to overcome the disability or to compensate for it. There is therefore a need not only for professional men and women who will define the structural or physiological deficit but also for well-trained teachers. All learning begins at home, so it is imperative that parents be encouraged to lead in this role, particularly in the early years, whilst medical and educational staff act as advisers. A wide range of technical aids are available for all types of disability and these should be employed in ways that take account of the changing needs of the child. Thus, splints need frequent modification and wheelchairs enlarging. Specially designed furniture can ease management at home and the house can be suitably modified to encourage independence of the handicapped child and ease the pressure on his family.

Children learn much from one another and group activities are helpful even for babies and toddlers. Pre-school playgroups, nursery schools and day nurseries have been available for many years, but their numbers remain inadequate and competition for places is intense. There is still a bias against the less proficient and a tendency to exclude the child with mobility problems or immature social behaviour patterns (wetting, soiling, poor concentration). The need for integration with normal children is now well recognized (Warnock, 1978) but many other issues of support for the handicapped child, his parents and his teachers in the educational setting designed for the normal child have to be solved and require imaginative staff, a flexible service and money.

The parents

The needs of parents merit as much consideration as those of the child and in certain circumstances may take precedence over them. Only stable parents can provide really effective care for their young and therefore the quality of their marriage, their economic resources and their domestic circumstances are all important. Understanding support of the wife by the husband, and vice versa, will often make the difference between success and failure in establishing the child in society and it is always worth drawing attention to the value of mutual help. Depression in one or both parents is common, particularly after they first realize what the future holds for them: it may be profound enough to impair significantly their ability to care for the child—occasionally physically but more often emotionally. Severe depression can lead to outright rejection of the child or, more subtly, to management problems which manifest themselves as poor co-operation with health and educational services or as behaviour disturbances in the child. Misunderstanding between husband and wife arises easily and can result in withdrawal of either marriage partner with all its possible consequences. It is therefore useful to encourage discussion of personal feelings of guilt, inadequacy or resentment in the hope of bringing about mutual consideration and support. Counting the assets in a marriage is as important as looking for the difficulties.

In the setting of a child-oriented service, it is easily forgotten that the needs of parents and children may be competitive and that the adults require some time for themselves and occasional privacy. Getting the balance right is difficult in families with normal children; it becomes crucial in those with a handicapped child (Pomeroy et al, 1978).

The siblings
The care of the handicapped is time-consuming and at times obsessional, so that brothers and sisters may miss out on their share of parental attention. Embarrassment, jealousy and resentment are common and can result in aggressive and even delinquent behaviour. It is never easy for parents to meet all the demands made on them, but they should be encouraged to look for opportunities to share the care of the handicapped child and to make time for their normal offspring as well as for themselves. A holiday without the disabled child can mend many strained relationships and make the family more able to handle the problem as a whole.

Services for handicapped children and their families
As has been pointed out in the Report of the Committee on Child Health Services (Court, 1976), no separate service has ever existed exclusively for the benefit of handicapped children. The Report identifies such children as those with special needs which should be met by the general child health services, with the primary health care team making the main health service contribution to the assessment and treatment of the majority of handicapped children. The primary care team should be supported by a district handicap team based on the district general hospital and able to draw on the resources which that can provide. Specialized medical, educational and social work expertise should be available to families of children with complex disorders, to co-ordinate treatment and management both at home and in the various educational establishments which the children might attend. Regional Assessment Centres should be available for the short-term investigation, diagnosis and assessment of children for whom district handicap teams lack the necessary facilities. Ongoing management should, where practicable, remain in the hands of the district team.

Whilst considerable progress has been made towards these developments, government has not accepted all the proposals made in the Court Report and much remains to be done at every level. The recommendation that primary care teams should be strengthened by 'general practitioner paediatricians' and 'child health visitors' who would widen their interest in child health in the community has not found favour and the consequence is that expertise is still not available at local level to resolve most problems of handicapped children where they arise. Although few appointments of consultant community paediatricians have been made, many clinical medical officers (see p. 180) have had further training and are at present undertaking this role. They provide a link with educational and social services in what is becoming an increasingly effective partnership.

The functions of an assessment centre

Separating assessment from treatment is never a satisfactory practice and, where it is attempted, both aspects of the management of the handicapped child tend to be less efficient. Sensitive appraisal of the multiplicity of issues takes time and the therapeutic approach must be capable of modification in the light of medical and social information which is not always available at a single session. These two functions consequently proceed together and can be considered under the following headings:
1. Medical diagnosis and intervention
2. Developmental assessment
3. Social analysis
4. Parent counselling
5. Teaching and training.

Medical diagnosis
A wide range of special skills is required and, whilst the centre needs a co-ordinator, it is unwise to think that one specialist should assume precedence over another. The paediatrician at the centre and paediatric staff from the community may all be involved in the diagnosis and analysis of developmental problems and in delineating the neurological component of conditions such as hydrocephalus, cerebral palsy, epilepsy or the myopathies. An orthopaedic surgeon is essential for the effective assessment and treatment of conditions with a musculo-skeletal component. The urologist participates in the management of the renal complications of children with spinal cord lesions. Both ophthalmologists and ENT specialists must be included in the team to ensure effective assessment of vision and hearing. As behavioural problems and disturbed family dynamics are frequent, the support of a child psychiatric unit and the child guidance service is crucial. Assessment services should be organized to complement other specialist services and not to compete with them. The choice of facilities used must remain at the discretion of the individual specialist. Thus, for example, a child with cerebral palsy may be seen by an ophthalmologist at the assessment centre and, whilst much of the orthoptic work is best done in that setting, he will clearly wish to correct a squint at his hospital ophthalmic unit.

Co-ordination is essential and is usually supervised by the paediatric and child health staff, who assume responsibility for making certain that every facet is covered and that the handling is sequential. They must ensure that social and educational issues receive consideration and that links with the organizations dealing with these aspects are firmly established. Poor communication between the various children's services is a cardinal sin when dealing with the handicapped, since only effective co-ordination of them all will make optimal habilitation possible.

The organization of an integrated programme is never easy. In most cases it is best to arrange recurrent reviews either at the assessment centre or at home. An associated residential unit for children and their parents is at times useful when they live at a distance from the centre, allowing the various aspects of the initial assessment to be compressed into one week.

Developmental assessment
Developmental status is determined concurrently by members of the multidisciplinary team and, in the very young, this is best undertaken during organized play. Critical observation in the playroom has been standard practice amongst teachers and psychologists for many years, but doctors still need to be encouraged to forsake their desks and examination couches. It is always useful to start any interview with a play session and to wean the child away from his mother's lap. The younger the child, the greater the need for modification of the test setting: though it often appears quite primitive to the untrained observer, obtaining reliable information about the skills and abilities of babies and toddlers requires a great deal of expertise. Degrees of function are determined by observing responses to varying stimuli and this is best done by involving two members of staff in the session. One will hold the child's interest and provide distraction if necessary, whilst the other will administer the stimulus. Both must be alert to observe the response. This arrangement is particularly appropriate for tests of vision and hearing but is also valuable for the orthopaedic surgeon or paediatrician who is interested in hand function and walking.

Only cursory delineation of function is possible in a consulting room and much more information is gained by observing children at play. Nursery provision is consequently an important element in any assessment centre and allows nursery nurses and therapists to gain a clear view of the child's developmental status and needs. Training and treatment programmes, as well as parent support and counselling, become more effective in this setting. With the help of the psychologist, nursery staff should be encouraged to record levels of achievement on scales such as those described by Griffiths (1954) and by Gunzburg (1963). Repeated observations can be made and the developmental progression charted. Demonstrating progressive maturation in this way is always reassuring to both parents and staff and encourages further effort by all concerned.

Particular attention is paid to comprehension and the production of speech. This involves medical personnel, psychologists and speech therapists: it is axiomatic that any child with a speech defect has one or more hearing tests until the staff is satisfied that hearing is normal.

Observation of behavioural characteristics is essential and should include notes on the predominant emotional state and whether the child is trusting or apprehensive, placid or aggressive, immobile or exploratory. Maturation brings with it an increasing ability to concentrate. Where this is delayed, as is often the case in children who are subsequently found to have educational difficulties, a short attention span frequently manifests itself as physical restlessness, a constant flitting from one activity to the next and a tendency to show disturbed sleep rhythms. These characteristics are often very taxing to parents and staff and may result in poor integration into the family and classroom.

Social analysis
A family's ability to rear a handicapped child may be impaired by adverse social influences and the more that professional staff are aware of the difficulties, the greater will be their ability to provide help and support. Prime responsibility for identifying the social issues rests with the specialist social worker, who should be contacted as soon after diagnosis as possible: with her assistance the parents may be helped to understand the implications of what they have been told and begin to plan for future management. She will be concerned about the quality of the support systems within the family, whether the parents show mutual understanding and whether help is available from relatives, neighbours or other agencies within the community. The economic status of the family is always relevant. The social worker will draw attention to the possibility of financial support from the Family Fund for particular items of need, and to the availability of the Attendance Allowance for children who need more than usual care, particularly at night. Children who are severely physically handicapped and immobile are entitled to a Mobility Allowance after the age of five years.

The quality of the housing needs consideration, from the points of view both of interior planning and the ease with which the family can manage their handicapped child at home, and of its geographical location. Convenience of access to helpful relatives can be as important as the ready availability of shopping precincts. The social worker will be in touch with the local authority housing department, as well as the occupational therapists in the social service department, who can recommend the installation of lifts, hoists, modified bathroom and toilet arrangements, and occasionally the addition of purpose-built accommodation. It must be stressed, however, that the provision of material support is not the only, or even the most important, function of those professional workers involved in the social analysis, for 'lending an ear', providing good counsel and becoming a friend are often the greatest needs.

Parent counselling
Of all the functions of an assessment centre, this is perhaps the most important and at times the most difficult. All staff members counsel during their individual sessions with the child and his parents, but co-ordination is essential and, in situations that are multifaceted with serious implications, this is assured by arranging a conference at which the staff discuss all aspects with the parents after the initial assessment has been completed. The conference may be repeated at times when particular management changes are being proposed, or at the request of the parents. It is vitally important to take account of the needs of every member of the family and to remember that occasionally parents require more consideration than their handicapped offspring. Nevertheless, the family

has to be looked at as a whole and it is useful to draw up a list of priorities and to attempt to resolve or modify each problem in turn. Urgent attention may sometimes be necessary in family crises precipitated by severe depression in either parent, imminent or actual marriage breakdown, or illness in other members of the family.

Parental ambivalence is an ever-present phenomenon which results in rational acceptance of the situation on one day and angry rejection the next. It becomes greater in situations of stress that often have only an indirect relationship to the handicapped child, and it is always helpful to elucidate the reasons for the additional pressures and to discuss them, preferably with both parents together. Inadequate support for the mother is all too frequent and both general practitioners and paediatricians have a golden opportunity to impress on the parents the importance of *shared care* in the context of the immediate family, where possible the extended family of aunts, uncles and grandparents and, eventually, the whole range of children's services. It is common experience that a united couple achieve acceptance of their handicapped child and stability for the family as a whole much more rapidly than those who are at cross purposes.

During the initial contact with parents, advice is best given repeatedly, because their anxiety levels are often too high for more than a few facts to register. Help should be provided in simple activities like feeding and postural control, graduating successively to toileting, dressing and other self-help skills. Information about aids and adaptations must be given by all staff, but particularly by the occupational therapist. The assessment centre staff can do much by arranging nursery groups for children who need the same therapeutic approach. Mothers are encouraged to join in these sessions and discuss mutual problems and their solution with one another. Although this does not relieve them of their burden, it counteracts the feelings of isolation by making them aware that they are not the only ones facing these difficulties. It also begins the process of allowing the mother some time to herself and this is gradually extended when the child finds a part-time or full-time place in a day nursery or nursery school. The development of parent workshops based in special schools, adult education institutes or research centres has been particularly useful and has given parents a teaching model with which to approach their own problems and their child's learning and behavioural difficulties (Voluntary Council for Handicapped Children 1979). Parents often comment that they derive greatest support from other parents of handicapped children and this becomes one of the main aims of the parent workshop, not least because it involves fathers as well as mothers.

Behavioural problems are common and need particular attention. Stressed parents react irritably and, in a subconscious desire to withdraw from the pressures of caring for their handicapped child, they may distance themselves from him emotionally or physically. This results in attention-seeking behaviour from the child, who may whine or cry as soon as the mother is out of sight or otherwise occupied. Problems are also created by parents who, in an understandable effort to compensate for the handicap, become overprotective and constantly available. The child then grows more than usually demanding, often to the detriment of other members of the family, and this eventually rebounds on them all when tolerance is finally at an end. Management instructions frequently repeated by members of staff can exacerbate these trends, which must be counteracted by drawing attention to the needs of all members of the family. An indulged toddler responds to frustration with a temper tantrum or by naughtiness and 'spoiling' him will adversely affect his ability to learn to integrate. Consideration of others has to be taught—even to the handicapped!

Parents walk a never-ending tightrope between giving frequent help to and demanding self-help from their children. The balance between the two can best be achieved in a setting of love, tolerance and encouragement. It is also important to remember that genuine praise provides powerful motivation and that success encourages further effort.

Genetic counselling should be part of a comprehensive counselling service. It is dependent on accurate medical diagnosis and aims at preventing the birth of children with handicapping disorders. Advances in biochemical and cytological techniques have made antenatal prediction and selective abortion a real possibility. However, geneticists often fail to appreciate that parents are also asking another series of questions with far-reaching implications. The question 'What is wrong with my child?' is inevitably followed by 'What is wrong with me/my wife/my husband?' The genetic counselling session is therefore one of urgent self-evaluation for parents and due regard must be paid to feelings of guilt and low self-esteem. The reaction that 'there is nothing wrong with my side of the family' is common and with it the implication that the other marriage partner carries the blame. This is seldom true and genetic counselling offers an exceptional opportunity to help parents to develop balanced attitudes to themselves, to their handicapped child and to one another. Discussion should not be confined to the possible risks to future offspring. It is also important to recognize that children form an important part of the biological and cultural continuum of life and that few couples attain full maturity without them. Children are as important to adults as adults are to children. For certain parents who wish for further children, adoption or artificial insemination can be considered, but care must be taken to determine the attitudes of both husband and wife and to allow them to investigate and discuss all aspects of any proposal made.

Teaching and training
Teaching parents about methods of stimulating children to improved developmental performance, and training the children themselves, are basic functions of the assessment centre staff. Indeed, it is important that the health, social service and education departments should clearly recognize the educational role of the centre, for remedial teaching commences in this setting and is subsequently continued in ordinary and special nurseries and schools run by the Education Department. It can be surprisingly difficult to get conventionally trained medical and other health staff to think of themselves as teachers. Those that do see their scope enlarge considerably and their work become more meaningful and afford them greater satisfaction. Teaching is the logical extension of healing. A physiotherapist seeking to improve hand function automatically shows interest in the acquisition of writing and encourages it by appropriate exercises. The overlapping roles of teachers and speech therapists have been

recognized for many years. In some countries, notably Hungary, remedial staff are trained to acquire a range of skills and are less specialized than staff in Western European countries. This approach should be encouraged elsewhere, as speech stimulation can be practised during sessions designed for improving mobility, and many everyday activities can be used to promote hand function. Assumption of the role of educator also changes the attitude to the handicapped child. Rather than doing things for him, the member of staff encourages the child to work for himself and so to become more independent.

Links with other children's services
The assessment centre must have good links with other children's services. The neonatologist will often be the first to detect a handicapping condition and at an agreed point the assessment centre will take on further supervision. Transfer of the child and his family will depend on the type and severity of the condition and individual needs. An occasional combined clinic is mutually useful.

Equally important is the link with playgroups, nursery schools and ultimately the whole sequence of educational establishments. This is best achieved by encouraging individual approaches, so that physiotherapists deal with their counterparts in the community, psychologists liaise with their colleagues in the schools, and so on. To be effective, information must be collated and shared. Discretion is essential but no professional worker can be sensitive to a family's needs without fairly detailed appreciation of the total situation. Every attempt should be made to identify and use local professional staff and services, though appropriately trained personnel are not always available and some travelling then becomes inevitable for children and parents. Well-organized transport arrangements are an essential prerequisite to full use of the facilities that have been created.

Playgroups and nursery schools
Nursery education is generally available for children from the age of two years but provision falls far short of the need. Arrangements for handicapped children require particular attention, with specialized programmes directed towards overcoming or compensating for their disabilities. Whilst these may appropriately be undertaken in ordinary nursery schools, their staff are not always trained in the special skills needed for the care and teaching of handicapped children, and the creation of special nurseries is highly desirable.

Pre-school playgroups established by committees of parents or by interested individuals usefully augment statutory provision, though they find it difficult to cope with children with serious disabilities. For these, the creation of a special form of playgroup—the opportunity group—has great advantages. It allows children with and without handicap to mix and brings parents of handicapped children together for mutual support. It is essential to provide such opportunity groups with the services of physio- and occupational therapists as well as social work support. The aim should be to provide a stable educational base which will subsequently allow the child to flourish in a non-specialist precinct school. This objective will not always be fulfilled but professional staff, and especially parents, are able to determine the degree of integration and where the child will best fit in.

Decision about further education is made in the light of progressive developmental advance and after full discussion with parents and staff. Full participation by parents is particularly important and will avoid the common situation where parents report acceptable social maturation, whilst teaching staff are aware of less than average progress in educational achievement.

Day and residential nurseries

Both day nurseries and residential nurseries are supervised by the social service department and their use nearly always reflects a pressing social need. Day nurseries are useful in the care of handicapped children whose parents need some relief for emotional reasons, or where the family makes unusual demands on the mother. Handicapped children are quite frequently cared for by single parents and financial necessity may make admission to a day nursery urgent.

Similar considerations may justify admission of a handicapped child to a residential nursery, though social problems are then usually more serious. There is often an imminent or actual family crisis which can only be met by lessening the burden on the parents until such time as they can again accept responsibility for the care of the handicapped child. The reasons range from parental illness or marital discord to serious financial and housing difficulties. Day and residential nurseries should, where practicable, be used interchangeably or sequentially. There are advantages in having both facilities on the same site, as it is clearly unsettling for children to have to adjust to new caring staff (surrogate parents) with any frequency. Fostering arrangements may be suitable for some handicapped children. They have the advantage of keeping the child in a more normal domestic setting but, as always, the choice of foster parents must be made with care and placement is not easy. Whatever the arrangements for day or residential care, it is important to ensure that satisfactory therapy, education and social support continue.

Hospital schools and the mental subnormality hospital

Many handicapped children require repeated admissions to hospital and education authorities have established schools in hospitals with children's departments. Both medical and nursing staff must be encouraged to recognize their importance and to form close links with the educational staff. Some teachers find it difficult to work in the hospital environment and they will need special consideration and help.

Severely mentally handicapped young children are increasingly admitted to long-stay mental subnormality hospitals for relief care only. It is unfortunate that these institutions, despite recent improvements, often have a clinical rather than a domestic atmosphere and attempts must be made to create more homelike surroundings. This requirement has obvious implications for accommodation, design, staffing and staff training. The greater the community support, particularly by assessment teams and social work departments, the less the need for admission, even of the most severely mentally handicapped children, though some long-term residential accommodation will always be required. Children admitted to these institutions for any length of time need careful appraisal of all their needs and, whilst many will go to hospital schools, some would benefit from attending appropriate special schools in the community. Strict demarcation of provision should always be avoided and effective inter-disciplinary liaison of all staff involved in the care of these children is as imperative as it is for those living in the community.

Housing

Mention has already been made of the importance of suitable housing for the handicapped. The presence of a handicapped child in a family materially affects the way that space in the home is used by everyone. The reduced mobility of this one member of the family encroaches on the main living area where the family spend most of their time. A wheelchair inevitably modifies the arrangement and type of furniture in a home, and the siting and height of shelves, switches, sinks and bathroom furniture all require attention. As the child's age and weight increase and the parents become older, accommodation on different levels becomes less and less acceptable, and the need for home extension on one level becomes important. In some areas, local authority housing departments have in recent years included purpose-built accommodation in new housing developments (e.g. the Habintech Scheme), where special housing is interspersed amongst conventional buildings to ensure that the handicapped child and his family are as integrated into the community as possible. Whilst this type of provision may represent an ideal, it is costly and not always appropriate. Social needs may make it advisable for a family to stay in their original house in a familiar environment, and it may then be possible to modify or extend this accommodation. Teamwork between parents, the local authority occupational therapist and the housing department is essential to find the best solution.

The needs of services for the handicapped

Clearly, if handicapped children and their families are to be effectively helped, the service itself needs consideration both at organizational and at professional level. Successive governments have introduced new legislation and provided additional resources to bring about better services. Health Authorities have gradually improved provision for the handicapped, but continued support and development remain high priorities. Little can be done without sympathetic understanding by the community as a whole and both the news media and voluntary organizations have an important part to play in disseminating information about needs and further advances. There is a continuing call for more and better trained staff at every level. Sustained effort is needed to provide further education for health, educational and social work staff. Courses, conferences and workshops do much to create new interest and develop alternative approaches.

Failure to meet the needs of institutions and particularly of their staff may induce disillusionment and despair, resulting in distancing and occasional withdrawal from the service. Professional staff nearly always try to do their best and it is essential to review their working conditions and consider their individual requirements and aspirations. It should not be forgotten that many—

especially caring staff and teachers—act as surrogate parents and that their needs are often very similar. It is consequently important to consider and encourage consideration in those who serve as well as those being served. Only in this way can an atmosphere of *mutual* satisfaction be created and the best interests of all be ensured.

REFERENCES

Court S D M (chairman) 1976 Fit for the future: Report of the Committee on Child Health Services. HMSO, London

Griffiths R 1954 The abilities of babies. University Press, London

Gunzburg H C 1963 Progress assessment charts. National Association for Mental Health, London

Parent Workshops Fact Sheet Number 9 1979 Voluntary Council for Handicapped Children, London

Pomeroy D, Fewtrell J, Butler N R, Gill R 1978 Handicapped children—their homes and life-styles: HDD Occasional Paper 4/78. Department of the Environment. HMSO, London

Warnock H M (chairman) 1978 Special educational needs: Report of the Committee of Enquiry into the Education of Handicapped Children and Young People. HMSO, London

Younghusband E, Birchall D, Davies R Pringle M L K 1970 Living with handicap. National Bureau for Co-operation in Child Care, London

Social work services for children

Introduction
Services to children can be considered in terms of their concern for the physical, the social, or the personal dimension of living. Each dimension interlocks with the other two and so in a sense to focus on one dimension in isolation is to give a misleading picture of a child's life. The potential for distortion can be seen in the recent growth in public demand for social workers to give substantial attention to the physical dimension of living. It is arguable that, whilst certain governmental and voluntary services rightly must focus on this dimension, the particular contribution of social work to the lives of citizens lies in affirming the equal importance of the social and personal dimensions of living and putting that affirmation into practice.

The provision of social work services for children is, like the provision of all social services, the product of a coming together of values held at individual and social levels, of resources available either immediately or within identifiable periods of time, of abilities to act in a sustained manner in relation to demands for service, and of a capacity to organize resources and abilities in ways which are relevant to the demands being made, while giving no serious offence to the values of the many people and institutions involved.

'Factual statements' about the existence of social work services for children can be very misleading if taken at face value. The organization of the social work services, and the policies and statutes which underpin them, serve as a framework within which instances of service are delivered. The form each instance actually takes is affected by a range of factors, the influence of which must be understood by anyone who wishes to make effective use of the services available. Critical to the form each instance of service takes is the way in which those providing the service can differ *first*, over what they notice in the situation they are working with, *second*, over the sense they make of what they notice, and *third*, over what they do in respect of the sense they make. Equally critical to the form a service takes is whether there are people who are able to make constructive and relevant use of what is actually being offered. It does not follow that because a service is available, it is usable in ways which are relevant to the condition of those who seek to use it. A service seemingly geared to meet the needs of the socially disadvantaged may in fact be meeting more the needs of the socially influential. Certain members of a family may be more acceptable to the providers of a service than are others: children may be either advantaged or disadvantaged relative to their parents in respect of the service they receive from a social worker. The opportunities offered to a child or his parents may not be usable by them because of the consequences of so doing for their self image or for the way other people treat them.

The present discussion of social work services for children will therefore begin by examining some of the focuses of concern which different practitioners and administrators might concentrate on as they seek to deliver such services. With these focuses available as pointers to the range of different approaches which social workers may make, the overall patterning of relevant local authority services will be detailed. To round off the picture of the current state of these services, we will look at some examples of the doubts and uncertainties about practice which are currently affecting the forms of service delivery.

The discussion will make use of the term 'social work services' as a way of reconciling the fact that in England and Wales the services in question are largely provided by 'Social Services Departments' whilst in Scotland the corresponding departments are 'Social Work Departments'.

Focuses of concern when providing social work services for children

Formulating focuses of concern

Concern for children is widespread throughout society. The forms it takes do, however, seem to be affected by the proximity between the children in question and the people expressing the concern. Thus our view of the service most appropriate for a child whom we hear about at a distance may be quite different from the view we are likely to hold if we know him face to face. We may, for example, be either more or less ready to recommend removing him from his parents if we have never seen him and his parents together, or if we have never explored with him what his parents mean to him.

Not only may the form taken by our concern reflect the degree of contact we have with the child and his circumstances, it may also be affected by the social context of that contact. If we meet the child in the classroom we may experience a rather different person from the one we meet in the consulting room, and in both cases the child met with may bear little resemblance to the one we will find if we get accepted into his home, or if we are so placed that we see him from day to day playing with other children. Each variation in our experience of a child's behaviour may affect the views we come to hold about the type of service he should receive. Each person who contacts him may claim, on the basis of that contact alone, to know 'the real child'.

Recommendations for making a given service available to a child should properly be based not only on our appreciation of his nature, but also on our appreciation of the nature of the service he is likely to receive. Disagreement over the 'correct' service to make available often arises not so much from different views about his nature and needs as from different views about the nature and relevance of the services actually available. Disagreement is particularly likely to occur when some of those making recommendations have personal experience of the services in question whilst others do not. It may be that the only truly relevant action to take in the case of certain children in need is to press for the development of services currently non-existent or seriously deficient in resources.

To correct for bias in planning and implementing services for children we need to be able to give due weight to information about all the facets of the child's life which are relevant to the issues which brought him to our attention. It is, therefore, of the utmost importance that we learn how to distinguish between issues which can be evaluated and planned for from a single viewpoint and issues which require perspectives on many facets of a child's life before an effective service can be made available to him.

One of the most frequently undervalued sources of information about a child's capacity to use a service is the child himself. Often it seems as if the child is the last person whose viewpoint is thought to be relevant to designing a service. The tendency to give overwhelming weight to the viewpoint of 'experts' when planning or implementing a service (often only one expert is involved in the latter case) needs to be replaced by ways of working which draw on information from as many people as possible who are in contact with the child in need (including the child himself). In part this entails appropriate forms of organizing for collaboration, but it also calls for changes in attitude (many parents, for example, seem to experience themselves as having little or nothing of value to offer when in the company of social workers or other 'authority figures'). Much of the criticism currently being directed at services for children seems to be about failure to make use of relevant sources of information and failure to involve in programmes of service people who are in daily contact with the children who are allegedly receiving the services.

Some major focuses of concern
Any feature of a child's life may become a focus of concern. It may well be that several features of his life may concern us at the same time. It is indeed arguable that we should be concerned for 'the whole child', on the grounds that each feature of his life resonates throughout the whole of his life.

In order to give some structure to our picture of social work services for children, the possible focuses of concern will be considered in three main categories: the child himself, the child in the family and the child in society. With the help of these categories, we will specify particular criteria on the basis of which a child may be thought to be able to use a social work service.

Focuses on the 'child himself'
The child may be viewed as an individual who displays the effects on himself of situations which he encounters. He may display these effects in three main ways.

First, he may show them in *physical terms*. The physical effects of situations are relatively easily observed and receive particular attention from the lay public, who tend not to realize how difficult such effects are to evaluate. People providing services which are concerned to do something about the physical effects on a child of his relations with his parents and others may however find themselves faced with uncertainty on the following counts: (a) they may be unable to arrive at a clear picture of how the effects came into being, whether by accident or intent; (b) in those cases when the effects occurred by intent, they may be unable to decide whether they are indicators of a violent life-style on the part of parents or other adults; and (c) in all cases they may be unable to decide whether serious positive measures to prevent a recurrence of physical effects may not have equally serious negative effects in other dimensions of the child's experience.

Second, the child may display the effects on himself of situations in *emotional terms*. A difficulty here lies in knowing what it is which is actually activating his behaviour. Seemingly similar behaviour displayed by a range of children may in fact derive from quite different sources. A child may truant from school because he cannot understand what is going on, because he is subject to bullying, because his friends truant, or because he is troubled about his life at home. Furthermore, his actions may be linked to a combination of such factors, with varying degrees of weighting being given from one child to another. Recommendations aiming at providing him with an appropriate service can be open to endless questioning, as different sources of recommendation make use of different ways of understanding the meaning of his behaviour.

Third, the child may be subject to situations which are *beyond his capacity to deal with*. Usually this state of affairs is associated with some form of handicap, physical, intellectual or emotional. There may be a tendency to offer him services specifically geared to the way he handles issues directly relating to his handicap. The possibility must always be borne in mind, however, that what he is seeking to develop is a greater capacity to experience and give expression to his handicap as part of an integrated life-style.

Focuses on the child in the family

Children are, of course, deeply rooted in the adults most constantly around them. Services for children are particularly concerned to give due weight to this rootedness. However, there are wide variations in the patterns of family interconnections which underpin the design and delivery of different services. These variations may reflect the range of awareness of the planners or providers of a service, the capacity of those delivering a service to work in terms of the interconnections actually holding between a child and his family, the willingness of members of a family to make use of a service in accordance with how they link up with the child or with each other, and so forth.

In terms of the interconnections which may affect the child in the family, services may be differentiated into three main directions. The *first* focuses on the effects of one or more family members on the child. Here services will be concerned with facilitating and controlling the contacts which the given family member (or members) has with the child. Problems may arise when one family member has effects on the child which conflict with the effects which another member has. On whom is the service to focus? Ideally a family-focused service will be provided which reconciles these differences of effect. In practice, a service may have to be designed where different providers of service work with different members of the family (for example, to handle the stresses on the service providers of split loyalties, or to ensure that the range of effects on the child is adequately catered for).

The *second* direction which might be taken is to focus services on those aspects of the family's social circumstances which directly or indirectly affect the child. Thus the family's capacity to obtain income may directly affect the child's access to basic necessities, or it may indirectly affect his well-being through the attitudes of other family members. The child may be similarly affected by such matters as the quality of housing and the range of services available (educational, health, leisure). Providing social services within these areas of living can produce conflicts with other providers of service; it can also involve lines of action which challenge widely held values (such as whether unmarried mothers should receive services to enable them to retain their children).

The effect which a child has on other members of his family constitutes the *third* possible direction for services focusing on the child in the family. A child may activate in his parents feelings and ideas which were first placed there during the parents' own childhood. Many parents express a desire not to repeat patterns of child raising which they experienced at the hands of their own parents, only to fall back on these very patterns as their own child seemingly challenges them to behave as the grandparents did. It may be that some parents bring out in their children the very behaviour which they displayed in relation to their own parents. The behaviour of children can often show with unsettling clarity the unresolved relationship problems in a family, with consequent defensive reactions on the part of the parents—for example, the child is assigned total responsibility for his delinquency or emotionally disturbed behaviour. Parents may seek to use children (often unconsciously) to disadvantage one another, or to hold their marriage together, and will be very upset if the child strives to act in terms of any needs of his own which conflict with these aims.

Children may also produce stressful effects on parents and other family members by bringing into the family the effects on them of extra-familial experiences. These experiences may arise out of the family's position in society: for example, the family's children may have access to limited and inadequate education, health and leisure services. A combination of family circumstances and social attitudes may have resulted in the child spending a period of his life away from home: on his return, the family members find themselves faced with a relative stranger whom they may try to turn into someone the child cannot be. The resulting conflict often proves too difficult to bear.

Children who enter families as strangers (as in fostering) inevitably raise feelings and thoughts which the family and the child may find difficult to cope with. A strong case can be argued for a direct social work service to foster parents. In those cases where the fostered child has a history of stressful relations with families, this service must be geared accordingly, with the aim of enabling foster parents to live with children who carry their distress about with them. Hopefully a successful experience of this kind will help to reduce the child's historically developed ways of reacting stressfully in the context of family life.

Services which make use of residential settings are most appropriately used by children who cannot help but generate acute stress in the types of family available to them. A child who experiences difficulties in relating to adults may well benefit from living in a residential setting which is sufficiently large to allow him opportunity to choose the adults he relates to, and to decide for himself and in his own good time what thoughts and feelings he shares with them.

In all instances where a child has effects on those around him, it is important to remember that at the same time the persons around him are having effects on the child. In order to justify focusing a given service on the people affected by the child we must be able to show that they can benefit from this attention and that, in part at least, the benefit is fedback to the child in the form of more productive attention from the people in question. We must beware of disadvantaging the child for the benefit of other people. The child is often a very poor advocate of his own position. Other people may tend to describe him in terms of the distress they experience in his presence. They may quite fail to look beyond the behaviour which has caused their distress, to seek out the distress which resides in him, and which gains expression through his offending behaviour. They may also fail to take note of how they compound that distress and its offending forms of expression by the very ways they express their distress in relation to him. Services concerned with the effects which children have on other people may therefore favour approaches to the child which minimize the opportunities available to him to experience and express the distress which lies within his offending behaviour. A just and effective service must be geared to bringing about a state of affairs where the distress of all involved is recognized and opportunities are provided for it to be experienced and expressed in ways which reduce it and replace the offending behaviour with more productive ways of relating to other people.

Focuses on the 'child in society'
The 'other people' who affect and are affected by a child may be contacted in the form of the socially influential, or in the form of members of organizations like schools, courts or the police. The child may also be subject to socially distributed attitudes towards such of his characteristics as social origin, place of residence and manner of speech or dress.

In respect of this dimension of living, services may focus on the effects of society on the child, on the effects of the child on society or on the values of society.

The opportunities for living productively which are provided by society in respect of a given child may be non-existent, inadequate, or positively stress-generating. Social work services for children may be geared to any or all these states of affairs. They may be designed to meet a previously unmet need, for example by providing opportunities for certain types of play in the form of playgroups or adventure playgrounds, or by providing day centres for the handicapped. Where services are inadequate they may aim to modify or supplement an existing service (which may not be provided by the social work service department), as when a social work service is provided within the context of a school, or a youth group is established for those who cannot conform to the standards of the generality of youth clubs. An example of a service which seeks to provide an alternative to more stress-producing ways of dealing with 'offending children' is intermediate treatment. Here the aim is to avoid the stress-producing effects of committal away from home and to do so by means of activities which teach the productive use of natural energies and interests.

Services concerned with the effects which the child has on society may take the form of advocating the child's viewpoint, of ensuring that recognition is given to his rights as a person, or of providing opportunities for members of society to enrich their understanding of the lives of children and of the effects which various features of society have on those lives. Services concerned with divergences between the values of the child and the values of society will be especially concerned to build bridges between children and society. They may take the form of services to existing services, of providing advice, or of consultancy. It should also be remembered that society is far from consistent in the way its various segments and individual members relate to children. Thus another aim of services concerned with divergences in values is to facilitate the growth of shared understandings about the lives of children, and to ensure that these understandings are expressed in ways which extend the opportunities available to children to experience more consistency and harmony in their lives.

The pattern of social work services for children

Legislative and organizational foundations
Social work services for children may be provided by local authorities and by voluntary organizations. Increasingly there is need for the two sources of service to work together. A variety of tendencies in contemporary society have favoured the coming under public control of many services which originated in the voluntary sector. Today voluntary organizations are increasingly seeking to develop services which extend the resources available to local authorities rather than replicate them. Examples include experimental forms of residential care and certain types of day care.

The local authority has the responsibility to provide certain services for children whose welfare might otherwise be at risk. Legislation and services have traditionally focused on (i) the care of orphaned children or those permanently deprived of normal home life, (ii) the adoption of children, (iii) children in need of temporary care and the development of foster care, (iv) children subject to cruelty, danger or neglect within the home and (v) children who have committed criminal offences. In England and Wales the Local Authority Social Services Act 1970 carried forward the local authority's power under the 1948 Children Act to receive children into care, and the requirement under the 1963 Children and Young Persons Act for the local authority to engage in such preventive measures as will 'diminish the need to receive children or keep them in care'. In Scotland, the Social Work (Scotland) Act 1968 requires the local authority to receive into care a child under the age of 17 who appears to be without a parent or guardian who can provide for his proper accommodation, maintenance and upbringing. Two other sections in the Act point to particular directions in which this care might proceed: 'It shall be the duty of that authority to ... afford him opportunity for the proper development of his character and abilities' and 'It shall be the duty of every local authority to promote social welfare by making available advice, guidance and assistance on such a scale as may be appropriate ... (in the case of) a person being a child under the age of eighteen to diminish the need to receive him or keep him in care.'

The local authority, police and the National Society for the Prevention of Cruelty to Children (Royal Scottish Society for the Prevention of Cruelty to Children in Scotland) have the authority to remove children and young persons up to the age of 17 from their homes and to bring them before a juvenile court (in Scotland, a Children's Hearing) for Care Proceedings. The Children and Young Persons Act 1969 requires that the court be satisfied that, first, the young person is in need of care or control which he is unlikely to receive unless an order is made and, second, that one of the following conditions applies in his case: (i) that his present upbringing is preventing his proper development, (ii) that he lives in a household where another child has suffered neglect, (iii) that he is in moral danger or beyond control, (iv) that he is not receiving adequate full-time education, or (v) that he has committed an offence. The Social Work (Scotland) Act 1968 lays down roughly the same requirements. The overall intent of the legislation is to achieve as much balance as possible between the rights of the parents and child and the views of those in authority concerning the child's best interests. The Children's Act 1975 emphasized that major concern should be given to the welfare of the child.

There is a critical distinction to be noted between the procedures involved when the local authority takes a child into care on a compulsory basis and when it receives him into care on a voluntary basis. If the child is placed in the care of the local authority, the authority has parental powers until such time as the relevant order is rescinded or the child reaches the age of 18. In all instances of voluntary care, the parents of the child are able to take him out of care whenever they are ready to do so. The differences in procedure for putting the two approaches into effect mean that it is much more difficult to take a child into care on a compulsory basis than it is on a voluntary one.

The Children and Young Persons Act 1969 sought to bring the juvenile offender within the range of services available to all children in need of care. Part I of the Act emphasizes the importance of keeping children out of the courts as far as possible. Residential services are organized on a regional basis under the general designation of 'Community Homes', thus blurring the boundary between 'Approved Schools' and 'Remand Homes' and other residential settings for children (in England and Wales). The Social Work (Scotland) Act 1968 established a new approach to the juvenile offender in the form of the Children's Hearing System, designed to provide services for children who, in the Children and Young Persons Act of 1963, are described as being in need of 'care, protection or control'.

In England and Wales, a juvenile court is empowered to make either a Supervision Order (to which an order for Intermediate Treatment may be added) or a Care Order, which transfers the legal custody of the child to the local authority. Under a Care Order the local authority has parental rights until the child's eighteenth birthday, but these can be revoked by a court on the application of parent, child or the local authority. Parental contributions towards the maintenance of children subject to Care Orders is obligatory.

Under 'criminal proceedings' a juvenile court can decide to: (i) discharge absolutely, (ii) discharge conditionally, (iii) bind over the offender and/or parents to keep the peace, (iv) fine the offender with or without an order for compensation/restitution, (v) commit the offender to a Detention Centre (if over 14), or (vi) to Borstal (if over 15), or (vii) to an Attendance Centre run by the police to provide a stated number of hours of training during the free time of the offender. Courts may add a requirement of 'Intermediate Treatment' within the context of a Supervision Order. The aim is that the offender will come willingly to accept whatever is offered under that heading and as a result the decision as to what form Intermediate Treatment should take in the case of a given young person is determined by those providing the service (see also p. 97).

The Social Work (Scotland) Act 1968 empowers a Children's Hearing to: (i) make a requirement of supervision (which may be augmented by a requirement of residence with a foster parent or in a Children's Home or a 'List D' School), or (ii) refer the child to the Education Authority for ascertainment for special schooling, or to the Social Work Department with a view to admission to hospital care or to the making of a guardianship order under the Mental Health (Scotland) Act 1960. When a 'requirement of supervision' is made (which places the child under the care of the local authority), it must be reviewed at least once a year by the Panel. Each specific Hearing should 'discuss in a concerned and informal way the difficulties of children, and provide the most appropriate measures of care and treatment for those who need them'. (Each Hearing has three members, including both sexes, one of whom acts as chairman: they are drawn from a panel whose members must have shown interest and aptitude and have had some training. The Hearing is serviced by a Reporter whose function is to identify and present appropriate cases.

Both the 1968 Social Work (Scotland) Act and the 1970 Local Authority Social Services Act (England and Wales) established departments which brought together social work services for children, the elderly, the mentally disturbed and the handicapped. In Scotland the probation service was additionally included. A major reason given for establishing comprehensive departments was that they would permit one social worker to provide all the services needed by all the members of a given family. In this way, it was argued, the services provided would interlock and be geared to the overall nature of the family's life. There are two flaws in the argument—first, the assumption that a single worker can do justice to the potentially manifold demands of the members of certain types of family and, second, that the difficulties which an individual child experiences in his life and displays through his behaviour originate in his family (and not in his school, in his immediate neighbourhood, or in society at large).

The provision of services for children since the passing of the two Acts has reflected the consequences of this flawed argument. A massive growth in demand for social work services has also affected the amount of service which can be provided. Evidence of the limits to certain services provided for children has recently appeared in the form of investigation into a number of instances of non-accidental injury to children. What this evidence seems to indicate is that social workers are finding the range of services demanded of them too great to control. Divisions of loyalty towards different members of the same family seem to have compounded their difficulties. The absence of consistent and practically meaningful guidelines from their employing agencies has also played a part.

At the same time it is becoming increasingly clear that services focusing on housing, education, employment, health, and supplementary benefits have as critical a part to play in the life problems of the clients of social services/social work departments as do those departments themselves. Perhaps even more fundamental is the question: 'What can the neighbourhood/community within which the client of a social worker lives, provide in the way of aids and assistance to help him cope with the problems so that he does not need to turn elsewhere?'

Caring for the child at home and away from home
The patterning of social work services for the child in the family may be classified into services for the child at home and services for the child away from home. Both types of service entail preceding and concurrent endeavours to identify and provide the service most relevant to the nature of the child and, where possible, his familial and social context.

The present section will examine, first, some features of the organization and practice of assessment. It will then go on to outline the main characteristics of services to the child who is living at home and of services to the child who is receiving care away from home.

Deciding the services to provide: assessment
It is widely accepted that decisions about which services to make available to a given child should be based on a detailed study of his circumstances. The purpose of the study is to give direction to the opportunities for experience and action which are subsequently and concurrently provided for the child.

Assessment studies are subject to much disagreement and confusion. A major source of difficulty resides in the wide range of concerns which may attract the attention of anyone engaged in assessing. As we have noted, many and indeed perhaps most children will give evidence of need for services covering many of these focuses. The services actually provided will have to be selective, and assessment inevitably entails giving priority to some focuses of concern over others.

Assessment is essentially concerned with knowing what to notice and how to go about noticing effectively. It cannot be separated from service provision (frequently called 'treatment' by social workers and others). Service provision entails being able to do something about what we have noticed. It should be possible to show how what we do is linked to what we have noticed, and how it is associated with outcomes which are consequent on our overall view of what will contribute most to resolving the issues which brought the child to our attention in the first place.

The process of noticing is obviously highly susceptible to the nature of the contact between the child and the assessor. It is to be expected that different assessors will notice different dimensions of the life of the child by virtue of relating to him from different standpoints and in different contexts. A child's behaviour can vary substantially from setting to setting, and from adult to adult.

Assessors may not find it easy to understand one another, or to arrive at a commonly agreed assessment.

The content of what is noticed inevitably reflects the personal abilities of the assessor, and the organizational resources of the context within which he is operating. At the personal level we may note the availability of skills in interviewing, in making sense of situations, and in enabling those interviewed to be 'who they are' in the presence of the interviewer (many interviewers seem unable to achieve this last condition with children). The 'philosophy of life' of the assessor is of prime importance—especially in terms of how far it reflects the nature of his fellow men, and how far it permits and indeed encourages individual differences in self-fulfilment. At the organizational level, interviewing can be affected by the availability of space and time, and of channels for exchanging information and views about information with other involved providers of services.

The part the person or persons being assessed play in the process of assessment is obviously critical, but it can be difficult to unravel. All too frequently assessment does not take adequate account of what the client notices in his life, and the sense *he* makes of what he does notice. Perhaps even less does assessment seek to ask what sense the client makes of the process of assessment itself.

An additional dilemma in assessment relates to the extent to which the assessors should carry their studies beyond the capacity of the available services to follow up what is noticed. The person studied may experience the process of assessment itself as the initial stage of service, and be led to expect that service will be continued according to the principles of elaborate concern which have informed assessment. If his expectations are too severely disappointed he may turn away from using the service which actually is available.

The organization of assessment is primarily concerned to bring the above factors under control. The initial stages of assessment for children are likely to be carried out under the auspices of a juvenile court in England and Wales, or a Children's Hearing in Scotland. Normally they will seek information about a child's nature and background from various sources, making particular use of social workers. When it is thought that the issue which brings the child to notice may point to complications in his life, he may be placed in an assessment centre for a period, when his behaviour will be available for observation under a variety of conditions and by a range of staff members. At some point the staff will formulate their views of his nature and these views, together with observations from outside sources (in particular, a social worker's view on life in the child's home), will be collated to produce a composite picture. Such a procedure, however, leaves a number of questions unanswered, not the least of which is uncertainty about what can be learned of a child's ability to live in one social context by observing him living in another. In particular, observing him in the residential context of an assessment centre may give little guidance about his capacity to make use of a service which is geared to his living at home.

Assessment may be said to have two faces. On the one hand it is concerned to identify the possible services a child might use. On the other hand it is concerned to identify which available service can be used by which child. There are settings in which both perspectives are carried out by the same providers of service: the child enters, for example, a residential setting and assessment is concerned with how best to meet his needs in the light of the known nature of the setting (although even here different members of the setting may differ in their views about what the setting can offer). In other contexts assessment is carried out by people other than those who provide the follow-on service—as when an assessment centre assesses a child's suitability for a Community Home (in England) or a List D School (in Scotland).

In the final analysis, it may be necessary to acknowledge that much assessment can do little more than prepare the way for the initial shape of follow-on service. The form the service takes will depend on too many unknown factors. Assessment may be able to indicate a child's capacity to make use of a given type of service but there can be no certainty that even what appears to be the type of service in question is actually encountered as such by the child. Nor can there be any prior certainty in the case of a great many children that they can or cannot make use of a given (and inevitably changing) environment as they grow into it and become transformed by their ongoing experience of it.

The major patterns of service for children

Children living at home. Services for children during the post-war years have tended to be planned and implemented on the basis that whenever possible the child should reside in the parental home. This policy seems to have been a product partly of unexamined assumptions and partly of conclusions drawn from implementing various approaches to child care. Perhaps the most influential of the unexamined assumptions has been the importance accorded to the blood tie between child and natural parent. The conclusions drawn from implementation have often tended to be largely reactive, so that even when they have been associated with research (and they have by no means always been so associated) the emotional effects of the findings have tended to give undue direction to the conclusions drawn from those findings. An extreme example of this tendency occurred in the early and mid-1950s, when research by Bowlby and others into the effects of maternal deprivation was used to argue the invariant necessity of maintaining an intensive contact between mother and child.

In the 1960s a more balanced appreciation of the effects of mother–child separation began to be disseminated. In 1962 Ainsworth summarized the effects in part as follows: (1) recovery from a single brief separation will be fairly prompt, although possibly leaving vulnerability to future stress; (2) relief from fairly prolonged deprivation can result in rapid and dramatic improvement, although socialization and possibly other aspects of personality functioning may be retarded; (3) severe deprivation beginning early and lasting as long as three years, usually has serious adverse effects; (4) in the first year the earlier that deprivation is relieved the better; (5) language, the ability for abstract thinking, and the capacity for attention seem to be more permanently affected than other functions.

At the same time the case for holding the family together was being made in increasingly temperate terms. According to Dinnage & Kellmer Pringle (1967) 'The ordinary family setting not only provides surprisingly much more stimulation when measured in time studies, it also provides one or a few people, who are regularly present and deeply interested in the infant, and who respond to his communications, so giving him an opportunity to learn early to distinguish, recognize and enjoy specific individuals, to make sense of the environment, and to acquire the sense of being able to influence it.'

Implementing legislation directed at regulating the relations which exist between parents and children can run into many difficulties. Three major sources of difficulty are: first, the assumptions made about the nature of the grounds used to justify taking a child into care, for example, overestimating the degree of parental cruelty or mental disorder; second, the range of resources available for child care, for example, the widespread lack of facilities for providing any but residential (and perhaps fostering) care which tends to favour separating child from parent; and third, insufficiencies in the legislation itself, as when the problems of children are almost wholly located in family relationships without adequate reference to the influences of such environmental factors as the attitudes of teachers, police officers, ministers, doctors and neighbours, or the impact of housing, shopping and leisure facilities, or the 'culture of childhood' as expressed locally by adults and children.

It has been argued that services to children should pay more attention to providing facilities which would allow children to live at home: for example, that an increase in day care facilities, by reducing the tensions experienced by a mother, might in turn reduce the likelihood that family tensions will be released on the child. It has also been argued that services should be more concerned to ensure that due weight be given to the rights of the parent who, because of social disadvantage, may lack access to channels for presenting his case, or lack the ability to make use of any channels to which he does gain access.

Arguments in favour of maintaining various types of parent–child contact must, however, be grounded on a clear appreciation of the limits and possibilities of such contacts. An understanding of effective patterns of parenting and how to achieve these in given types of family is required, as is a proper grasp of what to do to give the child a sense of personal continuity if he or she has to move from the parental home to, for example, a foster home and back again. The social worker who supervises a child in his own home must be constantly alert to the quality of parenting which the child is receiving and must possess the ability to work with members of the family to enrich their contacts with the child. It is tempting for the hard-pressed social worker (or any other provider of services in contact with the child and/or his family) to rest content with evidence which indicates that the child's life is free of serious incidents of violence, physical or emotional. However, it should be remembered that a child's personal world is the product of all his relationships with his family, and the effects of family strife or inadequate parenting can be hard to detect at any given time: it should also be remembered that violence is itself difficult to detect, especially with assurance, and that a broad approach to a family's life-style is more likely to give indications of things going wrong than a narrow one focusing perhaps on the child and his mother, or perhaps only on one or other of these (many social workers seem largely to ignore the child, and to focus their attention on the mother: the father can also be ignored as can other family members).

A strong case can be argued for social workers making more imaginative use than they usually do of ancillary services which might enable children to live at home. An extension of the Home Help Service can make it possible for some single parents (and perhaps especially fathers) to provide a viable home for younger children. Limited experiments have been made using peripatetic foster parents to enable children to remain in their own home. Day nurseries (and nursery schools) can also contribute to a general easing of the stress on parents for whom the need to look after a child throughout the day can prove too great a burden. The Day Nurseries and Child Minders Regulations Act 1948 requires registration with social work services departments. Lack of staff time amongst social workers seems to have led to the requisite supervision often being very cursory. A substantial amount of unregistered child-minding seems to indicate the very great need for this type of service. Adequate resources could well make possible an important development in this aspect of social work services for children living at home. In particular there is a need for social workers to be available to affirm the importance of emotional and intellectual stability and stimulation in many of the presently under-supervised (or even unsupervised) instances of child-minding, day nurseries, and pre-school playgroups.

For the emotionally disturbed child the Child Guidance Clinic can provide a way to increased family harmony. Much of the work here is linked to failure to attend school or behavioural difficulties at school. Whilst child disturbance is normally to be found associated with family conflict, difficulties at school may be linked to the organization and conduct of school staff and children at large. Child Guidance thus involves a substantial social perspective. Child Guidance teams include social workers (employed by the local authority) who may work with the family in the home as well as with school staff and others. Social workers may also be based in schools. Education Welfare Officers (employed by the Education Authority) may provide a variety of services to ensure that children benefit from the educational opportunities available to them.

Foster care. The 1948 Children Act specifies the responsibilities of the local authority with regard to boarding-out, adoption, and residential care. The authority is advised to board-out children whenever possible in preference to placing them in residential care.

The Boarding-out of Children Regulations 1955 define fostering in terms of the child living with foster parents in their dwelling as a member of the family. The Memorandum on Boarding-out issued by the Scottish Home Department in 1959 states 'Boarding-out is a great deal more than the finding of a house in which a child may be given a bed and board, kept reasonably clean, and sent regularly to school, it is, in its essential meaning, the creation of a home for the child.'

Creating a home for the child depends on the duration of the foster placement, on the attitudes of the child and his natural parents, on the ability of the foster parents to live with the child—and on his ability to live with them—and on the approach to fostering adopted by the local authority social services committee and their staff of social workers. The child in short-stay care should not become greatly attached to the foster parents, even if he is so inclined. The child in long-stay care is nowadays likely to arrive after a history of attempts to keep him in his family of origin. Frequently he will be deeply disturbed, when the foster parents may find themselves confronted with behaviour which only a trained adult could handle without upset.

The Boarding-out of Children Regulations (1955) and the Scottish Regulations (1959) govern all boarding-out by both local authorities and voluntary organizations. They require that before boarding-out a social worker shall make a written report on the physical conditions of the foster home, and on such characteristics of the foster parents as their religious persuasion, their physical and mental health, and any findings of guilt which might indicate their unsuitability to associate with a child. The Regulations require authorities to visit the child at set intervals, to review his progress at least once every six months, to arrange for regular medical and dental care and to move the child at once if his health, safety or morals are thought to be at risk. If the child is in care under section 1 of the 1948 Act the parents can insist on their right to have him returned on request. Children placed privately with foster parents are protected under the Children Act 1958 and the Children and Young Persons Act 1969: any persons acting as foster parents for more than six days to children not personally related to them are subject to inspection by the local authority.

The essential vulnerability of the foster parent renders many prone to fantasies concerning the loss of the child and the motives of child care officials. The power of the social worker to enter the home, and to comment upon the foster parents' style of child rearing, can be a ready source of negative attitudes. His acquaintance with the child's natural parents may lead the foster parents to treat him as an ally of the natural parents, to be rejected or manipulated in accordance with the problems they have about fostering another person's child. Interviews which he holds with the foster child in the absence of the foster parents may encourage them in the conviction that he is 'spying on' or 'setting the child against' them.

A skilled approach by the social worker can, however, make constructive use of these factors. The foster parents can be helped to face their fantasies. They can examine their feelings about the natural parents, and the social worker may be able to facilitate meetings between foster and natural parents. The social worker can use his extensive knowledge of the child's history and social background to make more understandable to the foster parents the child's otherwise easy to misunderstand behaviour. His interviews with the child can serve to help the child to come to terms with his foster parents. Provided the foster parents can be helped to feel involved, these interviews may result in a greater harmony between child and foster parents. For many children breakdown of a foster placement can be catastrophic, uncertain as they are of their natural parents' feeling for them. Often it is the child who most needs a stable foster home who does the most to ensure that his placement will break down.

Successful fostering seems to be associated with such factors as the following. The foster parents must be able to value the child 'for himself'. Fostering in order to resolve one's own family problems is unlikely to achieve anything but distress for all concerned. Ideally, the fostered child will receive satisfactions within the foster family's overall experience of satisfaction at having him live with them. Among the obstacles which may confront people interested in fostering are inappropriate housing, limited finance, lack of social work support and unhelpful public attitudes. A number of local authorities are seeking to develop new ways of overcoming these obstacles—for example, by paying suitable foster parents at a rate which allows them to provide a service free from financially avoidable deficiencies.

Under the Children Act 1948, the local authority is given the responsibility to oversee the well-being of children whose care and maintenance are undertaken for reward for a period exceeding one month by a person who is not a relative or guardian. Under the Adoption Act 1958, the authority has similar responsibilities and powers with respect to the 'protected child', that is, any child of compulsory school age or under who is placed by a third party with adults who are not relatives or guardians, and who do not receive any form of reward for the child's care and maintenance. In the case of children placed by their parents with adults without payment, the authority has no powers or responsibilities. In Scotland, the 1968 Act requires the local authority to visit a child who is fostered for a period of more than six days, providing that the overall period of fostering is not intended to last less than one month.

Adoption. The Adoption Acts of 1958, 1960 and 1964, and the Children and Young Persons Act 1975 consolidate earlier legislation. The Adoption Act of 1958 defines legal adoption as a process whereby 'all rights, duties, obligations, and liabilities of the parents or guardians of the infant in relation to the future custody, maintenance and education of the infant . . . shall be extinguished, and all such rights, duties, obligations, and liabilities shall rest in, and be exercisable by and enforceable against he adopter, as if the infant were a child born of the adopter in lawful wedlock'.

Adoption is possible in the case of all unmarried children under 18 years of age. Children may be placed for adoption by their own parents or legal guardians, by a third party, by a registered adoption society or by a local authority social services department. However, only a local authority or an adoption agency registered by a local authority may actually arrange for a child to be adopted. Adoption Orders may be made by a Juvenile, a County or a High Court (or in Scotland by a Sheriff Court), guided by the enquiries and reports of a guardian *ad litem* (in Scotland a *curator ad litem*), who is usually a social worker or a probation officer. The adopters must be the child's parents, or relatives over 21 or unrelated married couples where the husband is at least 25 and the wife is at least 21.

The Children and Young Persons Act 1975 requires local authorities to establish adoption agencies as an integral part of the work of the social services department. The period of probationary care under a guardian *ad litem* is extended from three to twelve months. Custodianship as an alternative to adoption is established: the custodian can be given powers over the person of the child without the assumption of full parenthood—in this way the interests of the child living under conditions of long-term fostering can be guarded. The Act permits the consent of the child's natural parents to be set aside when the child is abandoned or persistently ill-treated or where, in the view of the Court, parental consent is unreasonably withheld (the father of an illegitimate child must be informed of the child's proposed adoption but his consent is not required unless he has formally applied for custody under the Guardianship of Minors Act 1971). The Act also re-emphasizes the importance of foster care and the status of foster parents.

The 1958 Act states that except when the 'infant of school age or under' is to be adopted by a parent, the applicant for an adoption order must, at least three months before the date of the order, give notice in writing to the appropriate local authority of intention to apply to a court for an adoption order. The social services department then has the responsibility to arrange for the adoptive home to be visited and for the child to be supervised until the order is made. This responsibility can lead to complications. In the majority of cases the adoptive parents have already developed a good relation with the adoption agency, and the social worker can easily become an unwanted third party. Skilled intervention can help in certain instances, however, as when the adoptive parents welcome the opportunity to discuss matters they feel unable to raise with the adoption agency, although here again such discussion may lead to problems between the social services department and the adoption agency.

The Adoption Rules require the court to appoint a person who has the duty to safeguard the interests of the infant before the court. This guardian *ad litem* of the infant (in Scotland the *curator ad litem*) is required to investigate the circumstances of the adoption, to ascertain the physical and economic state of the applicants and their home, to interview all the people concerned, to make sure that all the necessary consents have been freely given and, whenever possible, to ascertain the infant's attitude towards the adoption.

The child for adoption is usually, but not always, illegitimate. The mother's feelings about retaining him or placing him for adoption are likely to be very mixed. Often the future is obscure and particularly if she is young, she may be unable to see her way to maintaining herself with a fatherless child. Alternatively, her youth and lack of experience may encourage undue optimism concerning her ability to bring up her child on her own. The parents of such young mothers may be deeply offended and refuse to help: however, the intelligent intervention of a skilled social worker can frequently tap latent reserves of family goodwill. The mother must explore these and other relevant aspects of her situation with the social worker, and must be helped to appreciate the irrevocable nature of adoption. If she decides on adoption, then when the child has been placed, and always after he is over the age of six weeks, the mother is asked to complete and sign a witnessed form of consent. The mother may specify the religion in which she desires the child to be brought up. Application for an adoption order cannot be considered by the Court unless the child has been continuously in the care of the prospective adoptive parents for at least three months. The three months cannot begin before the child is six weeks old.

Residential care. There are two conflicting sets of principles impinging on residential care. On the one hand there are the persistent themes of contemporary child care: to facilitate relations between children and their parents, to participate as far as possible in the everyday life of society, and to diminish the period spent in residence. On the other hand there is the responsibility to the handicapped and disturbed child to provide him with a regimen suited to his nature; there is also the obligation to satisfy the expectations of a society that classifies certain children as being in need of a form of care which is based on discipline and social constraints and which is aimed at rehabilitation. A reasonably comprehensive system of residential care must include establishments concerned with assessment; establishments concerned with providing 'the opportunity to live' to children whose nature prevents them from getting such opportunity in open society; establishments concerned with the care of children who, although not fostered or adopted, are perfectly capable of living in open society; and establishments designed to abate the anxiety and aggression felt by society against those children who break the law, or contravene certain strongly upheld customs.

Children who are classified as chiefly needing a caring regimen in which to grow up may be accommodated in hostels or in children's homes. Hostels enable the child to go out into the community for schooling or employment, and for leisure. The adolescent can benefit from hostel life, for he is at a stage of development which especially draws on experience in open society. Such accommodation is currently provided by certain local authorities and voluntary bodies for working boys and girls in care, and for adolescents on probation. On a somewhat similar basis the adolescent unmarried mother may enter a mother and baby home and there spend a number of weeks before and after the birth in a supportive atmosphere, where such difficult problems as whether to have the baby adopted and how to relate to parents can be explored and, hopefully, resolved.

Children's homes may variously offer the opportunity to participate in the life of open society. *The family group home* is located in a residential neighbourhood and is either purpose-built, or adapted from one or two council houses. Between six and 12 children are accommodated, normally in the charge of a married woman with a husband who goes out to work and who provides some 'masculine influence'; alternatively one or more housemothers may run the unit. A shortcoming of this fairly intensive type of care is that staff turnover can have an acute effect on the family group; and for a variety of reasons, staff turnover may be frequent.

The *large children's home* may be purpose-built or consist of a converted private dwelling house, often of substantial proportions. Up to 50 children may be accommodated, and regimens vary: some emphasize small group living, with units of six to 12 children being allocated a part of the building as their own, with a housemother in charge; others utilize the entire building as the child's basic unit of living. Contact with the community at large depends upon the type of child in residence, the geographical location of the establishment, and the principles of residential work observed by the staff, and in particular by the superintendent or warden in charge. Homes of this type are suited to children who need specialist regimens of care. They are being used increasingly to accommodate the seriously disturbed child who can thus be 'distributed' over a wide range of staff. The larger children's home offers staff a more varied way of life than the family group home, a promotion structure, and less stress in the event of staff sickness or resignation.

The *grouped cottage home* consists of a number of separate dwelling units each housing between eight and 20 children, and with a total population of as many as 300 or more. This pattern of residential life permits a family type atmosphere in the separate units, and may thus to some extent resemble the family group home. In general, grouped cottage homes have their own playing fields, assembly halls, sick bays, and sometimes chapels and swimming baths. The centralization of facilities may have two unfavourable consequences. First, the children are often almost wholly out of touch with the conditions of life in open society; and second, it is becoming increasingly difficult to find able staff who are prepared to live under the continuous oversight of seniors, and to accept the restricted opportunities for social life which the isolation of the establishment so frequently entails.

Children under the age of five who cannot be boarded out have tended to be treated as a special group. They may be placed in residential nurseries provided by local authorities or voluntary organizations. In the case of the infant and very young child no other setting may be able to provide the intensity of care needed. In general, however, the nursery approach has come to be regarded as too specialized for the somewhat older child: he benefits from contact with children of all ages, and the principles of nursery nursing are not always appropriate to his needs. Many are instead being placed in family group homes which provide whatever additional facilities are necessary.

Many children come into care at short notice. It is therefore not always possible to have a suitable foster placement ready for them. Children's homes also have their problems about taking on children at short notice. A home with a basic population of 'long-stay' residents would be seriously disturbed by a continuous turnover of short-stay children. The Children Act 1948 states that a local authority's residential accommodation must include separate provision for the temporary reception of children. Furthermore, facilities must be available for observing their physical and mental condition. Facilities for accommodating siblings together are especially difficult to arrange.

The *children's reception home* is intended to fulfil these requirements, although the use to which it is actually put varies with local policy. Some authorities place the majority of short-stay children directly into foster homes, whilst others, perhaps because of a different admission procedure, perhaps because of a shortage of foster homes, base their temporary reception on the reception home. Others again seek to leave the reception home free for more specialist functions by establishing short-stay children's homes. As the practice of residential care acquires a more systematic foundation of tested theory and practice, with links being established between forms of care and quality of need, the assessment facilities of the reception home will come to play an increasingly central part in the comprehensive service. Children who have come into care under conditions of acute crisis may need special forms of care rarely available to those living in children's and foster homes. The reception home can in principle provide a suitable protected environment, with the children being able to receive special schooling and psychiatric attention within the building.

Recent thinking about the residential care of delinquents, as exemplified by the Social Work (Scotland) Act 1968, the Report of the Seebohm Committee 1968, the Children and Young Persons Act 1969, and the Local Authority Social Services Act 1970, has tended to favour setting up a unified system of 'in care' provision to cover all children unable to reside with their natural parents. It is argued that so far as effective care and treatment are concerned the child who commits an offence, and even more so that child in moral danger, is in no essential respect different from other categories of child in care.

Education authorities have the responsibility of providing appropriate teaching for children who are handicapped physically, or who are of limited intelligence, or who are classified as being maladjusted. Authorities may provide facilities which enable the child to live at home; some children must however attend residential schools. Seriously disturbed children may go to specially designed units: a few end up in psychiatric hospitals.

After-care
Eventually the child in residential care returns to his parental home, or failing that enters some form of lodgings. The social services department has the responsibility of supporting him during this period. Ideally a social worker will have been working with both child and family to facilitate reintegration. Hopefully he will have become a point of reference for them all. This approach to after-care as simply one part of a comprehensive family service is implied in the Social Work (Scotland) Act 1968 and in the Local Authority Social Services Act 1970 (England and Wales).

Voluntary organizations have a long and substantial history of providing services to children. They have frequently pioneered forms of service which would otherwise have been unavailable. The early history of Dr Barnardo's or of the National Society for the Prevention of Cruelty to Children provides instances. With the growth of local authority social work services, many voluntary organizations have extensively rethought their activities into new and otherwise unavailable or imperfectly available directions. Thus the NSPCC has developed services to the battered child and battered wife, whilst Barnardo's are extending their commitment to services which facilitate children living in the parental home or with skilled long-term foster parents, or with adoptive parents prepared to provide a home for the older child.

Problems associated with providing social services for children
Current patterns of social work services for children are subject to a wide range of confusions and conflicts. These derive partly from the diversity of attitudes which are abroad in society today towards parent–child relationships, and partly from the ever-proliferating range of services which social workers are expected to provide. It is impossible to understand the forms taken by today's services unless we appreciate something of the doubts and uncertainties which lie within them. If social work is to have a viable future, some at least of these doubts and uncertainties must be resolved: in the process social work must change into unfamiliar, and perhaps unanticipated, forms.

The uncertainties and changing nature of social work services for children will be illustrated with reference to two central dimensions of practice.

Problems associated with the direction and control of relationships between adults and children
1. Adults are often not good at dealing with the effects which children have on them. Children would seem to have the power to move the residues of child-

hood experience in adults. If these residues are especially powerful the adult may react in a highly subjective manner. If he sees the child's actions as the product of the actions of one or more other people, he will defend the child against them (and thereby defend himself). If he sees the child as the source of the behaviour which disturbs him, or if, whilst acknowledging that the child is reacting to the behaviour of other people, he feels himself unable to defend the child from these people, he may either blame the child or blame the other people. However, whether he defends the child or whether he blames him, he is essentially engaged in defending himself from his own experience of distress: in neither instance is he concerned to enquire into the actual nature of the child's distress. Social workers are increasingly seeking to devise ways by which the processes of adult self-defence can be controlled to permit the provision of services more realistically geared to the total experience and need of the child.

2. The differences between the ways children and adults make sense of the world are often insufficiently appreciated by adults. One consequence is to make communication with children relatively ineffective. Adults must learn to give due weight to what children notice and how they use what they notice to convey accounts of what it is like to live in their world.

3. Children need to be children in relation to adults. They can only become who they are capable of becoming if an adult sets boundaries for their self-discovery and growth. These boundaries must be open to redefinition when the child grows beyond them. Social work with children calls for the social worker to establish creative limits in his relationship with them (i.e. to be able to stimulate them to action within boundaries which give them a sense of security). It also requires that he be able to show the child's parents ways by which they may, after their own fashion, relate productively to their children.

4. The vulnerability of children to what adults say and do is often not fully appreciated by adults. Confronted by an unperceptive adult they may respond not so much in terms of what he is referring to by his words or actions as in terms of the distress he is generating in them. Thus they may be aggressive towards him, or agree to anything he proposes, or lapse into total silence. Effective work with children entails being able to release and live with the feelings which children have. Their frequent incapacity to cope with their feelings makes them especially vulnerable when decisions about their future are being made. It is for this reason that certain children may be said to lack personal rights unless an adult advocates these rights on their behalf.

Problems associated with organizing services to children

Services to children may be organized at three levels. Each level is currently producing problems for social workers concerned with the needs of children.

1. At the level of the individual worker there is widespread uncertainty about where to draw the boundaries of legitimate practice. This uncertainty is concerned with, first, the range of activities which a social worker may be expected to carry out; and, second, the degree of detail and skill which should inform each of the activities which he does carry out. The recent tendency to promote so-called 'generic practice' has meant that virtually any type of service to a family experiencing problems in everyday living might be argued as legitimate for a

social worker. Certain categories of work have inevitably received more attention than others. Work with children has tended to be one such category. However, the quality of the work done has in a great many instances been affected by the social worker's awareness of how many other demands for service he is failing to meet.

Social work with all categories of person requiring service must be constructed within frameworks of legitimacy if it is to be effective. Many of these frameworks must be provided for the social worker. However, within the boundaries which define the limits of his practice he must be free to take courses of action which are appropriate to the circumstances in which he finds himself. The fluid and pressing nature of many of the problems of living which come his way is such that, without a substantial area of discretion, the social worker would be unable to make a relevant contribution.

Work with the child in the family highlights the dilemma which faces social work today over reconciling the need for boundaries with the need for discretion. A number of cases concerning physical damage and even death to children seem to have been associated with uncertainties on the part of social workers about the proper focuses of their concern, and with agency and social pressures to take on more activities than they were capable of doing effectively. Reaction to these cases tends to favour seeking to contain the actions of social workers within boundaries which would ensure that nothing was done by them unless they were certain of the outcome. The effect of such proposals would be to favour removing children to 'places of safety' on a far more substantial scale than at present. Children who have problems of living within the context of their natural family are inevitably 'at risk'. However, it is an essential part of living to be 'at risk': the issue here is not to eliminate the risk but to think through vigorously the amount of 'living at risk' which a given child and his family can maintain under reasonable control with the continuing assistance of social workers and other providers of services to the child in the family. At the same time social workers and other employees are being challenged over the rights of children and of parents (sometimes the rights in question ally children and parents, sometimes they set their interests against one another). Many of the duties and tasks of social workers give them a built-in advantage over their clients which the attitudes of their clients may compound. At present there are few formalized ways in which a dissatisfied client can appeal against the consequences for him of the work done by social workers.

2. The problems which face the agency organizing services for children are in part complementary to those which face the individual worker. Many agencies provide too little guidance to their staff about how to organize their practice. However, increasing attention is being given to establishing ways which permit and encourage practitioners to face the actual distresses of the child in the family whilst taking full account of the organizational and statutory limitations and the services which can be provided—for example, the function of the senior social worker in staff supervision is being developed, higher management are learning how to define the priorities of staff to maximize effectiveness, specialist jobs are being established at both practice and consultancy levels, and formalized approaches to staff collaboration are being worked out. An aspect of practice

which is calling for special attention is the allocation of financial support to families with children at risk—both the Children and Young Persons Act 1963 and the Social Work (Scotland) Act 1968 required social workers to provide financial aid to their clients if this would promote their welfare. The difficulty here is that financial aid can often function as a very short-term aid indeed, and can serve to protect both client and social worker from facing up to ways in which the client is generating his own difficulties. It can also serve to avoid the need to confront the extent to which the client's financial (and other) problems are affected by the policies of other institutions of society (such as Housing Departments or Social Security Departments) and of the conditions of society at large (e.g. the degree of unemployment in a given region).

3. In the past, and especially before the current upsurge of demand for multiple and often far-reaching services, a great many providers of service tended to operate with only marginal reference to the activities of other providers, even when these activities focused on the same recipients of service. This insularity was especially prevalent between agencies. Today such insularity is increasingly seen as a source of damaging effects on those in receipt of services. Benefit can be readily observed when the social work department collaborates with the housing department, or when teachers, general practitioners, health visitors and others join together with social workers in planning and carrying out a service to given children and their families.

This third aspect of organizing social services for children, ensuring effective practice between differentially based providers of service, may well come to be a major form of social work in the future. Amongst the activities involved will be the facilitating of collaborative practice in individual cases; setting up joint services for special categories of demand; establishing clearly recognized staff members who can act as channels for exchange of information between agencies, and as decision makers in respect of actions called for by the information exchanged; identifying standards of service appropriate to different categories of client and practitioner; and, of course, arriving at clear and acceptable decisions about the priorities to be observed by the different sections of the social work services involved.

Conclusion

This chapter on social work services for children has sought to give some indication of the immense complexity of the issues involved in the delivery of service, whilst at the same time giving some picture of the actual services delivered. Inevitably, in the space available, many important themes remain unmentioned.

Society has established social work services to provide certain types of service to children and their families. In so doing insufficient attention has been given to the feasibility of the ends which have been proposed or the relevance of the means which have been made available.

Social attitudes towards the provision of these services are highly confused and conflicting. Certain recommended services to children cannot be effectively provided because other social values make it impossible to do so. The child is all too frequently related to, not in his own right as a unique human person, but as a member of a family, social class, ethnic group, or 'problem category' (delinquent, mentally subnormal, physically handicapped) all of which activate negative attitudes of which he is the recipient. Society's attitudes to poverty, crime, promiscuity, emotional instability, social ineffectiveness, helplessness can all render ineffective a programme intended to benefit a child.

Over the past decade society has shown an increasing tendency to hand over to social workers those types of problem which arise out of confusions and conflicts in social attitudes. Social workers are then blamed when they fail to reduce the effects of such confusions and conflicts on their clientele. Many of the aims set for the social work services can only be carried through, if at all, when the whole of society contributes to the efforts which would be needed.

The individualization of the client in a largely antipathetic social context has traditionally been one of the major contributions of social work. This value is currently under question partly as a direct result of the pressure to provide services on a scale which precludes individualization, partly as an outcome of challenges about the effectiveness of individualization in achieving certain kinds of improvement in the condition of people (e.g. housing, financial benefits), and partly as a product of social policies which require social workers to provide services which reduce the likelihood that behaviour by the recipients of the services will cause distress for other members of society. Especially when the protected members of society are the socially influential, this leaves the social worker faced with children and adults whose expressions of their own distress he must control and play down.

Social workers are divided amongst themselves over virtually every possible priority in practice. They work with the concerns of all manner of people, who from their various standpoints are equally at odds, one with another, about what to notice, what sense to make of what is noticed, and what to do about the sense made. In sum, social work reflects the many doubts and uncertainties of contemporary society about how men should live, and those who look to social workers for service must expect to meet with the consequence of these confusions and conflicts.

FURTHER READING

1. About children
Writings on the nature and background of children which can shed light on possible focuses of concern for social work services for children have multiplied in recent years. The following raise many of the fundamental issues.

Bowlby J 1951 Maternal care and mental health. WHO, Geneva
Bowlby J 1965 Child care and the growth of love. Penguin, Harmondsworth. Contains 2 chapters by Ainsworth on the adverse effects of maternal deprivation
Bruner J 1975 The relevance of education. Penguin, Harmondsworth
Carter J (ed) 1974 The maltreated child. Priory Press, London
Davie R, Butler N, Goldstein H 1972 From birth to seven. Longman, and the National Children's Bureau, London
Department of Health and Social Security 1972 The 'battered baby syndrome'. HMSO, London
George V, Wilding P 1972 Motherless families. Routledge & Kegan Paul, London
Holman R (ed) 1970 Socially deprived families in Britain. Bedford Square Press, London
Howells J 1974 Remember Maria. Butterworth, London
Kempe R S, Kempe C H 1978 Child abuse. Fontana/Open Books, London
Marsden D 1969 Mothers alone: poverty and the fatherless family. Allen Lane, London

Morgan P 1975 Child care, sense and fable. Temple Smith, London
Pringle M L K 1974 The needs of children. Hutchinson, London
Ren J 1975 Children in danger. Penguin, Harmondsworth
Rutter M 1972 Maternal deprivation reassessed. Penguin, Harmondsworth
Rutter M 1975 Helping troubled children. Penguin, Harmondsworth
Wedge P, Prosser H 1973 Born to fail. Arrow Books, and National Children's Bureau, London
Winnicott D W 1969 The child, the family and the outside world. Penguin, Harmondsworth
Wolff S 1974 Children under stress. Penguin, Harmondsworth

2. About the provision of social work services for children

Writings in this area tend to focus on concerns which are associated with (a) ways of classifying children who might share common needs and therefore might be able to use a common service, for example the maltreated child, or the handicapped child; (b) ways of providing services which have a core of common characteristics for all children, for example foster care, residential care; and (c) ways of planning, organizing and delivering services.

Balbernie R 1966 Residential work with children. Pergamon Press, Oxford
Beedell C 1970 Residential life with children. Routledge & Kegan Paul, London
Berlins M, Wansell G 1974 Caught in the act. Penguin, Harmondsworth
Berry J 1972 Social work with children. Routledge & Kegan Paul, London
Berry J 1975 Daily experience in residential life. Routledge & Kegan Paul, London
Brunel Institute of Organisation and Social Studies 1972 Social services departments. Heinemann, London
Central Council for Education and Training in Social Work 1978 Good enough parenting. Study 1. CCETSW, London
Davies B, Barton A, McMillan I 1972 Variations in children's services amongst British urban authorities. Bell, London
Dinnage R, Pringle M L K 1967 Foster home care: facts and fallacies. Longman, and the National Children's Bureau, London
Dinnage R, Pringle M L K 1967 Residential child care: facts and fallacies. Longman, and the National Children's Bureau, London
Dockar-Drysdale B 1968 Therapy in child care. Longman, London
Donnison D, Chapman W 1974 Social policy and administration. Allen & Unwin, London
Fabian Society 1970 The fifth social service. Fabian Society, London
Franklin A W (ed) 1975 Concerning child abuse. Churchill Livingstone, Edinburgh
George V N 1970 Foster care: theory and practice. Routledge & Kegan Paul, London
Heywood J S, Allen B K 1971 Financial help in social work. University Press, Manchester
Holgate E (ed) 1972 Communicating with children. Longman, London
Holman R 1973 Trading in children. Routledge & Kegan Paul, London
Jordan W 1972 The social worker in family situations. Routledge & Kegan Paul, London
King R, Raynes N, Tizzard I 1971 Patterns of residential care. Routledge & Kegan Paul, London
Laycock A L 1970 Adolescence and social work. Routledge & Kegan Paul, London
Oswin M 1974 Empty hours: weekend life of handicapped children in institutions. Penguin, Harmondsworth
Packman J 1975 The child's generation. Blackwell, Oxford
Parfit J 1972 Spotlight on physical and mental assessment. National Children's Bureau, London
Parfit J 1972 Spotlight on services for the young handicapped child. National Children's Bureau, London
Parker R A 1966 Decision in child care: a study of prediction in fostering. Allen & Unwin, London
Pringle M L K 1967 Adoption, facts and fallacies. Longman, and the National Children's Bureau, London
Pringle M L K 1968 Caring for children. Longman and the National Children's Bureau, London
Rodgers B, Stevenson J 1973 A new portrait of social work. Heinemann, London
Timms N (ed) 1973 The receiving end: consumer accounts of social help for children. Routledge & Kegan Paul, London

3. About legislation and policy

Social work services for children are grounded on legislation and policy, although as has been previously indicated in themselves legislation and policy give only limited guidance about the service which might be received in a given setting. The following are some major documents, in order of publication.

Children and Young Persons Act 1963	HMSO, London
The child, the family and the young offender 1965	HMSO, London
Social work and the community 1967	HMSO, Edinburgh
Children in trouble 1968	HMSO, London
Report of the Committee on the Local Authority and Allied Personal Services (Seebohm Report) 1968	HMSO, London
The Social Work (Scotland) Act 1968	HMSO, London
Children and Young Persons Act 1969	HMSO, London
Goldstein J, Freud A, Solnit A 1973 Beyond the best interests of the child	The Free Press, New York
The Local Authority Social Services Act 1974	HMSO, London
Report on the Committee of Inquiry into the care and supervision provided in relation to Maria Colwell 1974	HMSO, London
Report of the Committee of Inquiry into the consideration given and the steps taken towards securing the welfare of Richard Clark by Perth Town Council and other bodies or persons concerned 1975	HMSO, Edinburgh
Terry J 1976 A guide to the Children Act 1975	Sweet & Maxwell, London
Hoggett B 1977 Parents and children	Sweet & Maxwell, London

For an extremely thorough survey of relevant reading, reference should be made to:

Sainsbury E E 1977 The personal social services. Pitman, London

Part Five: Health and School

The School Health Service: organization

Historical development

It has been appreciated for several hundred years that there is a connection between the physical condition of children and their capacity to benefit from education. The idea that schoolchildren should be medically examined was published in Germany 200 years ago (Frank, 1780) and school doctors were appointed in Sweden as early as 1840. Towards the end of the nineteenth century there was considerable interest in school health throughout Europe and services were started in several countries including France, Germany and Russia. In Britain, school inspections were started in advance of legislation by a few enlightened local authorities.

The education of handicapped children was the subject of laws that were enacted in the closing years of the last century. Under the Elementary Education (Blind and Deaf Children) Act 1893 parents were obliged to submit their children for education and local authorities had a duty to provide or support suitable schools. The Elementary Education (Defective and Epileptic Children) Act 1899 was permissive but although the powers that it conferred were not applied in many areas, it was noteworthy because the work of ascertaining whether or not children were defective or epileptic was given to a qualified Medical Officer approved by the Education Department—the first time in this country that a doctor had been given statutory powers in connection with school administration.

The impetus to mandatory medical examinations came from public concern about the large number of army recruits for the Boer War who were found to be physically unfit. A Royal Commission on Physical Training (Scotland) in 1903 reviewed arrangements for physical training in schools and recommended medical inspection, not only for remedial purposes but also to obtain information about the health of schoolchildren. In England, an Interdepartmental Committee on Physical Deterioration was appointed 'to inquire into the health and physique of the people, to indicate the causes of such physical deterioration as exists and to make recommendations as to the means by which it can be most effectively diminished'. In its report, published in 1904, eight of the 53 recommendations concerned schoolchildren. One was that 'a systematized Medical Inspection of schoolchildren should be imposed as a public duty on every school authority'. As a result of this and a subsequent enquiry by the President of the Board of Education (1905), two important pieces of legislation were enacted by

Parliament. They were the Education (Provision of Meals) Act 1906 and the Education (Administrative Provisions) Act 1907. The latter ordered local authorities 'to provide for the medical inspection of children immediately before, or at the time of, or as soon as possible after their admission to a public elementary school'. In the same year a circular from the Board of Education indicated that three examinations of each child during this school life would be required (Circular 576, 1907).

In some European countries, school doctors were at first preoccupied with premises and the material conditions in which children were taught. Environmental hygiene has continued to be a concern of school health personnel but in Britain the service, from its inception, has been centred on the medical examination. A schedule of inspection and detailed notes for the inspecting officer which emphasized nutrition, hygiene and infectious disease were circulated (Circular 582, 1908). These remained the most important considerations for several decades and, even though there was a gradual improvement in the health of children, it was stated as late as 1921 that in London on average about 8 per cent of children were always absent on account of illness. Of those away for three months or more, rheumatism, heart disease and chorea were responsible for 21 per cent, tuberculosis for 20 per cent and nervous disorders, anaemia and ringworm for 7 per cent each (Annual Report of the Chief Medical Officer of the Board of Education for the year 1921).

The discovery of defects without facilities for treatment has a very doubtful value and laws were passed to permit local authorities to provide suitable care. A duty to make adequate arrangements to attend to the health of children in public elementary schools was first imposed by the Education Act 1918 and an obligation to ensure that pupils receive medical and dental treatment was restated in the Education Act 1944. A significant treatment role continued to be played by the School Health Service until the inception of the National Health Service in 1948 when, with the exception of dental treatment, the need declined.

As a consequence of the great reduction in the amount of serious illness in childhood during the past 30 years, the usefulness of routine medical inspections has been frequently questioned and their content and timing have been reappraised. Although the majority of children are physically well, many present educational problems due to intellectual subnormality, emotional illness, speech disorders and other conditions and the emphasis of school medical work has shifted towards their management. Considerable interest has also developed in the identification and care of handicapped children.

Objectives

The purpose of a School Health Service is to help to ensure that every child is able to derive full benefit from his education. This entails the prevention of disease in healthy children, making certain that ill children get appropriate treatment, caring for handicapped children and bringing medical expertise to learning problems. Of these component parts it is the last which is the essentially unique function and may be called educational medicine.

The School Health Service in Britain has failed to develop this distinct and specialized role and generally there appears to have been no clear understanding of the aims of educational medicine. A definition of the agreed objectives states that they are 'to maintain the health of schoolchildren, to identify and treat the handicapped and, by working closely with teachers and psychologists, to promote the study and understanding of the area where sensory, physical, intellectual, emotional and cultural factors merge and contribute as variables to specific learning disabilities and to general educational failure or success' (Scottish Home and Health Department, 1973).

The fundamental purposes of the School Health Service are consistent with those of paediatrics of which it forms an important part. Furthermore, they are in harmony with those of other professions concerned with the development and care of children. Their aims are to help individual children and to improve the quality of society, both now and for the future. Implicit in the latter is a political duty in the sense that politics is the exercise of public responsibility. Such a role demands not only technical expertise but also vision and hope.

Administration and legislative framework
In most western countries except Germany and the United States, authority over the School Health Service lies with the legislative body of the entire state. This has always been so in Britain where school health is a Secretary of State's responsibility. Before April 1st 1974, the School Health Service was provided by education departments, but this was changed by the National Health Service Reorganization Act, 1973 and the service now operates within the National Health Service as an integral part of it. In this and succeeding paragraphs, the arrangements in England are described: there are variations, for the most part of a minor nature, in other parts of the United Kingdom.

The duties and powers of local education authorities with respect to medical activities had been mostly derived from the Education Act 1944 and these were transferred to the National Health Service. The latter now has a statutory duty to provide for the medical inspection of pupils at maintained schools but although parents were formerly obliged to allow their children to be examined, this is no longer so. With the consent of the parent, free medical treatment can be arranged on school premises and in some areas this service is still available but in many others it is no longer considered to be necessary and is not provided. Parents have a legal right to be present at examinations and this is exercised by most parents of school entrants but with diminishing frequency as their children get older.

Medical officers may be authorized to inspect the body and clothing of children to find out if they are clean and verminous children may be excluded from school. Examinations may be undertaken to ascertain whether the health of children would be prejudiced by employment and others are done in connection with the supply of free milk for children between seven and 12 years, under the provisions of the Education (Milk) Act 1971.

There are specific duties concerned with handicapped children. The Education Act 1944, Section 34, requires local education authorities to ascertain which children in their area need special educational treatment. In England and Wales provided that the children have reached the age of two years, their parents may be obliged to submit them for examination by a medical officer. Equally they may request the local education authority to arrange for an examination to be carried out if they think that their child requires special education. They have a right to notice of the examination, to be present at it and to be informed of the result. A form (Form SE5) stating the nature and extent of any disability of mind or body may be used. There is machinery for parents to appeal to the Secretary of State against a decision that their child requires special education. In Scotland, education authorities may examine children from birth and have a statutory duty to do so in the case of children over five years. It has been recommended recently that the laws should be appropriately amended to give local education authorities the power to require not just a medical examination, but a multiprofessional assessment of children of any age from birth onwards and that parents should have a legal right to require local education authorities to provide such assessment (Warnock, 1978).

Although formal procedures exist there has, in recent years, been an increasing use of informal admission to special schools and classes. This has arisen for a number of reasons, not least the growth of developmental screening of pre-school children and the use of multidisciplinary assessment centres. Furthermore, the Education (Handicapped Children) Act 1970, which discontinued the classification of children as unsuitable for school because of ineducability, removed the need for formal ascertainment of a large group of children. The trend towards informal placement seems likely to continue, but it has been acknowledged that enforceable procedures will still be needed in a small minority of cases.

Regulations govern the qualifications of doctors who examine subnormal children. Unless he is a psychiatrist working in a Child Guidance Clinic, a doctor employed to examine children who may be educationally subnormal must first have attended an approved postgraduate course and must have spent a probationary period of six months assisting a qualified medical officer. Formerly the report of an approved medical officer stating the category of handicap was made directly to the local education authority but it is now recommended that this advice should be given by an experienced educational psychologist or adviser in special education after he has seen the child and received medical and other information (Department of Education and Science Circular 2/75).

The Employment Medical Advisory Service Act 1972 imposed a statutory duty on doctors employed in the School Health Service to provide information about pupils. An examination of the child is not obligatory and much of the information is gleaned from records. Advice about children with disabilities had been given to the Youth Employment Services for many years but the Act regularized the practice.

Regulations (Training of Teachers Regulations, 1967) require student teachers to be examined before admission to training colleges to ensure that they are in good health and teachers on first appointment may be required to satisfy the Secretary of State of their health and physical capacity for teaching (Schools Regulations, 1959). These examinations have generally been undertaken by the staff of the School Health Service. Certain diseases developing in teachers are notifiable to the Department of Education and Science.

Recruitment and training of personnel

The work required of the School Health Service by law is very diverse. Medical inspection is the biggest single item and this, together with the examination of children prior to employment and for the allocation of free milk, constitutes a form of primary paediatric care. The skill and training needed for these tasks are not as extensive as those required for providing advice about handicapped pupils and consultation about learning disorders. The latter demands a greater knowledge of paediatrics and does not differ in nature from other types of secondary care. Opinions about the employment of teachers should be the work of an occupational health service rather than of experts in child health and medical help in the planning and supervision of school premises belongs to the field of environmental medicine. It can be stated with justice that the School Health Service is not a single entity and for this reason a unitary approach to recruitment and training is inappropriate.

The School Health Service has been largely staffed by salaried medical officers. Most of them were engaged whole-time by the local authorities and subsequently transferred to the National Health Service, but in recent years an increasing proportion of doctors, including family practitioners, have been employed part-time. Any person with a medical qualification is entitled to work in the British School Health Service and the same is true in the Low Countries. In most other parts of Western Europe the service is staffed by paediatricians or doctors with special training.

Medical employees of the School Health Service have not enjoyed high status or prestige within their profession and their salaries are relatively low. There has been, and still is, a tendency for posts to be used as the first step on a ladder leading to a career in administrative and preventive medicine. As in the United States, school health work attracts many who do not wish to follow it as a life career. In Britain some are promoted to senior clinical posts in child health in which they gain a great deal of experience with handicapped children, but there is no clear progression or training for these jobs and in the past they have been isolated from the mainstream of paediatrics. It was suggested by the Committee on Child Health Services (Court, 1976) that the primary care work of the School Health Service should be done by 'general practitioner paediatricians' and that medical services for the handicapped child and advice about those with difficult learning disorders should come within the remit of 'consultant community paediatricians'. The government has not accepted these proposals at the time of writing and there are still many uncertainties about future staffing of the School Health Service.

Training needed

A *Proposed Report on Educational Qualifications of School Physicians* (1953) suggested that they should have an 'understanding of others, ability to select and help develop subordinates, ability to evaluate and improve accepted procedures, adaptability, a friendly but dignified manner, a liking for people and particularly children and an aptitude for preventive medicine. As important as any other personal quality is the personality and skill that will facilitate co-operative relationships with private practitioners.'

In the United States, it has been stated that 'Medical School teaching curricula allow little or no opportunity to acquaint the undergraduate student with school health problems' and that 'Residency training programs are ordinarily so hospital-based that the average graduate has had little or no preparation for dealing with this important aspect of child care' (Medovy, 1965). The same is true in Britain. More could probably be done at the undergraduate stage in most medical schools but essential education by experience must take place after graduation. It has been suggested that training for school health work should include, in addition to clinical paediatrics, at least a year spent in a full-time working apprenticeship within schools (Senn, 1965).

Doctors undertaking work in child health, including school health, need not only aptitude, sympathy and experience in dealing with children and their parents but also an understanding of the concepts of developmental medicine and a knowledge of the achievements of normal children at different ages. Competence in administering screening tests of development and in supervising tests of hearing and vision are required of them. They need to know how illness relates to attainment and how to identify handicapped children. Insight into the difficulties of social pathology and deviant behaviour is necessary and they require a tolerant and flexible approach to the particular problems of adolescence.

Some school doctors hold a Diploma in Public Health or a Diploma in Child Health but in the past there was no comprehensive postgraduate course for them. Specific training in the 'ascertainment' of mentally handicapped children was undertaken at four-week courses organized by the University of London jointly with the National Association for Mental Health but their emphasis was on the diagnosis of mental subnormality and the use of intelligence tests. In recent years several universities have run approved courses for school doctors that are more broadly based.

There has been an increasing use by local education authorities of National Health Service centres with facilities for the diagnosis and assessment of children with handicaps affecting educational progress (DES and DHSS, 1972). It is recognized that hospital-based assessment may be necessary for some children with severe or complex disorders but it is not suitable for all those who require special educational provision and it has been recommended that multiprofessional assessment should usually take place at a centre within the community other than a hospital (Warnock, 1978). Paediatricians should be employed in both types of centre and will require an understanding of the School Health Service and of educational medicine. They will need to know about paediatric neurology, behavioural science, ophthalmology and audiology and about educational philosophy and practice. These subjects have been incorporated into the programmes of training for consultant paediatricians to an increasing extent in recent years.

Other professions
Personnel from many other health professions besides medicine are employed in the School Health Service. The most numerous are nurses and more than half of them have a Health Visitor's Certificate. Health visitors have a particular responsibility for health education and for family counselling and health super-

vision. Nurses without this qualification should only be employed in clinics, special boarding schools or on specialist duties.

There are no special training programmes for ancillary medical staff employed in the School Health Service. There is, however, an obligation on the employing authority to engage only those therapists and technicians who have officially recognized qualifications.

Communication and records
Educational medicine cannot be practised in isolation and its effectiveness depends on co-operation with other professions concerned with the education and care of children. An increase in mutual confidence and reliance between the professions and a willingness to communicate within the educational team are needed. Unless these are developed, doctors will never fully understand the extent and nature of learning problems and the important contribution that they are able to make will be lost.

In practice there are usually personal contacts between senior education officers concerned with policy and Area Specialists in Community Medicine (Child Health), from whom local educational authorities have a statutory right to advice. The care of individual children and other day-to-day management decisions are usually delegated to senior clinical medical officers and to deputy or assistant education officers and much depends upon easy, informal communication between them.

The school doctor has three main directions of communication. His most important contact is with teachers: he normally meets the head teacher of any school in which he is conducting an inspection and frequently has the opportunity to talk to class teachers about individual children. Good relationships are facilitated by continuity of service in an area by one doctor.

It is important that school doctors should avoid isolation from their own profession and that they should liaise closely with family practitioners. Difficulties have arisen in the past about conflicting opinions and arrangements for referral for treatment. Such differences are not surprising when two sets of doctors are both providing primary care, and especially if there is little opportunity for personal contact. In order to avoid misunderstandings about referral for specialist opinion, the British Medical Association has recommended a form and procedure of referral for non-urgent cases that enables family practitioners to make alternative arrangements for their patients if they so wish.

Contacts with hospital specialist services, especially in paediatrics, ophthalmology, otorhinolaryngology and orthopaedics, are also important. In many areas arrangements have been made for copies of letters about consultations and hospital in-patient treatment to be sent from hospitals to school doctors. This practice facilitates understanding, helps to reduce inappropriate referral and ensures that specialist advice is applied for the child's benefit in his education. It has been recommended that it should occur as a matter of course (Warnock, 1978).

Much routine documentation is based on the use of standard forms and these are inevitably open to criticism because they tend to direct the content of examinations. The basic school health record used for every child is called Form

10M and an entry is made in it at all school medical inspections. It consists of a quarto-sized folding card and is printed out with boxed sections for various items of identification, history and examination. The card follows the child if he moves from one town to another.

Opinions about handicapped children are often conveyed on a series of forms recommended by the Department of Education and Science and known as the SE forms procedure. Medical reports are contained on Form SE2 in England and Wales and Form SE3 in Scotland. They have pages for disabilities of vision, hearing, speech and language, motor function, physical health, behaviour and emotional development and intellectual development. Apart from the last, each has sections enabling a description of the problem, its diagnosis and prognosis and the teaching and management implications to be recorded. There has been criticism that the forms do not provide adequately for contributions by child psychiatrists and other health professionals and it has been proposed that they should be revised and that their use should become mandatory (Warnock, 1978). A short medical certificate prescribed under the Education Act is referred to as Form SE5 (replacing the former Statutory Form IHP).

Medical forms are also required for the communication of opinions to the Employment Medical Advisory Service. These give a brief statement of the diagnosis and in broad terms the implications for employment.

All these formal procedures are undoubtedly useful and necessary but they cannot replace inter-professional discussion and consultation in the difficult case. In the School Health Service personal contact is no less important than in any other branch of medicine.

Resources and cost

A School Health Service costs money and uses skilled manpower. There is a relationship, though not necessarily a direct one, between the service provided and the resources used. In most countries the entire cost is met from taxes levied either locally or centrally, or by a combination of the two, but in some, for example France, the parents make a contribution.

Inflation and the different levels of service provided make comparisons difficult. In the financial year 1976-7 the net cost of the School Health Service to local authorities in England and Wales was £55 280 000 and this excluded capital expenditure (DHSS, Health Service Costing Returns, year ended 31.3.77: published 1979). It was a small proportion of the total health budget but it was, nevertheless, a substantial sum of money and whether it was worthwhile expenditure is a matter of opinion rather than of ascertained fact.

Careful analysis of the cost-productiveness of school health services has been urged (Nader, 1974) but it is an enormously complex problem. In order to be useful, separate analyses of the many diverse activities of the service would have to be made. An attempt to cost the School Entrance Examination in 1969 showed that the amount spent in staff salaries to complete the inspection of 1020 children was £593 so that the cost of inspecting each child is relatively low (Grant, 1970).

Criticism of the preventive child health services in Britain has been directed against their use of scarce medical and nursing personnel. In England and Wales in 1972 a whole-time equivalent of 985 medical officers and 3312 nurses was employed (DES, 1974). This approximates to one doctor and three nurses per seven to eight thousand pupils. In addition, the whole-time equivalent of 62 ophthalmic specialists and 17 other specialists was used, together with speech therapists, audiometricians, chiropodists, orthoptists and physiotherapists. This is a considerable body of trained personnel and their value is such that the usefulness of the tasks they are asked to do should be constantly under review.

The buildings and capital equipment used by the School Health Service are relatively unsophisticated compared to those required for other health service activities. Much of the work is rightly done in schools and often in multipurpose rooms. Special premises for school clinics often serve as centres from which the service operates and as venues for specialist clinics.

Relationship to other medical services

The School Health Service in Britain developed in isolation from other branches of medicine although co-ordination within public health departments was urged from the outset. Despite this, it remained separate from infant welfare for many years. During the past few decades, medical officers have commonly held joint appointments in both services and the same premises have been used for infant and school clinics.

The separation from the family practitioner and hospital paediatric services was understandable because they were both largely concerned with the treatment of childhood infections and their purpose was, therefore, different from that of the School Health Service. In recent years there has been a change in the pattern of morbidity and the importance of developmental paediatrics has been generally recognized so that there is now a greater confluence of interest among those providing medical services for children than at any time during this century. In these new circumstances, administrative unification of the National Health Service was timely and the proposition that all services for children should be represented in each paediatric divisional committee was appropriate (Scottish Home and Health Department, 1973).

REFERENCES

Board of Education, Circular 576. Memorandum on Medical Inspection of Children in Public Elementary Schools, Under Section 13 of the Education (Administrative Provisions) Act, 1907
Board of Education Circular 582. Education (Administrative Provisions) Act, 1907, Section 13, Schedule of Medical Inspection, 1908
Chief Medical Officer of the Board of Education 1922 Annual Report for the Year 1921. HMSO, London.
Chief Medical Officer of the Department of Education and Science 1974 The Health of the School Child, 1971–72. HMSO, London
Court, S D M (chairman) 1976 Fit for the future: The Report of the Committee on Child Health Services, HMSO, London
Department of Education and Science, Circular 2/75. (1975) HMSO, London
Department of Education and Science and Department of Health and Social Security. Working Party on Collaboration. First Report of School Health Service Sub-Committee (1972) HMSO, London
DHSS, Health Service Costing Returns 1976/77: published 1979
Education (Provision of Meals) Act 1906 HMSO, London
Education (Administrative Provisions) Act 1907 HMSO, London
Education Act 1918 HMSO, London

Education Act 1944 HMSO, London
Education (Handicapped Children) Act (1970) HMSO, London
Education (Milk) Act 1971 HMSO, London
Elementary Education (Blind and Deaf Children) Act 1893 HMSO London
Elementary Education (Defective and Epileptic Children) Act 1899 HMSO, London
Employment Medical Advisory Service Act 1972 HMSO, London
Frank J P 1780 'Eine Vollständige medizinische Politzei'
Grant G L 1970 Medical services and the school entrant's examination. Medical Officer 123: 189–193
Medovy H 1965 Symposium on school health problems. Pediatric Clinics of North America 12: 851–1109
Nader P R 1974 The school health service: making primary care effective. Pediatric Clinics of North America 21: 57–73
National Health Service Reorganisation Act 1973 HMSO, London
Proposed Report on Educational Qualifications of School Physicians 1953 American Journal of Public Health 43: 75–82
Report of the Interdepartmental Committee on Physical Deterioration 1904 HMSO, London
Report of the Interdepartmental Committee on Medical Inspection and Feeding of Children attending Public Elementary Schools 1905 HMSO, London
Report of the Royal Commission on Physical Training (Scotland) 1903 HMSO, London
Schools Regulations 1959 HMSO, London
Scottish Home and Health Department 1973 Towards an integrated Child Health Service HMSO, Edinburgh
Senn M J E 1965 The role, prerequisites and training of the school physician. Pediatric Clinics of North America 12: 1039–1056
Training of teachers regulations 1967 HMSO, London
Warnock H M (chairman) 1978 Special educational needs: The Report of the Committee of Enquiry into the Education of Handicapped Children and Young People HMSO, London

The School Health Service: methods

The purpose of this chapter is to review the methods generally used by the School Health Service in helping to ensure that every child is able to derive full benefit from his education. It concerns only those activities that involve children directly and not those such as environmental hygiene and teachers' health examinations that have often been undertaken by school doctors. The discussion is based on the premise that the supervision of the health of schoolchildren is a part of developmental paediatrics and that the unique contribution of the School Health Service is to study the medical aspects of learning problems.

School medical inspection
This, by far the largest item of school health activity, has been carried out routinely and with relatively little modification since the inception of the service. It is undertaken wherever school health is practised and, although the recommended number of examinations varies from country to country, universal examination of school entrants is regarded as an essential minimum. The school medical inspection has, nevertheless, been referred to as an anachronism and the comment made that, 'in an age of free medical care, generally good nutrition and a shortage of doctors, the search for defects among children of school age is hard to justify' (Lancet, 1966). Furthermore, it has been stated that the pressure of ritual and perfunctory examinations makes it impossible to engage in other worthwhile activities. The question is one of priorities; whether the use of this traditional method accomplishes more with the time and facilities available than could be achieved in other ways.

Place of inspection. The majority of school medical examinations take place in schools. This has the advantages that the children feel more comfortable in familiar surroundings and that personal contacts between the school doctor and the teaching staff are facilitated. Ideally, examinations should be conducted in a room set aside for the purpose and affording privacy and quietness. The unfortunate truth is that many examinations take place in head teachers' rooms, assembly halls, gymnasia or even cloakrooms. They interfere with the normal life of the school and for this reason are not always unreservedly welcomed by the staff. Even where medical rooms have been planned in new schools, it is not unusual for them to be used for other purposes. The examination is, therefore, likely to be subject to physical constraints due to its location.

Duration. A further limitation is imposed by the time that can be devoted to each child. After morning assembly and breaks have been taken into account, no more than two and a half hours are available in each session. During this time between 12 and 20 children are inspected. This means that on average each child has a consultation of no more than 10 minutes. In practice it is often much less because any child with problems is inevitably given a greater share of the time. The accusation that examinations are perfunctory and that they are conducted in unsatisfactory circumstances is therefore substantially true and it may be doubted whether any useful purpose can be served by them.

Purpose. The reason for the school medical inspection has been officially stated as 'not primarily to examine a child for defects but to identify those children with defects which may adversely affect their education and to offset these adverse effects by ensuring early and continued treatment and/or by providing special educational facilities' (DES and DHSS, 1972). The difficulty is that in practice it is impossible to avoid paying equal attention to all defects, whether or not they have educational implications. In other words, the health and educational functions of the examinations cannot readily be separated. The essence of any consultation is the medical history and, although questionnaire histories can be obtained, they are not entirely satisfactory nor are they conducive to the necessary personal interaction. In well-organized areas, records of the past and family medical history and of the outcome of previous developmental examinations are available but, even if these are helpful, the difficulty remains of obtaining an appropriate history within the space of two or three minutes. Many school doctors settle for a single general question such as: 'Is your child well?' but perhaps they should be asking a few more specific questions. If the child is to be examined in the time available, the most that could be routinely asked would be a handful of educationally orientated questions such as: 'Does your child have any trouble with his eyes, ears or speech? Is he able to run and to get about as well as other children? Does he show undue clumsiness in his movements? Is his behaviour difficult or unusual and does he get on well with other children?'

In medical practice the clinical examination is usually directed towards confirmation or otherwise of the provisional conclusions reached after a history has been taken. The lack of an adequate history leaves the school doctor to cast around looking for abnormalities that he has little reason to believe are present. He often has to do this without the aid of an examination couch, even if there is time to lie the patient down. The surprising thing is not that relevant defects are missed but that so many are found.

Results. Despite the difficulties, a considerable number of abnormalities are noted. It has been stated, for example, that at the initial examination 14 to 15 per cent of children have defects and that between 20 and 50 per cent of them are not being treated (Cohen, 1964). Many are trivial but in one survey 2.5 per cent of children were referred to a hospital specialist and three quarters of these required investigation or treatment (Horner, 1967). The most commonly found unknown defects are of vision; these are significant from an educational point of view but most could be detected by a simple screening procedure alone. Other important conditions are identified occasionally and it is probable that this will continue to happen unless and until there is universal examination of pre-school children.

Even if very few defects are found, it can be reasonably argued that the routine inspection is worthwhile. Taylor (1961) places first in his list of reasons for continuing the examinations that the mothers wish it and this is undoubtedly true. The degree of parental appreciation of these brief inspections is remarkable and presumably stems from the need of many parents for reassurance about their child's health. In so far as their short meeting with the school doctor helps to foster their pride in the child, it makes a positive contribution to his care. Whether most school doctors have time to enhance this positive aspect of the examination with a little health education is doubtful but it should be at least a theoretical objective.

The recurrent criticism of the school medical inspection is not of the concept of health and developmental examinations of children but of their content and duration. Traditional methods of examination fail to detect significant neuropsychiatric conditions that have been shown to be present in many school children (Rutter et al, 1970). It has been suggested that at the entrant examination there should be a review of the child's state of growth and development with special reference to sensory and neurological development and that what is known about the child should be collectively considered by the child health staff so that teachers can be appropriately advised (Court, 1976). It is acknowledged that examinations of this kind would each take 20 to 30 minutes, i.e. substantially longer than is generally the case at present. In the short term this would have to be achieved with the same number of doctors and would, therefore, necessitate a reduction in the total number of examinations.

Selection. In most areas all children are examined immediately before or shortly after their admission to school but there is a policy of selection with respect to the examination of children in other age groups. Although selection procedures have been advocated and adopted there is no general agreement about the way that they should be operated. Often the children to be examined are selected at a health conference of head teacher, doctor and nurse. Many methods of selection do not save much time. For example, Horner (1966) found that in 52 per cent of children positive symptoms were reported on a questionnaire and this method is, therefore, ineffective. He commented that when the number selected exceeds 40 per cent of the total, the argument in favour of selection begins to lose its force because some of the time saved is taken up by the selection procedure. Another method is to select the school rather than the individual pupils. Asher (1967) thought that the yield of treatable defects in residential areas was so low as to make routine examination unjustifiable and suggested that the time saved should be spent on necessitous children and on improved follow-up. For the school leaver examinations, linkage to an adolescent health counselling service and selection based on self-referral could be considered.

Selection for medical examination may be based satisfactorily upon a regular review by a school nurse. It has been recommended that the school entrant examination should again be statutory and that at the age of approximately 13 years each child should have a private interview with a school doctor. During each of his school years up to the age of 13 to 14 years he should be seen by the school nurse for a health care interview and the screening tests outlined below (Court, 1976).

Follow-up. Many of the 15 per cent of children found to have defects at routine medical inspections require follow-up to ensure that appropriate action has been taken. There is some evidence that this is not carried out very assiduously and that potentially serious defects may be left without supervision or treatment (Asher, 1967). This failure might be due to the pressures to undertake other examinations.

Special inspections. In some areas of Britain, politicians decided that priority should be given to the examination of many children in order that they could be legally provided with free milk. An enormous amount of time was spent on this exercise which was generally unnecessary. Moreover, an additional load was placed on the service at a time when increased demands were being made because of the expansion of nursery provision. Other inspections that tend to waste effort are those of children of 14 years and over who are seeking part-time employment. Didsbury (1964) found that less than one in every thousand children examined was considered unfit. In contrast, the far more important supply of medical information to the Employment Medical Advisory Service can be based on past records. Provided that these have been well kept and that basic screening tests have been completed, it would be reasonable to dispense with many special medical inspections. In some countries, for example, France and Italy, but not in Britain, special examinations take place after intercurrent illness and before the child returns to school.

Screening tests

The School Health Service undertakes a number of screening procedures and these are mostly carried out by school nurses. Some, such as those for vision and hearing, have direct relevance to learning, while others, such as for growth and urinary infections, are of peripheral importance to schools. The frequency, timing and techniques used vary from area to area but their purpose is the same, namely, to pick out those children who require further expert examination. The screening tests should not in themselves be regarded as definitive diagnostic tests.

Screening tests of vision

It has been recommended that tests of visual acuity should be undertaken annually in all primary and secondary schools and in special schools (Committee of Enquiry into the Education of Visually Handicapped Children, 1972; Court, 1976). This frequency of testing is not achieved in most schools but it is, nevertheless, desirable. The tests are usually part of the work of school nurses but occasionally they are done by nursing assistants or other ancillary personnel. It is important that whoever does them should have had at least a minimum training.

The examination should commence with a brief external inspection of the eyes before proceeding to the test of acuity. For the latter, the most commonly used method is the Snellen chart which requires the recognition of letters. Good illumination and a measured 20-feet distance between the child and the chart are needed but these standards cannot always be achieved in older school buildings. For this reason some services use apparatus such as the Keystone Vision Screener which gives standard illumination and can be used in small rooms. For younger children the Snellen picture chart or the E test may be used but the test that has gained considerable popularity is the Stycar test, which involves matching rather than naming of letters (Sheridan, 1960). Each eye should be tested separately and faulty occlusion is an occasional source of error. Children with squint, nystagmus or defects of acuity of 6/9 or more should be referred for further examination.

Colour vision should be tested, especially in boys but also in girls, at some time during their school life so that defects are known before career choice. With the fairly recent use of teaching methods dependent on colour, there may be a case for testing at school entry although it is a time-consuming procedure with young children. The traditional method of testing is by the recognition of numbers or the tracing of lines on Ishihara charts. These are not quite so sensitive as the tests used in the transport industry and any child opting for this type of career should be offered a more sophisticated examination.

Screening tests of hearing

Most children have their hearing tested by a health visitor, using distraction methods, in the first year of life. Although this is not absolutely reliable, the majority of children with deafness which is either congenital or acquired in early infancy have been identified by the time that they reach school. The commonest remaining cause of hearing loss is middle ear infection and this may occur at any time but especially in early childhood. Since the educational implications are considerable, a screening test of hearing at the time of school entry is highly desirable. This can be done by use of a forced whisper test or a word test but many areas now employ pure-tone audiometric sweep tests.

All the tests require the use of a reasonably quiet room. They are done either by paramedical staff who have training in audiometry or by health visitor/school nurses, some of whom have attended special courses.

Failure to hear 20 decibels with either ear is an indication for examination of the ears, nose and throat and, in the absence of an easily remediable condition, referral for specialist advice.

At present most children have a single audiometric examination during their school life but a case can be made for the test to be repeated and it has been recommended that each child should have his hearing tested by a school nurse twice during primary education (Court, 1976).

Monitoring growth

Paediatricians are 'measuring doctors' and the reason that so much importance is attached to accurate records of height and weight is that variations in the pattern of growth of children are among the best indices of things going wrong. Growth may be affected, not only by physical disease, but also by emotional upset.

There is no reason why accurate measurements of standing height and nude weight cannot be obtained in schools and the cost of providing suitable scales and a stadiometer is far outweighed by their value. It is, however, of very little use to record heights and weights routinely unless they are compared with each other, with norms for children of the same age and sex and especially with previous measurements of the same child. In the opinion of the author, every school child should have a centile chart on which his growth can be recorded and annual measurements of height and weight by the school nurse have been recommended (Court, 1976). This would give a far better indication of the need for medical examination than many of the selection methods now used.

Screening for other disorders
It it possible to offer screening tests for a wide variety of disorders. Some involve the use of medical personnel, others need laboratory facilities and all place extra burdens on the nursing staff. Most do not have any direct relevance to education.

School screening programmes to detect adolescent idiopathic scoliosis are becoming commoner in Britain (British Medical Journal, 1979). Withnell (1958) commended routine surveys by chiropodists and thought that the detection of scoliosis could be within the competence of the school nurse. Similar inspections to detect hernia have been suggested. Screening of girls for urinary abnormalities using dip slide and test stick methods has been undertaken (Silverberg et al, 1973). Many of the screening procedures that have been advocated are reasonable but whether or not they should be adopted depends on such factors as the availability of personnel. They should not be allowed to detract from the essential function of the School Health Service which is to assist education.

Control of infection

Immunization
Immunoprophylaxis is routinely offered by the School Health Service to protect children against diphtheria, tetanus, poliomyelitis and rubella. Parents are asked to sign consent forms and the children of those who agree receive the vaccine at school.

About the time of school entry and sometimes at a separate session immediately after the medical inspection, children who have received triple antigen or diphtheria and tetanus immunization in infancy are offered a reinforcing dose of diphtheria and tetanus toxoid. Those who have not been protected previously are given a primary course of three doses of diphtheria and tetanus toxoid. Reinforcing doses of tetanus toxoid are given at minor ailment clinics after injuries and additional doses are offered to adolescent boys participating in sports such as rugby in which there is a risk of field injuries. There are very few adverse reactions to the vaccine although a few children develop a sore arm and slight malaise due to hyperimmunity.

Oral poliomyelitis vaccine (Sabin) is offered at school entry and given at the same time as the diphtheria and tetanus toxoid. A single trivalent dose is used for those who have been protected and the remainder are immunized with a primary course of three doses. In this country trivalent vaccine is usually employed for primary as well as for reinforcing doses, although for the former a sequence of three doses of monovalent vaccines may be used.

In some areas a single injection of live attenuated measles virus vaccine is offered to those children who have neither had the disease nor been previously immunized. Children with a history of allergy, convulsions or immune deficiency disease and those on immuno-suppressant therapy are excluded. There is a distinct morbidity associated with this procedure and rarely there are major encephalopathic reactions. The justification for using the vaccine is that its side-effects are significantly less than those following the natural infection. Gamma-globulin is sometimes used concurrently with the vaccine to reduce the risk of reaction.

Rubella vaccine is offered to all schoolgirls between the ages of 10 and 14 years, irrespective of whether there is a past history of the disease. Approximately 60 to 80 per cent of girls are already immune at the time that they receive the vaccine and for them the procedure is unnecessary, but it is impracticable to determine the immune status of all girls prior to immunization. Serious side-effects of the vaccine occur very infrequently although there is occasional malaise and arthropathy.

Official policy in Britain is to offer a tuberculin test to all children at 13 years followed by BCG vaccination of those who have a negative reaction. Heaf tests are commonly used to determine tuberculin sensitivity and those who require it are protected with a single intradermal dose of freeze-dried vaccine. Side-effects are rare except for local ulceration and adenopathy and the incidence of these depends to some extent on the skill of the operator.

Some children receive BCG earlier in childhood because in a few areas there is routine vaccination of all neonates and of immigrant children at the time of school entry. In addition, children who are contacts of patients with tuberculosis are normally protected with BCG. The reason for the usual practice of offering the vaccine in adolescence is to afford maximum tuberculin sensitivity at the time the young person enters employment when the risk of infection is greatest. A contrary argument is that post-primary tuberculous infections in early childhood are so serious and still sufficiently numerous in our urban centres that BCG vaccine should be given to all infants. In many parts of the country the number of notified cases of tuberculosis has fallen and the need to continue routine BCG vaccination of all children has become questionable.

Infectious disease

School closure because of serious infections such as diphtheria or poliomyelitis is now very rare, although there are still occasional small localized outbreaks. The most common notifiable infection in school children is measles. Since the introduction of measles vaccination the incidence has declined but there is at present a lack of parental enthusiasm for the vaccine and many children are unprotected.

Once measles has been controlled, the main infection problems in schools will arise from lack of hand hygiene. Gastrointestinal infections, particularly with *Shigella sonnei* and type-specific coliform bacteria, are still a common problem in nursery classes. Many of the children have minimal symptoms but some become quite ill and there is always the anxiety that they will carry an infection home to more vulnerable siblings. The normal practice is to exclude children until there is clinical recovery and three rectal swab or stool examinations have proved negative. Hand washing is emphasized and appropriate handbasins are an important part of nursery equipment. Deficiencies of hand hygiene are the cause of fairly frequent infestations with threadworms in nurseries and primary schools.

Another problem arising from lack of hand and toilet hygiene is occasional outbreaks of infective hepatitis. Surveillance of classes for early signs of jaundice and the administration of gammaglobulin to close contacts is undertaken by the staff of the School Health Service.

The arrival during the 1960s and early 1970s of a substantial number of children from tropical countries gave rise to concern about possible importation of exotic diseases. There is an increased risk of infection, not only because of the occurrence of these diseases in their countries of origin but also because the immigrant child may be more susceptible to disease after his arrival here. In fact, the anxiety was misplaced and there was no evidence of any substantial outbreak of infection in schools originating from a recently arrived immigrant child. Vigilance may still be required, however, as it is in the case of children who go on overseas holidays or educational visits.

Few immigrant children are admitted to school within two weeks of arrival here and the risk that they are incubating an acute infection is therefore negligible. Special medical inspections, including tuberculin surveys and screening for intestinal pathogens and soil-transmitted helminths, have been undertaken (Thompson et al, 1972; Archer et al, 1965). The primary purpose of these inspections is to identify treatable conditions for the benefit of the particular children.

A recurrent task of school doctors is surveillance of children who have been exposed to the risk of tuberculosis through a member of the staff or an older pupil. Contacts are tuberculin tested at school and arrangements are made for those with positive reactions to have a chest X-ray. In these circumstances there is close liaison with local chest clinics.

Control of cleanliness

Hygiene inspections are carried out periodically by school nurses or assistant nurses. Their purpose is to identify children with skin infections and ectoparasitic infestation, especially pediculosis capitis. The latter still occurs in approximately 4 per cent of the school population inspected and in central urban areas the incidence is substantially higher. Head lice spread quickly among children because it takes only nine or ten days for the eggs to hatch and the larval form has matured and is laying further eggs after another two weeks. Unless they are detected promptly, children develop heavy infestations, frequently resulting in discomfort and impetigo in themselves and spread of lice to others. Infestations are usually family affairs and the problem cannot be tackled exclusively within schools. The School Health Service does, however, provide treatment facilities for children.

In some areas cleansing orders are issued to parents and children are excluded from school. Unfortunately, these children are often the very ones who can least afford to miss school and since their infestations often drag on for a long time and frequently recur, they may suffer significant educational disadvantage. In practice, it is unnecessary to exclude children, provided that it is certain the child has had an effective insecticidal shampoo. A recent problem has been the resistance of lice to gamma benzene hexachloride and DDT but this has been overcome by the use of 0.5 per cent Malathion shampoos. In order to ensure that children have been adequately cleansed it is preferable that treatment should be provided at local clinics rather than at cleansing stations.

Scabies infestations increased very greatly among schoolchildren during the 1960s and have continued at a fairly high level. As in the case of head louse infestation, there is no need to exclude children provided that there has been an adequate application of benzoyl benzoate or an equivalent substance.

Many children are found to have impetigo and plantar warts and these are generally treated at minor ailment clinics. Ringworm is also a problem in some areas.

Health education

In their everyday practice all good clinicians influence attitudes to disease and impart some knowledge about health to their patients. School doctors have additional responsibilities for health education although these are not always clearly defined. They do, nevertheless, regard it as an essential part of their job.

The importance of health education has been recognized from the inception of the School Health Service. Initially there was an emphasis on factual instruction about nutrition and personal hygiene but in recent times a very broad approach has been encouraged (Report of a Joint Committee of the Central and Scottish Health Services Councils, 1964). Its purpose is to equip children to understand and value health and to make effective and appropriate use of health services. Furthermore, it is concerned not only with information but also with the 'formation of attitudes which are favourable to personal and community health and to changes in attitudes if these are not satisfactory' (Dalzell-Ward, 1975). There is a clear intention to modify behaviour and to reduce anxiety and irrational beliefs about disease (see Ch. 6). In order to achieve these ends, children require factual instruction and personal contact with someone who is not only sincere and positive in his attitudes to health but also a competent teacher. School doctors have a role in assisting professional teachers in these tasks.

School doctors and health visitors vary in their ability to teach and it is usually inappropriate for them to assume a solo role in the classroom. They can usefully be involved in discussion with senior pupils and their teachers and should make themselves available for questions. There is a very wide range of subjects that may be discussed because it is not simply a matter of talking about personal hygiene and nutrition. The discussion may include ecological questions, population control and child rearing, smoking, alcohol and other addictions and indeed the health aspects of almost any biological or social issue.

Some schools have specialist teachers of health education but a proposal to have them in Scotland was turned down. In schools without specialist teachers there are often designated organizers who ensure the exposure of pupils to health education during the course of other classes. It has been asserted that programmes should be directed by qualified health educators functioning in consultation and co-operation with school personnel, parents, students, physicians and health agencies in the community (Committee on School Health of the American Academy of Pediatrics, 1978).

Health visitors have a special concern for health education and there are about 300 Health Education Officers in post who have attended Health Education Council Courses. Many school doctors have made sincere but usually sporadic efforts and it is fair to say that in most areas they have lacked co-ordination. Just as local education authorities have curriculum advisers in other subjects, so they require a senior doctor to give advice on questions of health education.

There is at present a considerable unmet need for the involvement of doctors in teacher-training. Hygiene does not have sufficient standing in the curricula of training colleges and important subjects such as care of the handicapped are often dealt with only as special options for a few students. It has now been recommended that all courses of initial teacher training should include a special education element (Warnock, 1978) and that health education should be part of every elementary and secondary teacher's training programme (Committee on School Health of the American Academy of Pediatrics, 1978).

School Health Service clinics

Minor ailment clinics
In most countries the School Health Service is prohibited from engaging in treatment other than First Aid. This is not so in Britain and many areas have minor ailment clinics although their numbers have dwindled. In some ways they are a relic of the past and their function is being taken over by treatment facilities provided at health centres. There are, nevertheless, several million attendances annually.

Work in the clinics is done by clinic nurses under the supervision of the school doctor and treatment of small injuries, skin infections, etc. is undertaken. This is useful in that it minimizes loss of school time and provides a convenient minor accident service for schools.

Specialist clinics
Specialist consultations are arranged in some local school health clinics. They are mostly to deal with visual problems or ear, nose and throat defects but other specialties are represented. There are differing views about the merits of these arrangements. On the one hand the clinics may be more convenient for the public and the specialist sees the child in his community setting. The contrary arguments are that they take an undue amount of consultant time, are less efficient because of lack of support facilities and can lead to confusion of records.

Child guidance services

At present child psychiatric services are inadequate because only a very small proportion of children get professional help when they need it. School doctors and educational psychologists are asked to advise schoolteachers about children who exhibit difficult behaviour and the latter increasingly give direct help through School Psychological Services provided by local education authorities. In many cases answers can be given after a simple examination in a school or clinic but there are others who need more prolonged investigation. These children are referred to child guidance clinics of which there are approximately 500 throughout England and Wales. Unfortunately they have developed in a fragmented fashion and their distribution is very uneven. This had led to the recommendation that there should be integration of the child psychiatric services (Court, 1976).

Education authorities turn to the clinics for recommendations about the education of children who are maladjusted. The latter is an administrative category encompassing children with abnormal relationships towards other people or their environment. It implies, therefore, a constellation of symptoms which may or may not have a specific medical significance and it certainly does not constitute an adequate psychiatric diagnosis. The lack of a clear definition of maladaptive behaviour leads to great variations in the demand for child guidance services. Much depends upon the tolerance of teachers and parents and the prevailing view of what is unacceptable conduct.

In sharp contrast to most school health activities, the time devoted to children attending child guidance clinics is considerable and the number examined is very small relative to the staffs employed. The Underwood Committee (Report of the Committee on Maladjusted Children, 1955) recommended that there should be one child psychiatrist, two educational psychologists and three psychiatric social workers per 45 000 schoolchildren. This pattern of staffing has been adopted in most areas, although the actual numbers of each profession vary from place to place and are often grossly deficient.

It has been argued that more clinics and more staff are required because the service is not meeting present demands and many children are not receiving the treatment that they need. On the other hand, the expectations of those referring children are often unrealistic, in that many of the problems arise out of social deprivation and are not susceptible to cure in a medical sense. The value of the clinics in most cases is in establishing a diagnosis upon which rational management can be based.

Care of the handicapped

This is a problem of enormous importance to the School Health Service (see Ch. 17). School doctors have a special role in the care of handicapped children but many other agencies and professions may be involved and optimum results are obtained by a co-operative multidisciplinary approach to each child's problems. The services involved are very costly and for this as well as for humanitarian reasons their use should be efficiently organized.

Disabilities may come to light in a wide variety of ways. They may be diagnosed antenatally or become evident at or shortly after birth. Some are the result of illness in childhood and an increasing proportion are due to accidental and non-accidental trauma. The age at which handicapping conditions are identified has been reduced because of the growth of developmental screening of preschool children. There are, nevertheless, still many children with moderate degrees of educational subnormality which is not recognized until after they have failed to make progress in a normal school.

Tests in infancy can measure the rate of development and can lead to the diagnosis of a number of disabilities but it is impossible to be certain about mild degrees of mental subnormality. Illingworth (1972) has stated that there never will be a high correlation between developmental assessment in infancy and subsequent intellectual achievement. There are, therefore, bound to be a number of children about whom there is significant doubt and it is often useful to observe them in nursery classes or assessment units.

District Handicap Teams consisting of members from a number of professions have been set up in many areas. The creation of a team in each health district has been accepted in principle by the government (DHSS, 1978) and its intended location was the District General Hospital (Court, 1976). A contrary view that 'multiprofessional assessment should usually take place at a centre within the community other than a hospital' was put forward by another committee, clearly suspicious of the predominant medical role in assessment (Warnock, 1978).

In the past, limited assessments have been provided away from hospitals by school doctors who have generally provided a good account of children's abilities but unfortunately they did not always investigate the causes of disabilities that they found. There has not, therefore, been a preventive approach to handicapping conditions in children. The reasons for this deficiency have been the lack of access by school doctors to diagnostic facilities and their relative professional isolation. Siting assessment units at a distance from hospitals capable of the necessary diagnostic investigation will, in the opinion of the author, tend to perpetuate the isolation and lack of preventive approach so unsatisfactory in the old system.

The purpose of assessment is to define a child's disability, to determine its cause and to decide about management. It is not a once-for-all procedure and there is a need for continuous review. Parents are entitled to an adequate and structured system of follow-up and in the case of children attending special schools or units, this is best provided at school. It has been stated that 'the school *is* the responsible treatment agent and other resource people will be helpful to children and the school to the degree that their input is seen as being consistent with what schools and society see as important for all children' (Schoenwetter, 1974). Subsequent to the initial diagnostic assessment, staff from the Assessment Centres should therefore seek to provide a continuity of service in schools.

Learning disorders
The special contribution to be made by the School Health Service is in the elucidation and management of the medical aspects of learning disorders. School failure may occur for a number of reasons, some medical, others educational and many of them social. There are obvious differences between the professions in their approaches to these problems but there is common ground in that most agree that they should be looked at in the context of child development as a whole.

The School Health Service has concerned itself with the identification of the large group of children who fail because of intellectual subnormality and of those children who have sensory defects. There is an emergent need for school doctors to be concerned with the minor neurological disorders that so often constitute major educational handicaps. Although the medical contribution is to the study of biological components in learning, these cannot be separated from psychological and socio-cultural factors. Walzer & Richmond (1973) reviewed the work of many investigators who 'reported a significant association between neurological disorder and gross psychiatric disturbances in children', thus tending to confirm the interdependence of biology, behaviour and culture.

It has been suggested that 'an emphasis on continuing assessment of function in an educational context, rather than an etiological orientation, will be most productive' (Berkson, 1973). Others have said that 'the assessment and management of hyperactive children of school age should be directed towards behavioural and psycho-educational factors and remediation techniques primarily rather than medical and neurological investigations' (Kenny et al, 1971). These methods are, however, unsatisfactory because they are empirical and make little contribution to understanding the nature of underlying problems or to the overwhelmingly important question of prevention. Furthermore, if they are employed to the exclusion of a biological approach, remediable conditions are likely to be overlooked. It is a function of school doctors to assert the need for a search to be made for physical factors in all learning disorders and to collaborate in their total appraisal. The methods of medical diagnosis and research can be applied to these problems with profit.

REFERENCES

Archer D M, Bamford F N, Lees E 1965 Helminth infestations in immigrant children. British Medical Journal ii: 1517–1519
Asher P 1967 One thousand school children. Medical Officer 117: 327–329
Berkson G 1973 Learning, a theoretical perspective. Pediatric Clinics of North America 20: 543–548
British Medical Journal 1979 Adolescent idiopathic scoliosis. British Medical Journal i: 1446
Cohen H M 1964 School years. Journal of the Royal Institute of Public Health and Hygiene 27: 256–264
Committee of Enquiry into the Education of Visually Handicapped Children 1972 The education of the visually handicapped. HMSO, London
Committee on School Health of the American Academy of Pediatrics 1978 Health education. Pediatrics 62: 117
Court S D M (chairman) 1976 Fit for the future: Report of the Committee on Child Health Services. HMSO, London
Dalzell-Ward A J 1975 A textbook of health education. Tavistock Publications, London
Department of Education and Science and Department of Health and Social Security Working Party on Collaboration 1972 The First Report of School Health Service Sub-Committee. HMSO, London
Department of Health and Social Security 1978 Circular H.C. (78)5. HMSO, London
Didsbury B 1964 The school health service and the family doctor. Lancet i: 101–104
Horner J S 1966 The selection of children for school medical inspection. Medical Officer 115: 29–34
Horner J S 1967 School medical inspections and the family doctor. Lancet ii: 882–885
Illingworth R S 1972 The development of the infant and young child, normal and abnormal, 5th edn. Churchill Livingstone, Edinburgh

Kenny T J, Clemmens R L, Hudson B W, Lentz G A, Cicci R, Nair P 1971 Characteristics of children referred because of hyperactivity. Journal of Pediatrics 79: 618–622
Lancet 1966 Anachronism at school. Lancet i: 587
Report of the Committee on Maladjusted Children (Underwood Report) 1955 HMSO, London
Report of a Joint Committee of the Central and Scottish Health Services Councils 1964 Health education. HMSO, London
Rutter M, Graham P, Yule W 1970 Neuropsychiatric study in childhood. Clinics in Developmental Medicine Nos. 35/36. Spastics International Medical Publications and Heinemann, London
Schoenwetter C D 1974 The school health service, review and commentary. Pediatric Clinics of North America 21: 75–80
Sheridan M D 1960 Manual for the Stycar Vision Test. National Foundation for Educational Research, London
Silverberg D A, Allard M J, Ulan R A, Beamish W E, Lentle B C, McPhee M S, Grace M G 1973 City-wide screening for urinary abnormalities in girls. Canadian Medical Association Journal 109: 981–985
Taylor G B 1961 The routine medical inspection. Medical Officer 105: 48–49
Thompson R G, Hutchison J G P, Johnston N M 1972 Survey of intestinal pathogens from immigrant children. British Medical Journal i: 591–594
Walzer S, Richmond J B 1973 The epidemiology of learning disorders. Pediatric Clinics of North America 20: 549–565
Warnock H M (chairman) 1978 Special educational needs: The Report of the Committee of Enquiry into the Education of Handicapped Children and Young People. HMSO, London
Withnell A 1958 The value of the routine school medical examination. Medical Officer 99: 31–36

The handicapped child in school

This chapter looks at the problems that arise in relation to the education of handicapped children, and describes some of the special arrangements that health and education authorities and schools in England and Wales make in order to help them.

Handicapped pupils

Under the 1944 Education Act parents have a responsibility for seeing that, from the age of five years, their child, even if he is handicapped, receives efficient full-time education suitable to his age, ability and aptitude. At the same time local education authorities have a duty to ensure that 'special educational treatment' (i.e. education by special methods) is made available within special schools or in other ways for children who suffer from 'any disability of mind or body'. The authorities have an additional duty to ascertain which particular children aged five or over need special education and to satisfy themselves that the children are receiving it. If they so wish, they may do this for any child from the age of two, but they are not bound to do so.

As a guide to the kind of special educational treatment that authorities are required to make available, and in order to achieve some standardization of arrangements throughout the country, regulations have been passed (The Handicapped Pupils and Special Schools Regulations, 1959: SI No. 365) defining 10 categories of handicapped pupils in educational terms (see Appendix). Special schools have been established for pupils in each category.

The Department of Education and Science (DES) publishes annual statistics showing the number of these special schools and the number and ages of the pupils attending them (see Tables 17.1 and 17.2). In Table 17.3 the total number of children ascertained as handicapped pupils is shown, according to their principal handicap: it includes children awaiting special education (9313) as well as those receiving it in special classes in ordinary schools (20 670) and at home.

The total number of handicapped pupils represents 1.8 per cent of the school population and falls far short of the number of handicapped children of school age wherever they may be educated. This discrepancy arises, in part, from the lack of any widely adopted criteria as to what constitutes a handicap to development in children of school age, but largely from the traditional tendency in educational circles to equate handicap in pupils with the need for full-time special educational treatment in a special school. For teachers in ordinary schools who

HEALTH AND SCHOOL

Table 17.1 Types of special school and their full-time pupils: England and Wales, 1976 (January)

Category of pupils	Number of schools	Number of pupils
Blind	17	990
Partially sighted	17	1553
Blind and partially sighted	2	231
Deaf	24	2057
Partially hearing	6	628
Deaf and partially hearing	21	2247
Deaf and partially sighted	1	169
Physically handicapped	95	6911
Delicate	52	4036
Physically handicapped and delicate	64	5751
Delicate and maladjusted	6	486
Maladjusted*	177	7044
Educationally subnormal:		
medium	539	61 223
severe	388	25 453
medium and severe	26	3571
Epileptic	6	631
Suffering from speech defect	5	204
Multiple handicaps	14	958
Pupils in hospital special schools	159	9466
Total	1619	133 609

* Including autistic

have the care, as well as the education, of children with a wide range of handicapping conditions, and for those who have to provide supporting services to teachers, pupils and their parents, a broader concept of handicap is required. Even when the criterion of handicap is the need for some kind of practical intervention, the total number of handicapped children of school age is many times greater than the number of handicapped pupils in special schools.

Table 17.2 Full-time handicapped pupils in special schools by age and sex: England and Wales, 1976 (January)

Age	Number of boys	Number of girls	Total
2	270	215	485
3	598	453	1051
4	1380	1043	2423
5	2549	1830	4379
6	3337	2199	5536
7	4350	2838	7188
8	5405	3426	8831
9	6384	4231	10 615
10	7590	4628	12 218
11	8659	5172	13 831
12	9273	5777	15 050
13	9697	6039	15 736
14	9142	5850	14 992
15	8635	5616	14 251
16	3162	2101	5263
17	551	431	982
18	246	195	441
19+	180	157	337
Total	81 408	52 201	133 609

Table 17.3 Numbers of handicapped pupils receiving and awaiting special education, by principal category: England and Wales, 1976 (January)

Category of pupils	Number of pupils
Blind	1235
Partially sighted	2349
Deaf	4237
Partially hearing	5865
Physically handicapped	15 885
Delicate	6627
Maladjusted*	20 400
Educationally subnormal:	
medium	81 344
severe	34 591
Epileptic	1429
Suffering from speech defect	2142
Total	176 104

* Including autistic

In a recent series of studies of schoolchildren aged nine to 11, and aged 14 years (Rutter et al, 1970b; Graham & Rutter, 1973; Yule et al, 1974; Rutter et al, 1975; Berger et al, 1975), handicap was defined strictly in functional terms which implied the need for practical intervention. All the children were examined individually before being assessed as handicapped in one or more of the following ways:

1. by *intellectual retardation*, i.e. a scale score on the Wechsler Intelligence Scale for Children of two standard deviations or more below the mean (average) scale score of all children in a control group;

2. by *educational backwardness*, i.e. with a reading accuracy or comprehension which was 28 months or more below the child's chronological age;

3. by *psychiatric disorder*, i.e. an abnormality of behaviour, emotions or relationships which was sufficiently marked and sufficiently prolonged to cause a handicap to the child himself and/or distress or disturbance in the family or community, and which was continuing up to the time of assessment;

4. by *chronic physical disorder*, lasting at least one year, present during the 12 months preceding assessment, and associated with persisting or recurrent handicap of some kind.

Relevant data from these studies are summarized in Table 17.4 and 17.5. They show that 14 per cent of nine- to 11-year-old children living in rural or semi-rural areas are likely to have either a moderate or a severe disorder causing educational concern and needing some form of special medical, educational and/or management help, usually in school as well as at home. In inner-city areas of large conurbations the proportion of handicapped children may approach 20 per cent because the rates of educational backwardness and psychiatric disorder are two or three times as high as in rural areas (Table 17.5).

This prevalence rate is less than the sum of the rates for the four major handicapping conditions set out in Table 17.4 because some children have more than one disorder. It is fashionable to regard all handicapped children as having multiple disabilities and to suppose that the simple, single disability is a rarity

Table 17.4 Prevalence of four handicapping conditions of educational concern and of moderate or severe intensity. Age-specific rates per 1000 children in a population of 2199 children aged nine to 11 years (Isle of Wight). Note: This table differs from that given by Rutter et al (1970b) in that only physically handicapped children with moderate or severe disability are included; figures for the other handicaps are unchanged

	Intellectual retardation	Educational backwardness	Psychiatric disorder	Physical handicap	Rate per 1000
One handicap only	3.6	46.4	36.4	16.9	103.3
Two handicaps:					
Intellectual +	—	12.7	0.5	0.5	
Educational +	12.7	—	10.0	1.4	26.5
Psychiatric +	0.5	10.0	—	1.4	
Physical +	0.5	1.4	1.4	—	
Three handicaps:					
Int + Ed + Psych	2.3	2.3	2.3	—	
Int + Ed + Physic	4.1	4.1	—	4.1	7.8
Int + Psych + Physic	1.4	—	1.4	1.4	
Ed + Psych + Physic	—	—	—	—	
All four handicaps	1.8	1.8	1.8	1.8	1.8
Total with each handicap*	26.4	78.7	53.7	27.3	138.9

*Computed

(Younghusband et al, 1970). Whilst it is common knowledge that among the children attending special schools for physically handicapped and for educationally subnormal pupils there are many who have two or more handicapping conditions, they represent a select group. There have been very few reliable studies of handicapped children in a total child population and in the cross-sectional survey of the Isle of Wight children (Rutter et al, 1970b) it was the exception rather than the rule to find a child with more than one well-defined disorder of significant severity (Table 17.4). Once handicapped, a child is certainly at risk of additional handicaps, especially educational backwardness and psychiatric disorder, and this possibility should always be a prominent factor guiding parents and teachers and their professional advisers in the care of the child.

It cannot be assumed that the same rate of handicap will be found in older and younger schoolchildren as in the nine- to 11-year-old group. However, the

Table 17.5 Prevalence of three handicapping conditions of educational concern and of moderate or severe intensity. Age-specific rates per 100 children in two population groups (Isle of Wight and London)

Population group	Educational backwardness (%)	Specific reading retardation* (%)	Psychiatric disorder (%)
Isle of Wight 10-year-olds	8.3	3.9	12.0
London 10-year-olds	19.0	9.9	25.4

*Specific reading retardation was defined as an attainment on either accuracy or comprehension which was 28 months or more below the level predicted on the basis of each child's age and short WISC IQ (Rutter et al, 1970b).

indications are that the rate may be less in five-year-old children only in so far as epilepsy is less common and the definition of educational backwardness is not appropriate (see p. 315). In 14-year-old children it is likely to be higher because of the increased rates of educational backwardness and psychiatric disorder (Graham & Rutter, 1973; Yule et al, 1974).

Classification and numbers of handicapped schoolchildren

The use of legally defined categories of handicapped pupils and matching special schools has served a purpose in building the institutional foundations of a special education service. It has achieved this by focusing attention on selected groups of children with different kinds of disorder, some more specific than others but all of them creating educational disadvantage. However, this has proved to be a crude method of meeting the special educational and treatment needs of individual children. Particularly, the categories 'delicate', 'educationally subnormal' and 'maladjusted' include children with such diverse needs that these cannot be conveyed in a single catchphrase. Similar criticisms have been made in the past (Scottish Education Department, 1944; Ministry of Education, 1955; Younghusband et al, 1970) but it has always been assumed that categories of one kind or another are required for administrative reasons. Consequently, controversy has centred round the question of whether to have more or fewer categories rather than whether to have any at all.

Legal education categories have serious drawbacks in addition to the one mentioned above. One of these is that they create a dilemma of definition. As the rationale for categories rests upon the identification of specific subgroups of handicapped children within a larger undefined or ill-defined group for whom education authorities should plan more selective special education, advances in special education logically create a need for more categories not fewer, for more educational definition not less. For instance, serious problems arise when authorities are required by law to provide schools for children with handicapping disorders such as acute dyslexia and autism when these remain undefined (Chronically Sick and Disabled Persons Act 1970). Yet it is exceedingly difficult to define handicap in precise legal terms that are meaningful, not only educationally but also medically and socially. The present definition of an epileptic pupil is a case in point (see Appendix). It raises the whole issue of whether it is ever in the overall interests of a child that one aspect of handicap among several should be subject to legal definition independently of the others.

The corollary to more definitions for the convenience of educational administration is more labelling of handicapped children, a practice further compounded by the irresistible tendency for more categories to lead to more special schools with intake restricted to children with the defined handicap. Educational labels have a tendency to stick long after the child has ceased to require special education. Whereas common-language descriptive adjectives, for example blind, physically handicapped, may be appropriate at any age, those newly coined for special education purposes are not: for instance, maladjusted has acquired connotations beyond educational significance which may be unhelpful to a school leaver, whilst to refer to a parent as being 'educationally subnormal, like her child' (a not uncommonly heard remark) is absurd.

To avoid these drawbacks a more sophisticated system of providing a child with special education is required, one which depends upon a child's personal, educational, therapeutic and management needs being accurately specified and the range of educational, medical and child care facilities in each special school being described. This was the basis of an experiment sponsored by the Department of Education and Science (1973). Since then, as a result of their enquiries into the education of handicapped children and young people, the Warnock Committee (1978) have recommended that the statutory categories of handicapped pupils should be replaced by a system for recording the special educational requirements of individual children based on a detailed profile of their needs.

Table 17.6 A classification of handicap

Functional handicap	Underlying disorder
Somatic (physical)	Cardiovascular disorder
	Respiratory disease
	Asthma
	Diabetes
	Epilepsy
	Other physical conditions
Motor	Cerebral palsy
	Spinal palsy
	Other neuromuscular disorders (with lesion at or below the brain stem)
	Orthopaedic conditions
Visual	Severe partial or total loss of sight
Communication	Severe partial or total loss of hearing
	Specific language disorder
	Speech defect
Learning	Specific reading retardation
	Intellectual retardation:
	mild
	severe
	Autism
Behavioural	Neurotic disorder
	Conduct disorder (with or without neurosis)
	Others

There remains a need however for a classification of handicap which is epidemiologically feasible and rational as a basis for planning special education and supporting health services. It has to indicate broadly the nature of the educational expertise and therapeutic facility each handicap requires and it has to be expressed in terms that are meaningful to professionals and public alike and do not stigmatize the child. The classification set out in Table 17.6 attempts to meet these conditions. It is not exhaustive, nor is it consistently scientific, but it is practical for service planning. It is essentially a functional classification: it refers to the six principal functions in which a child may be handicapped and it lists important or relatively common childhood disorders that may produce such handicaps. For this reason social handicap does not feature in the classification. Whereas a child is often described as being socially handicapped, family circumstances and environment only act as external obstacles to normal function. They may predispose or contribute to dysfunction and sometimes cause it, especially in learning and behaviour, but they are not in themselves an intrinsic functional disability.

Local education authorities also need to know the number of children for whom special education of various kinds is to be provided. Prevalence rates of disorders causing handicap, even when adjusted for children of school age, are not adequate for education planning purposes because not all children with a given disorder are handicapped to the extent of needing treatment or special education, and such rates do not take account of the fact that more than one disorder may occur in one child. What education authorities require are prevalence rates of children, among primary and secondary school populations separately, who need special services, and according to whether they need the full range that is usually provided in special schools, or certain facilities only that could perhaps be offered in an ordinary school.

The figures shown in Tables 17.7A and 17.7B can only be regarded as approximate prevalence rates. They have been compiled from the few studies known to the writer which produced reliable data regarding the severity of the

Table 17.7A Estimated prevalences of children with six functional handicaps of educational and medical concern and of moderate or severe intensity: age-specific rates per 1000 nursery school children, aged three and four years

Handicap	Rate per 1000 needing education and medical care
Somatic	2.0
Motor	4.2
Visual	0.4
Communication:	
hearing	2.0
language/speech	2.2
Learning	4.1
Behavioural	28.0

handicap and the child's school placement. They refer only to children with moderate or severe handicap, whose ability to participate in all classroom and school activities will consequently be limited and who will require either special education or regular health care (including nursing) or both, in school. In Table 17.7A, which refers to children at an age when they do not normally attend a school, the figures in the second column indicate the proportion of children requiring education, either part-time or full-time, as well as regular medical care whatever school or unit they may attend. In Table 17.7B, columns (c) and (d) indicate the distribution of handicapped children between ordinary schools and special schools. In so far as the figures are based upon current or recent practice, the special schools in column (d) would be those at present designated according to the category of handicapped pupil they admit; matching these categories to the functional handicaps presents no problem. The rates for children attending ordinary schools are likely to be minimal because of the stringent criteria of severity and because there are children who are educationally retarded and not shown in the table but have neither specific reading retardation nor intellectual retardation. The rates for children attending special schools are likely to be maximal since no allowance has been made for the possibility of

Table 17.7B Estimated prevalences of children with six functional handicaps of educational and medical concern and of moderate or severe intensity: age-specific rates per 1000 children attending Infant Schools, Junior Schools and Secondary Schools

School (age group)	Handicap (a)	Total rate per 1000 in need of special education and medical care (b)	Rates per 1000 children attending Ordinary school (c)	Special school (d)
Infant school children (aged 5–7 years)	Somatic (incl. epilepsy)	20.7	20.5	0.2
	Motor	6.0	3.6	1.5
	Visual	1.1	0.4	0.7
	Communication: hearing	2.5	1.7	0.8
	language and speech	10.8	10.3	0.5
	Learning	26.8	10.4	11.1
	Behavioural	28.0	27.8	0.2
Junior school children (aged 8–12 years)	Somatic (incl. epilepsy)	29.4	6.9	0.7
	Motor	6.0	3.6	1.5
	Visual	1.1	0.4	0.7
	Communication: hearing	1.8	1.3	0.5
	language and speech	3.2	2.8	0.4
	Learning	63.1	44.4	13.4
	Behavioural	45.0	28.2	0.9
Secondary school children (aged 13–16 years)	Somatic (incl. epilepsy)	29.4	26.9	0.7
	Motor	6.0	3.6	1.5
	Visual	1.1	0.4	0.7
	Communication: hearing	1.8	1.3	0.5
	language	0.8	0.4	0.4
	Learning	63.1	44.4	13.4
	Behavioural	90.0	56.4	0.9

Note. The figures in columns (c) and (d) do not always add up to that in column (b) because some children have more than one major handicap. The principal overlaps occur when severe intellectual retardation accompanies a neurological disorder (e.g. cerebral palsy, epilepsy, blindness) and governs school placement; and when children with a behavioural handicap have specific reading retardation (as happens in approximately one third of cases).

a proportion of them being able to attend ordinary schools, given the necessary supporting health services.

Health and education authorities need to carry out their own surveys, since the prevalence of some disorders is known to vary between different geographical areas (Laurence et al, 1968) as well as between inner-city and rural communities and between social classes (Davie et al, 1972; Akesson, 1974; Rutter et al, 1975; Berger et al, 1975).

Recognition and investigation

Recognition
The nature and severity of the disorder causing a schoolchild to be handicapped will often determine how soon he receives special education. Severe congenital malformations are almost invariably noticed within the first few days of life,

either by the mother and her attendants or as a result of a neonatal paediatric examination. Less serious abnormalities are usually detected during the preschool years, particularly by the health visitor, the general practitioner or the doctor in a child health clinic. Notable exceptions may be congenital malformations of the heart and genito-urinary disorders. The former, in the absence of symptoms, would only be picked up on routine medical examination associated with developmental surveillance or on routine auscultation in the event of an illness for which the family doctor is consulted. Brimblecombe et al (1975), in an exhaustive follow-up study of over 25 000 births, found one child whose congenital heart defect passed unnoticed until the age of five years.

Nevertheless, physical abnormalities are rarely missed, and their early recognition results in early investigation and treatment. When treatment has not been entirely successful in overcoming the handicap, and even if this is not immediately apparent to the teacher, there is seldom any reluctance on the part of the parent to tell either the infant school teacher or the school doctor. If special education is required by these children it is arranged with minimum delay.

The same cannot be said so confidently of sensory, psychiatric and neurological disorders, which may handicap a child in his learning and behaviour control. Quite serious impairment of hearing may not be discovered until it is found to be a cause of educational retardation. Such delay in recognition has usually been due to the child's not having undergone routine developmental testing, including a hearing test, at between the ages of nine months and five years; but sometimes loss of hearing, particularly when it is intermittent (as in 'glue ear'), is missed in spite of serial testing. Screening tests for high-tone deafness are not always effective and the signs and problems created by this handicap are not sufficiently appreciated by parents and teachers.

Alternatively, severe loss of hearing may be diagnosed and treated when it does not exist. This may happen in the case of a child who makes very slow progress in speech development or who fails to talk by the age of three or four years (Renfrew & Murphy, 1964; Rutter & Martin, 1972). These children present complex problems in diagnosis that may not be resolved before they enter school. The majority are likely to be mentally handicapped, unless they have a specific developmental speech disorder or infantile psychosis (autism).

It may still happen that the full extent of a child's mental handicap is not recognized until he goes to school. Prevalence rates for 'severe subnormality' (IQ < 50) in children aged 0 to four years are almost invariably lower than those reported in older age groups (Tizard, 1964; Birch et al, 1970; Kushlick & Cox, 1973). Exceptionally, a child with severe cerebral palsy may mistakenly be judged to be severely mentally retarded.

Instances of children with severe handicaps failing to receive the special education they need because of delay or confusion in the diagnosis are fortunately becoming more rare. It is the disorders of seemingly mild or only moderate severity whose recognition is a matter of more concern, and not only because of the much greater number of children involved. Borderline or mild mental retardation, minimal cerebral palsy, slight impairment of hearing, petit mal epilepsy with infrequent 'turns', or a minor degree of neurodevelopmental disorder (a term that summarizes a complex of signs without excluding the possibility of a developmental rather than pathological aetiology)—any of these may very easily pass unnoticed by the unsuspecting parent or teacher. The school doctor's medical examination is often not sufficiently searching to detect them. Moreover, even when parents are aware of intellectual retardation or petit mal, they may keep this knowledge to themselves. Yet the handicaps these mild disorders pose in a child's development may be disproportionately great, although this is only recognized when educational failure or disturbed behaviour have set in.

A system of identifying children who may need special education that is largely dependent upon the referral of individual children as and when their teachers feel they can no longer effectively help them, results often in unnecessary postponement of special education. Failure to adopt epidemiological methods for their identification is to deny education authorities the data that are a prerequisite for forward planning of special education facilities, as well as to miss opportunities teachers might otherwise have had for preventive educational intervention. The widespread use of serial developmental surveillance procedures in the health care of pre-school children (see Ch. 6) offers an opportunity to apply such methods. The introduction of neurodevelopmental tests into the medical interview of every child on entry to school at the age of five, that is now the practice of a number of school doctors, also adds a new dimension to the early recognition of children needing special education.

Investigation and assessment
In so far as a child in school has a handicap which was recognized at a young age, it is likely that his primary or presenting disorder will have been thoroughly investigated by a paediatrician or other specialist in hospital. It does not always follow that an assessment will have been made of other functions, especially vision, hearing and language, that might seem to be unrelated to the principal disorder. The establishment of assessment centres for handicapped children has added immensely to the breadth of investigation and encouraged a holistic approach to the care of young handicapped children (Sheridan, 1962; Ministry of Health, 1968). This has come about as a result of the combination of psychological, educational and social expertise with paediatric skill and experience, that has been a feature of such centres. Many paediatricians are now keenly aware that the diagnosis of disability, followed by assessment of handicap and treatment when indicated, meets only a proportion of the total needs of the child. The importance of behavioural and educational difficulties is better understood: it is recognized that, whilst these take longer to sort out than most medical problems, their initial evaluation is the better for having been carried out with reference to the medical background, and that all need continual review in the light of the development and maturation of the child and of his response to a co-ordinated programme of therapy, care and special education.

Assessment centres that include a nursery group in charge of a trained nursery school teacher with experience of handicapped children meet these requirements to some extent but they cannot do so for any length of time if, primarily, they have to serve an initial diagnostic and assessment function. Some centres have no nursery group and some health districts have no assessment centre. Education authorities have reacted to this situation by opening their own 'observation', 'diagnostic' or 'assessment' units. The exact number of these at present is not known. The main object of the units has been to provide a setting in which children could be observed over a period of time to allow an unhurried educational assessment to be made by teachers and educational psychologists with medical participation (DES, 1970). These units quickly ran into the same difficulties as the health service assessment centres in maintaining ready access to their diagnostic and assessment facilities. Waiting lists for admission grew because of a reluctance to discharge children from what had, in effect, become a therapeutic experience by the time initial diagnosis and assessment had been completed. This situation was exacerbated but not caused by a shortage of places for nursery and infant school children in special schools, and of special educational expertise in ordinary infant schools. The units also found difficulty in obtaining the necessary support from school psychological and school health services; the medical support suffered from being out of contact with paediatric and child psychiatric services.

A rationalization of the overall arrangements for the diagnosis and assessment of young handicapped children living within the common geographical boundary of health and education authorities, and of social service departments of local authorities, is urgently needed (Whitmore, 1969). What the early years of trial and error have shown is that arrangements for the diagnosis and assessment of young handicapped children must not be separated without very good reason from arrangements for their treatment, and that treatment must be viewed in educational as well as medical terms. There is more to a handicapped child than his medical disorder, and more to his special education than what is conventionally provided in special schools. There is a clear need for a centre in each local authority area which handicapped children can attend from a young age, if necessary daily or less frequently, and where there is a recognizable educational as well as medical component to developmental and social care. More recent experience in Exeter (Brimblecombe, 1974) has shown the additional benefit to the child and his parents of incorporating social services, including short-term residential facilities. Such centres would supplement rather than replace health service assessment centres, and both should co-ordinate their services with those of the education authority's special schools. There is now a real prospect of health, education and social service authorities co-operating to provide some common facilities for handicapped children. District handicap teams, as described by the Court Committee (1976) in their recommendations for child health services, have been accepted in principle and are beginning to be set up with staff contributed by the three services; and many of the recommendations of the Warnock Committee (1978) on special education, though not yet accepted, are complementary to the concept of unified, comprehensive services for handicapped children.

Role of the doctor
Health service assessment centres have been used almost exclusively for the investigation of young handicapped children. In the drive to identify disability as early as possible, the spotlight has naturally turned to the very young child.

After the newborn period, parents and health visitors are usually the first to notice a child's handicap, often a sensori-motor defect, and it is they who seek help. Even when physical signs first appear in a child attending school, it is the parent who takes the initiative and she turns to the family doctor. In contrast, the commonest handicaps first recognized in junior school children are educational retardation and behaviour disorder. More often it is the teacher rather than the parent who feels or appreciates the need for investigation and possible special education: and the teacher usually refers the child first to the educational psychologist.

A full medical examination is no less important for backward and disturbed children than for those presenting with physical signs. At least one in seven have physical handicaps also and among those with mental retardation the proportion is even higher (Rutter et al 1970b). For this reason a medical examination has been an essential feature in the procedure for obtaining special education for a child. In fact, not only have education authorities the power to require a child to be examined by a doctor so that they may be advised if the child has 'a disability of mind or body'; they have come to depend upon the doctor to advise them into which category of handicapped pupil the child should be placed, and this amounts to a prescription for special education.

The predominant role of the doctor in ascertainment has not been altogether satisfactory. It has often been a cause for dissension between school doctors and educational psychologists: only recently has it come to be accepted that it is professionally inappropriate for doctors to make educational decisions on behalf of an education authority. It has led to a misrepresentation of the function of a doctor in relation to handicapped schoolchildren; it has cast him in the role of controller of admissions to special schools; it has fostered the erroneous idea that medical examination is only necessary when formal ascertainment of a child as a handicapped pupil is required, and it has thus contributed to the reluctance of teachers to refer educationally retarded children for medical investigation unless they have themselves been of the opinion that the child needs to attend a special school for educationally subnormal pupils. In addition, it has bedevilled professional relationships between the doctor and his 'patient' (parent) when his certification of the child as a handicapped pupil has allowed the education authority to place the child in a special school against the parents' wishes. Mentally retarded schoolchildren have usually been at the centre of these disputes (see p. 335) yet the parents of such children are the very ones who are in great need of continuing support.

In a circular issued by the Department of Education and Science (1975), attention was drawn to the importance of the contribution of teachers and psychologists as well as of doctors in the assessment of handicapped children and the need for all three to work together in arriving at decisions entailing a combination of treatment and special education. The intention of the circular was to bring about a gradual re-allocation of responsibilities between medical and educational personnel in a way that is consistent with their professional experience and, through the introduction of a new set of special education (SE) forms, to influence the quality and range of the assessment of these children. These aims and the accompanying procedures have been generally welcomed by the teaching profession and supported by the multidisciplinary Warnock Committee (1978), though it is feared by some that any attempt to apply the Committee's rather rigid concept of five stages of assessment might be confusing and in many ways counter-productive.

It is generally the school doctor who carries out the medical examinations of schoolchildren needing special education, except in the case of maladjusted pupils and those with sensory handicap (see below). He also has the task of supervising the treatment and health care of handicapped children in whatever school they attend, and of advising their teachers. He can provide better continuity in this care if he works in both the pre-school and the school health services of the authority and if he is involved in the work of the assessment centre.

The school doctor is better able to provide a competent service if he has received an appropriate training. Some have sought to obtain this but it is a matter for concern that, save in one respect only, doctors employed in the school health service have not been required to have any special qualifications or experience. The single exception is for doctors called upon to examine mentally and educationally retarded children whom local education authorities have had in mind to formally ascertain as educationally subnormal pupils (as set out in Section 34 of the Education Act 1944). These doctors must have attended approved courses of instruction and practice in such examinations; a number of university departments of child health now organize these courses on a day-release basis (DES, 1974b; DHSS, 1975).

There continues to be a very real need for doctors knowledgeable about educational medicine and competent in the care of handicapped children in school but in future they will surely need to have undergone a period of postgraduate training in this field of paediatrics (see Ch. 15). Because problems of learning and behaviour predominate among the handicaps of schoolchildren, training should contain a considerable content of child neurology and psychiatry. It should also aim to establish an understanding of the role of psychologists in school (DES, 1968a; Whitmore, 1972). The adjacent realms of child neurology and child psychology are not sharply differentiated and paediatrician and psychologist should each be aware of his own limitations and learn when the special skills of the other need to be invoked. They have to build up a working relationship based upon professional equality.

Special arrangements in school
Some of the special arrangements made for handicapped children when they reach school age are of a general kind that apply to all handicapped children, notably for instance special schools and specialist supporting staff; others are more specifically designed for children with particular handicaps.

Special schools and special classes
The origins of special schools largely reside in the efforts of parents of handicapped children and other keenly interested and committed individuals to obtain better educational arrangements than were current in their time for children with particular handicapping disorders. In bygone years this led inevitably to

the opening of private special units or schools and the segregation of handicapped children in institutions according to their handicap or disorder, for example blindness, physical handicap, mental handicap, epilepsy (Pritchard, 1963). The separation of these children from the normal population also met with the general approval of the public for social reasons, at a time when society was rather more rejecting of its 'lame ducks' than it is today (Kershaw, 1973). So successful was this method that, in spite of the advent of local education authorities with legal obligations to provide their own arrangements for special education, it has continued to be used to this day in extending special education to other groups of handicapped children, for example by the Spastics Society for children with cerebral palsy and by the Society for Autistic Children.

More than 20 years ago the Ministry of Education (1954) forthrightly declared: 'No handicapped pupil should be sent to a special school who can be satisfactorily educated in an ordinary school.' The Achilles heel of this axiom proved to be the ambiguity of the phrase 'can be'. Did this refer to the education the child could achieve as a result of being a pupil like any other child in the school, or to what the school could achieve in adapting to the educational needs of the child? In any case, the pronouncement was overshadowed by the subsequent preoccupation of the Ministry in the building of special schools (for the programming and financing of which it had a major responsibility) and its failure to gather statistics about handicapped children in ordinary schools comparable to those obtained annually about handicapped pupils in special schools.

Thus, past expediences have exerted a considerable influence on present-day educational provision (Ministry of Education, 1956; National Union of Teachers, 1964; Kershaw, 1973; Henderson, 1974).

The concept that special education is synonymous with education in a special school has taken firm root, as shown by the three-fold increase in the number of special schools since 1946 and the four-fold increase in the number of children attending them over a period during which the school population increased by only two thirds.

Now there are signs of renewed interest in catering specifically for handicapped children in ordinary schools. 'In a variety of ways the barriers are coming down within and around special education' (DES, 1973) and integration is the watchward. The trend was first seen in the 1960s when many classes and units for children with impaired hearing were opened, mostly in primary schools (DES, 1967). It received impetus from special surveys (e.g. Rutter et al, 1970b) which reminded people how many handicapped children there were in ordinary schools, some of them being severely handicapped, and from the response of local education authorities to the initiative of parents of children with congenital deformities due to thalidomide in campaigning for ordinary school placement for most of their children (DES, 1964 and 1972a). The impetus has been maintained by a greater understanding of the issues involved, as a result of detailed studies of physically handicapped children in both ordinary and special schools (Pringle & Fiddes, 1970; Wilson, 1970; McMichael, 1971; Anderson, 1973; Tew, 1973) and of mentally handicapped children fostered in community settings rather than isolated institutions (Tizard, 1964); by the challenge to change presented by the experience of Scandinavian countries (Melchior, 1968;

Grunewald, 1971; Anderson, 1971); by local experiments in integration (Conway, 1968; Peirse, 1973); and by the greater interest shown this time by education departments in central government in stimulating dialogue and supporting research projects (DES, 1973; Scottish Education Department, 1975) and in collecting information about handicapped children attending special classes in ordinary schools. The picture is emerging of very uneven organization of special classes for children with different handicaps. In 1976, 2.9 per cent of children with somatic and motor handicaps whom education authorities had placed in schools as handicapped pupils were in special classes in ordinary schools, compared with 30 per cent of children with communication handicap and 10 per cent of behaviourally handicapped children. Nevertheless, that year 12 per cent of all handicapped pupils in schools were attending ordinary schools.

An extension of these facilities would be one way of augmenting the special education services in areas having little provision. In the past there have been very wide ranges in the regional rates of handicapped pupils in each category (DES, 1966). A number of explanations have been put forward, including shortage of professional staff, lack of funds and policy decisions by education authorities. To these could be added a reluctance to use residential special schools when no day special school is available. This is another aspect of the issues associated with the school placement of handicapped children. Whereas only 9 per cent of children in special schools and classes because of learning handicap were residential pupils in 1976, the comparable figure for those with communication handicap was 11 per cent, for those with somatic and motor handicap 32 per cent, and for children with behaviour disorder 25 per cent. The more special the school the more uncommon and sheltered the environment, and the more likely it is to be residential in order to be viable; yet many physically handicapped children will have spent long periods in hospital in pre-school years. Little is known about the effects of these less tangible and immeasurable features of special school education. The indiscriminate use of residential special schools for some physically handicapped children has been criticized and clear criteria for such placements have been suggested (Rackham, 1975).

The debate on integration versus segregation continues (DES, 1971, 1972b, 1974a; Pless, 1969; Joint Council for the Education of Handicapped Children, 1975; Scottish Education Department, 1975) but if and when Section 10 of the Education Act 1976 is implemented there will be a further shift of emphasis in special education towards integration. Section 10 requires local education authorities to arrange for the special education of all handicapped pupils to be given in county and voluntary schools, except where this is impracticable, incompatible with efficient instruction in the schools or involves unreasonable public expenditure. However, the day on which Section 10 will come into force has not yet (1980) been appointed by the government. In the meantime, there is likely to be a continuing increase and improvement in the facilities for special education of handicapped children in ordinary schools without any significant reduction in the provision of special schools, for the report of the Warnock Committee (1978) is expected to have a major influence on special education. Strongly advocating a much wider general framework for special education than the present statutory concept and the idea that special education be viewed as additional or supplementary rather than separate or alternative provision, the report at the same time confirms unequivocally the need for special schools for certain groups of handicapped children.

Within this context it is the function of those who plan and man the child health services to provide the necessary facilities for handicapped children where they are needed and to avoid introducing therapeutic considerations too prominently in the case for special schools. It is tempting to argue that the concentration of medical facilities in a few special schools ensures the most 'efficient' and 'economical' use of these resources for handicapped children, and is therefore one justification for teaching the children in separate schools from normal children. Yet no study has ever been made of the comparative cost-effectiveness of different methods of providing therapeutic services to handicapped children in various kinds of school, balanced against the overall developmental interests of the child; and there is a point at which these must take precedence over the maximum efficiency in the use of resources. In strictly medical terms, the recurrent interruption in the continuity of certain forms of health care, for example the treatment of epilepsy, physiotherapy, or psychiatric management, caused by school holidays can be a serious disadvantage in concentrating resources in special schools, especially residential schools.

The basic needs of every handicapped child in terms of education and social development are those of all children (Pringle & Fiddes, 1970) and the advantages to him of their being realistically met in the company of all children nearly always outweigh the disadvantages. Once it is accepted that these, and not medical treatment, are the long-term factors governing school placement, teachers can explore ways of adapting the educational and social arrangements in their schools to meet the additional needs of children with functional handicaps, and the latter can be relieved of the burden of having to measure up to the requirements of the school in order to remain within it. It is in this context that health care has to be arranged; rarely, and only then episodically, may it need to take precedence.

Specialist supporting staff

The health care of handicapped children in school is an essential component of educational medicine and a task that falls pre-eminently to doctors and nurses in whose special training and experience this work should have been included. The services of other paediatricians and specialists are required according to the underlying disorder from which the child suffers. All have a role in the treatment and care of the child but they have a responsibility also, in the interests of the child, to keep the teacher informed about his medical state and management in so far as such information is necessary for the proper teaching and care of the child in school.

This raises problems of confidentiality which may be very difficult to resolve, and are perhaps becoming greater as a result of the tendency for 'personal services' to become depersonalized as they are increasingly managed by large authorities. Some doctors believe that the interests of handicapped children are better served by maintaining strict medical confidentiality but this is questionable when a child's safety in school is at stake, as it may be for instance if unbeknown to a teacher he is liable to have a major convulsion. It is easier to avoid than to overcome these problems and any doctor concerned with handicapped schoolchildren should work always in collaboration with, and never in isolation from, their teachers, just as much as with their parents. Parents almost invariably appreciate the advantage this holds for their child and welcome medical information being given to teachers once the reasons are explained. The importance of continual dialogue between doctor and teacher, and the risks involved in underrating this, have been clearly shown in the case of children with epilepsy, diabetes, spina bifida and some other disorders (Laurence, 1971; McMichael, 1971; Watson, 1972; Anderson, 1973; Holdsworth & Whitmore, 1974; Tyrrell, 1975) but they apply to children with every form of handicap.

Arrangements for children with somatic and motor handicaps
In the terminology of categories (see Appendix), children with somatic handicaps are referred to as delicate pupils, and the special schools they attend have traditionally been known as 'open-air schools'. This was originally an apt description, as one of their hallmarks was classrooms and rest sheds open to the fresh air; they were commonly residential and situated on the coast. They were used especially for poor, undernourished city children suffering from physical debility and respiratory disease, and their regimen provided for an hour's rest and three meals every day, even when they only admitted day pupils (Ministry of Education, 1952). Now premises and regimens are like those of other schools, though they still provide a sheltered environment. Only a minority of children attend because of failure to thrive and these children are frail because of medical disorders, for example cystic fibrosis, diabetes, congenital malformation of the heart, haemophilia, rather than debilitated from poverty and undernourishment. Children with chronic bronchitis and asthma predominate, but increasing numbers are admitted with a diagnosis of 'nervous debility', having found the ordinary school overwhelming, and more and more children with neuromuscular and orthopaedic disorders use the schools. In some schools as many as one third of the children may have motor handicaps (Lowden & Walker, 1975).

Again in the terminology of categories, children with motor handicaps are referred to as physically handicapped and attend special schools for such pupils. Cerebral palsy and spina bifida are the two commonest disorders (in the ratio of 2 : 1) necessitating a child's admission, followed by muscular dystrophy and congenital limb deformity. However, in addition, these schools have always been considered as providing an alternative placement for children with congenital heart disorder and haemophilia, thus serving in part the function of schools for the delicate. For this reason, and because all the disorders mentioned above appear among physically handicapped children in ordinary schools, arrangements for children with somatic and motor handicaps are dealt with under one heading in this chapter.

In 1976, 64 per cent of delicate pupils receiving special education were in schools catering only for delicate children, whilst 45 per cent of physically handicapped pupils were in schools solely for the physically handicapped. The principal difference between schools for the delicate and schools for the physically handicapped is that the latter are designed more specifically for motor handicapped children. They are built with wide circulation areas and doors, with slopes rather than occasional steps, and a lift as well as stairs to upper floors to permit mobility of children in wheelchairs; a few of the schools are built only at ground level. They also have well-equipped physiotherapy departments, often including a hydrotherapy pool. Schools for delicate pupils have physiotherapy available but often only on a sessional basis. Both types of school have a full-time nurse on the staff, and more than one if the school accepts boarders. The children are registered with their own family doctor, or with the school's general practitioner if they are residential; they will usually be attending a hospital consultant at home, although some schools arrange for consultants to visit the school. Speech therapy is usually available in both kinds of schools, though seldom full-time.

The responsibility for maintaining health surveillance of the children rests largely with the school doctor; general practitioners rarely provide health supervision of a child's chronic handicapping disorder and hospital consultants rarely have time to examine the child and talk to his parents and teachers as often as supervision requires. The school doctor has to ensure that educational factors are not overlooked by those who have to treat the child and that medical aspects of the disorder and treatment receive full consideration in the education of the child. This continuity of care is difficult to achieve when the school doctor has only an advisory role, without personal clinical responsibility for the child. Exceptionally, the general practitioner to a school will assume a school doctor role, but this is not a solution for children attending day schools. A doctor who knows both the child and his teachers may be in the best position to judge the need for and supervise restrictions on physical activities in school; unnecessary restrictions might then be avoided (Dawkins & Reid, 1965; Brown, 1966; Holdsworth & Whitmore, 1974). A school may sometimes be a more appropriate place to treat certain disorders, for example epilepsy or asthma, than either health centre or hospital.

Nursing and treatment demands in school may be greatest from children with spinal palsy. They include the management of urinary and faecal incontinence, the prevention and treatment of urinary infection, trophic ulcers and obesity, and the oversight of Spitz-Holter and other valves. Henderson (1968) has described the nursing and medical care of these children in school and Nash (1969) has discussed ways in which teachers can co-operate in their health care. Intensive and regular physiotherapy is most needed by children with cerebral palsy and spina bifida, although its efficacy may be overrated (Wright & Nicholson, 1973): as with speech therapy, the mother's contribution can be invaluable. These children, and those with congenital limb deformities, may need a variety of aids, including walking aids, wheelchairs and powered or conventional prostheses (Blockey, 1971; Holt et al, 1972).

A survey carried out in 1969 revealed over 10 000 children in ordinary schools whom school doctors had classified locally as physically handicapped (DES, 1972a). Two thirds of them were in primary schools, although the rate for primary and secondary schools was the same: 1.2 per 1000. All but a few of the children were in ordinary classes with their peers; special classes for physically handicapped children in ordinary schools have not been developed to the extent reported in Denmark (Melchior, 1968). As the range of disabilities is as great among these children as among those in special schools, so is the range of nursing and treatment facilities required. A quarter of them were using a wheelchair, walking aid or prosthesis; 607 were incontinent, of whom 262 wore appliances. The survey showed that 60 per cent of the schools attended by the children were receiving a visit from the school nurse less frequently than once a month, and almost as many were visited by the school doctor only once a year or less often, so that the short-fall in services is considerable.

Failure or inability to organize the services that are needed in ordinary schools is one reason for physically handicapped children having to go to special schools. Another reason is restriction on mobility, due either to the severity of the child's handicap or, as often as not, to the limitations of the design of the school. Travel to school does not create a problem save in remote rural areas: education authorities have power to pay for the transport of any child to an ordinary or a special school, if need be. The time that such transport takes to a day school may be the determining factor in attendance at a special residential school. The presence of an additional handicap also makes special school placement necessary for some children; these other handicaps occur more often than is realized in severely motor handicapped children (Pringle & Fiddes, 1970; Smithells, 1973; Tew, 1973).

The severity of somatic disorders, or the frequency with which symptoms recur, are the main considerations in sending a somatic-handicapped child to a special school. The educational and health care problems of asthmatic children have received particular attention in a number of recent studies (Graham et al, 1967; Dawson et al, 1969; Mitchell & Dawson, 1973; Miller et al, 1975).

Local education authorities have been able to pay for asthmatic schoolchildren to receive special educational treatment in Switzerland. The effect of such treatment on the frequency of attacks has sometimes been disappointing (Smith, 1970).

Most of the estimated 6000 schoolchildren who have diabetes mellitus attend their local school; a minority attend special schools for delicate children and there is hostel accommodation for about 100 children. In these hostels children and their parents soon learn the discipline and routine of the diabetic life and thereafter return to their own schools.

It has been estimated that approximately 1200 schoolboys in Britain have haemophilia or Christmas disease but at any time only one in six is in a special school. What happens to these children during their school years is crucial, since severe crippling is most likely to occur before adolescence: the prompt treatment of bleeding is essential. As not all primary schools are sufficiently close to a special centre for the treatment of haemophilia for this to happen, Britten and her colleagues (Britten et al, 1966) recommended the establishment of a special school for haemophiliac boys in association with a hospital treatment centre. So far this has not materialized, but one special school for physically handicapped children in Alton, Hampshire, has special experience in the treatment of haemophilia and works closely with the special treatment centre at Oxford.

With epilepsy occurring in seven children per 1000 aged five to 14 years, there are probably close on 67 000 children with epilepsy in school. Only 2 per cent of these are in special schools, mostly schools for physically handicapped or educationally subnormal pupils. Six hundred and thirty-one are in the six special schools for children with epilepsy; this group of children are very severely handicapped by the frequency and severity of their seizures and by learning and behaviour handicaps (Ministry of Education, 1962). Children with epilepsy who remain in their own schools also have considerable difficulties. Seizures that occur in school premises trouble nearly half of them but the incidence of learning and behaviour disorders far exceeds that in other children (Gastaut, 1964; Rutter et al, 1970a; Bagley, 1971; Holdsworth & Whitmore, 1974; Stores, 1978). The frequency with which a child's epilepsy is not revealed to his teachers, the latter's unfamiliarity with and misconceptions about the disorder and its potential handicap to the child, and the additional problems for the child arising from his treatment and his restrictions in school, again indicate the need for considerably more health care in ordinary schools.

At any time there are approximately 2300 schoolchildren who are not at school but receive part-time home tuition. Half these children are physically handicapped. There are many reasons why they have not been attending a school but in most cases this form of special education is not satisfactory and the health care of the children is frequently inadequate (DES, 1964, 1972b).

Arrangements for children with visual handicaps
Children with a severe visual handicap will be examined by an ophthalmologist before arrangements are made for their education. The methods of special education vary according to the child's visual acuity: he may be classified as either partially sighted or blind. At the same time the ophthalmologist will consider whether the child should be registered under the National Assistance Act 1948 as blind or partially sighted for the purposes of receiving welfare services. Problems have arisen in the past from a child being ascertained as a partially sighted pupil but registered as a blind person.

Few 'blind' children are totally without sight but they are regarded as blind educationally if their visual acuity is not sufficient for them to be taught by methods dependent upon sight. This is almost invariably the case when visual acuity is below 3/60 on the Snellen test. Blind pupils then require special education from trained teachers of the blind and they need to learn Braille as soon as possible.

There is less certainty about the Snellen test rating of visual acuity that differentiates the partially sighted pupil. In the classroom the child needs to be able to see print on a blackboard and on wall charts as well as in books, and whilst various lenses and low visual aids may partly compensate for his defect, his ability under such circumstances to profit from teaching in an ordinary classroom will depend very much on other factors, such as his personality and intelligence and his teacher's understanding of his handicap and patience and help in dealing with it.

Special committees set up in Scotland, and in England and Wales, have recently reported on the education of visually handicapped children, and on criteria that might be used in making educational recommendations (Scottish Education Department, 1969; DES, 1972c).

The characteristics and abilities of blind and partially sighted schoolchildren, and their educational needs, have also been described by Fine (1968), Smith & James (1968), Watts (1972) and Lansdown (1969, 1975). The effect of a squint on a child's education has been reviewed by Haskell (1966) and by Alberman et al (1971). The trend has been towards the education of blind and partially sighted children in separate special schools. In 1976, 85 per cent of the blind pupils receiving special education were in schools for blind children only, whilst 70 per cent of the partially sighted pupils were in schools taking only partially sighted children. There was one school for children who were deaf and partially sighted.

Arrangements for children with communication handicaps
There are more children with impaired hearing than with speech and language disorder who need special arrangements in school. Their handicaps are best investigated in audiology clinics, staffed by an otologist, paediatrician or school doctor, psychologist, teacher of the deaf and audiometrician, any one of whom may be a trained audiologist (Reed, 1971). These clinics are organized in hospitals, in schools or in independent premises but there are still too few of them; Ear, Nose and Throat Departments of hospitals are seldom so staffed and equipped as to serve the function of an audiology clinic.

As with visually impaired children, so the hearing impaired rarely suffer from total loss of function. Educationally, the difference between deaf and partially hearing children has hinged upon the level of the child's naturally acquired speech and language. When a child has virtually neither of these he is regarded as a deaf pupil, requiring education by trained teachers of the deaf. Their methods of special education are principally oral, the child learning to understand their spoken words from visual (lip-reading) and tactile cues. The value and need for manual methods of communication (finger-spelling and signing) in the education of deaf children remains a matter of keen professional argument (DES, 1968b).

If the child has sufficient hearing acuity to have acquired a modicum of speech and to serve as a basis for aural learning, he will be classified as a partially hearing pupil and be taught by a teacher of the deaf using auditory methods. The child has to wear a single or binaural hearing aid and the classroom needs to be fitted with an induction-loop system. Lip-reading is also an important aid to his understanding spoken language. The special arrangements that can be made for hearing-impaired children in school have been described in detail by Ewing (1960), Dale (1967) and Watson (1967).

Medresco hearing aids, including behind-the-ear models, are supplied free through the National Health Service but a commercial aid can be provided for schoolchildren with severe loss of hearing who cannot benefit from the standard range of aids. School doctors as well as teachers of the deaf have a responsibility to ensure that teachers are familiar with the use and care of hearing aids when they have a hearing-handicapped child in their class. A high proportion of aids have been found to be unreliable (DES, 1969).

More children have been supplied with a hearing aid than have been ascertained as deaf or partially hearing pupils. Whether they need to attend a special school or special class, or remain in their own class in an ordinary school, depends upon many other factors than the degree of hearing loss. It is generally agreed that a loss of about 55 decibels or more necessitates education in a special school or unit (Sheridan, 1972; Peckham et al, 1972). The child with a loss of hearing for high tones is particularly vulnerable in school in respect of both his learning and his behaviour. There is one special residential school in England for deaf children who also have severe behaviour disorder.

Most children with speech defects when they first enter school at the age of five have achieved normal, intelligible speech before they move into the junior school at seven or eight (DES, 1966). A small proportion, perhaps seven or eight per 1000 (Ingram, 1963; Rutter et al, 1970a), have continuing severe speech or language disorders although their hearing is normal. The features of these children have recently been reported by Sheridan (1973): they have to be distinguished from other non-communicating children (Minski & Shepherd, 1970). There are five special residential schools for children with severe speech and language disorder; their education presents great difficulties and they make only slow progress (Rose, 1973; Petrie, 1975).

Arrangements for children with learning handicap
Learning handicap is manifest and usually measured as reading retardation but this is very commonly accompanied by retardation in other educational tasks, such as spelling and arithmetic. Whether reading handicap is expressed as reading backwardness (see p. 315) or as specific reading retardation (see footnote to Table 17.5), more than 80 per cent of children so handicapped are likely to be in ordinary schools. Clearly, arrangements for the special educational help of learning handicapped children need to be more plentiful in ordinary schools than special schools.

Education statistics show 12 904 children in England and Wales as receiving full-time special education in special classes in ordinary schools in 1976 (DES, 1976). This figure only represents the number whom education authorities have ascertained as educationally subnormal pupils; many more who would have been needing special help with their learning would have been given remedial reading for a session or more each week, or have been placed in 'progress', 'remedial', 'tutorial' or 'opportunity' classes for part of their time in school. The variety of arrangements for slow learners in secondary schools have been recorded by Her Majesty's Inspectors of Schools (DES, 1971). The progress of some junior schoolchildren for whom similar arrangements were made has also been recorded (Mannix, 1972).

Arrangements in school for children with dyslexia have again become the subject of educational debate. Argument has mainly centred round whether a syndrome of specific developmental dyslexia with a special aetiology, as postulated by certain neurologists (Critchley, 1964), really exists. The opposing view has been that severe reading difficulties are associated with a whole variety of factors, any one of which may operate singly or in combination in a given child, and that the particular combination of features said to be characteristic of children with specific developmental dyslexia occurs only in a very small number of children at one end of the continuum of reading disorders. The Advisory Committee on Handicapped Children (of the DES) suggested in their report on the matter (1972d) that the term 'specific reading difficulty' should be used instead of dyslexia or specific developmental dyslexia in describing the disability of children whose reading attainments are significantly below the standard which their abilities in other directions would lead one to expect; they advised that remedial teaching, geared to the needs of the child as determined by full investigation, should be organized in ordinary schools and in a few remedial education centres.

A Word Blind Centre for Dyslexic Children was opened in London by the Invalid Children's Aid Association between 1965 and 1974 as an experimental and research unit for the assessment and treatment of dyslexia. Ninety-eight boys were studied and the findings supported the view that some reading and spelling disorders are constitutionally determined but that varying aetiological factors were associated with different patterns of reading disability (Naidoo, 1972). The study also showed that such help or remedial tuition as the boys had received was inadequate. The Association had earlier published advice on the teaching of children with specific dyslexia (Franklin & Naidoo, 1970).

Intellectual retardation is closely associated in people's minds with educational retardation, so much so that educational subnormality and mental subnormality are commonly regarded as synonymous. This of course is not so. Intellectual retardation is only one of many reasons for a child being backward in his school work and needing special education, whilst mental subnormality (and severe subnormality) in children is an expression of intellectual retardation in terms of social prognosis. The importance that in the past has been attached to a child's IQ in reaching educational decisions, and especially the use of the cut-off IQs of 70 and 50 as principal criteria respectively for admission to a school for educationally subnormal pupils and classification as severely subnormal, has fostered this misconception. It is often overlooked that almost as many intellectually retarded children may be found in ordinary schools as in special schools, and one quarter to one third of children in schools for the educationally subnormal are not intellectually retarded ($IQ<70$). Understandably, parents have sometimes accepted that their child is backward in school but objected to his going to a special school as an educationally subnormal pupil because 'he is not mental'.

Parents have always had a right of appeal to the Secretary of State for Education against decisions of education authorities to place handicapped children in special schools. This right may be exercised whatever the nature of the child's handicap but the very great majority of appeals in the past were made in respect of educationally subnormal children, especially those who had some degree of intellectual retardation (DES, 1972a; Ministry of Education, 1962). Until 1970 it was possible for education authorities to exclude a child from receiving teaching in school or at home: as a result of investigation the authority could conclude that the child was so mentally handicapped as to be incapable of receiving education. The health authority then offered the child a place in a training centre. As a result of the Education (Handicapped Children) Act 1970 local education authorities are no longer able to make exceptions in meeting their legal responsibility to provide all children with education according to their age, ability and aptitude, and what were health authority training centres for severely subnormal children have become education authority special schools for severely educationally subnormal pupils (DES, 1972a). Within the last three years a number of experiments have been taking place in mixing severely mentally handicapped children with mildly educationally subnormal children in special schools (Nicholls, 1975) and in providing special education for them in special classes in ordinary school (Peirse, 1973). These mentally handicapped children are among the most seriously learning handicapped of all children, and they have high rates of associated somatic and motor handicaps (Marshall, 1967): some 6000 attend hospital schools (Mittler & Woodward, 1966).

Arrangements for children with behaviour handicap
The present practice is for child psychiatrists, as directors of child guidance and child psychiatric clinics, to make recommendations for children with behaviour disorders who need to attend special schools for maladjusted pupils. This recommendation will be made following full investigation and assessment by the teams, which include a social worker and either an educational psychologist, or a clinical psychologist.

Schools for maladjusted children were mostly residential but more day schools have been opened during the last decade. All the schools are small, taking on average 50 to 60 children, and they have a high staff/child ratio. Some schools are well supported by a visiting psychiatrist and psychologist, and occasionally by a psychotherapist; a few have the part-time services of a social worker. The organization and special education in day schools in London has been described by Lansdown (1970); the residential treatment of maladjusted pupils has been discussed by Hamblin (1975) and the heads of some schools have written of their own schools (Wills, 1960; Lenhoff, 1966).

Most schools for maladjusted children aim at being therapeutic communities, tolerant and accepting of behaviour that has frequently been such as to cause the child's exclusion from his own school. Initially fewer educational demands are made on him; educational failure is a prominent feature of many children with behaviour disorders (Rutter et al, 1970a; Varlaam, 1974). Nevertheless, remedial education is seen as an important method of treatment. Roe (1965) attempted to evaluate the effect on children's educational progress and behaviour development of attending day and residential schools. This was in the nature of a pilot study and her findings were inconclusive, though they demonstrated the difficulty in making generalizations in this field.

The number of children ascertained as maladjusted pupils in 1976 in England and Wales (20 878) is equivalent to a rate of 2.2 per 1000 schoolchildren, which is only a fraction of the rate of behaviour handicap requiring special attention in school (see Table 17.7B). As for children with learning handicap, the urgent need is for more special arrangements in ordinary schools. Most maladjusted children must be treated by people other than professionals who work in child psychiatric clinics but the latter need to give their advice and time in support of teachers. Tizard (1973) has called for an extension of remedial education and behaviour modification techniques in the classroom. A major research study in Newcastle is engaged in exploring the use of certain preventive and interventive measures in ordinary schools by specialist and teaching staff together (Kolvin et al, 1975). Webb (1967) has convincingly shown how teachers can help young children with behaviour disorders which first appear or spill over from home in the Infant School. Boxall (1973) has been studying the value of organizing small groups of children ('nurture groups') in infant schools, in which young children with seriously unsocialized behaviour related to impoverished early experiences are helped to re-learn from restorative experiences and developmental opportunities provided by a teacher and helper, guided by a psychologist.

The special education of overactive (hyperkinetic) young children in whom there is evidence of brain damage presents even greater problems. Special teaching methods have been described that aim at creating a learning situation which is not too stimulating for these children, who have great difficulty in concentrating (Cruickshank et al, 1961; Maier, 1970). Wilson (1967) has compared special arrangements seen in schools in the United States with those in England.

Autistic children are handicapped in many of the ways characteristic of children with learning and behaviour disorders, including distractability and overactivity. Several special schools for autistic children have been opened during recent years but the progress in development and in learning made by the children is usually very slow (Bartak & Rutter, 1973).

Appendix: education, England and Wales*

Categories of handicapped pupils
(a) *Blind pupils*, that is to say, pupils who have no sight or whose sight is or is likely to become so defective that they require education by methods not involving the use of sight.
(b) *Partially sighted pupils*, that is to say, pupils who by reason of defective vision cannot follow the normal regime of ordinary schools without detriment to their sight or to their educational development, but can be educated by special methods involving the use of sight.
(c) *Deaf pupils*, that is to say, pupils with impaired hearing who require education by methods suitable for pupils with little or no naturally acquired speech or language.
(d) *Partially hearing pupils*, that is to say, pupils with impaired hearing whose development of speech and language, even if retarded, is following a normal pattern, and who require for their education special arrangements or facilities though not necessarily all the educational methods used for deaf pupils.
(e) *Educationally subnormal pupils*, that is to say, pupils who, by reason of limited ability or other conditions resulting in educational retardation, require some specialized form of education wholly or partly in substitution for the education normally given in ordinary schools.

* Extract from *The Handicapped Pupils and Special Schools Regulations*, 1959, No. 365 as *amended* by The Handicapped Pupils and Special Schools Amending Regulations, 1962, No. 2073.

(f) *Epileptic pupils*, that is to say, pupils who by reason of epilepsy cannot be educated under the normal regime of ordinary schools without detriment to themselves or other pupils.
(g) *Maladjusted pupils*, that is to say, pupils who show evidence of emotional instability or psychological disturbance and require special educational treatment in order to effect their personal, social or educational readjustment.
(h) *Physically handicapped pupils*, that is to say, pupils not suffering solely from a defect of sight or hearing who by reason of disease or crippling defect cannot, without detriment to their health or educational development, be satisfactorily educated under the normal regime of ordinary schools.
(i) *Pupils suffering from speech defect*, that is to say, pupils who on account of defect or lack of speech not due to deafness require special educational treatment.
(j) *Delicate pupils*, that is to say, pupils not falling under any category in this regulation, who by reason of impaired physical condition need a change of environment or cannot, without risk to their health or educational development, be educated under the normal regime of ordinary schools.

REFERENCES

Akesson H O 1974 Geographical differences in the prevalence of mental deficiency. *British Journal of Psychiatry* 125: 542–546
Alberman E D, Butler N R, Gardiner P A 1971 Children with squints, Practitioner 206: 501–506
Anderson E M 1971 Making ordinary schools special. Guidelines for Teachers, No. 10. College of Special Education, London
Anderson E M 1973 The disabled schoolchild. Methuen, London
Bagley C 1971 The social psychology of the child with epilepsy. Routledge & Kegan Paul, London
Bartak L, Rutter M 1973 Special educational treatment of autistic children. Journal of Child Psychology and Psychiatry 14: 161–179 and 241–270
Berger M, Yule W, Rutter M 1975 The prevalence of specific reading retardation. British Journal of Psychiatry 126: 510–519
Birch H G, Richardson S A, Baird D, Horobin G, Illsley R 1970. Mental subnormality in the community. Williams & Wilkins, Baltimore
Blockey N J 1971 Aids for crippled children. Developmental Medicine and Child Neurology 13: 216–227
Boxall M 1973 Multiple deprivation: An experiment in nurture. Occasional Papers of the Division of Education and Child Psychology of the British Psychological Society, Spring, 91–113
Brimblecombe F S W 1974 Exeter project for handicapped children. British Medical Journal iv: 706–709
Brimblecombe F S W, Vowles M, Pethybridge R J 1975 Congenital malformations in Devon: their incidence, age and primary source of detection. In: Bridging in health (Nuffield Provincial Hospitals Trust) Oxford University Press, London
Britten M I, Spooner R J, Dormandy K M, Biggs R 1966 The haemophilic boy in school. British Medical Journal, ii: 224–228
Brown A 1966 Physical education for spastics. Special Education 55: 15–17
Butler N 1969 Children at risk. Concern, No 3. National Bureau for Co-operation in Child Care, London
Conway E S 1968 An experiment in integration. Education 132: 227
Court S D M (chairman) 1976 Fit for the future: Report of the Committee on Child Health Services. HMSO, London
Critchley M 1964 Developmental Dyslexia. Heinemann, London
Cruickshank W, Bentzen F, Ratzeburg F, Tannhauser M 1961 The teaching method for brain injured and hyperactive children. University Press, Syracuse

Dale D M C 1967 Deaf children at home and at school. University Press, London
Davie R, Butler N, Goldstein H 1972 From birth to seven. Longman, London
Dawkins J M S V, Reid J J A 1965 School children undertaking restricted physical education. Medical Officer 114: 71–73
Dawson B, Horobin G, Illsley R, Mitchell R 1969 A survey of childhood asthma in Aberdeen. Lancet i: 827–830
Department of Education and Science 1964 Report of the Chief Medical Officer, 1962–1963. HMSO London
Department of Education and Science 1966 Report of the Chief Medical Officer, 1964–1965. HMSO, London
Department of Education and Science 1967 Units for partially hearing pupils. Education Survey 1. HMSO, London
Department of Education and Science 1968a Psychologists in education services (Summerfield Report). HMSO, London
Department of Education and Science 1968b the education of deaf children. HMSO, London
Department of Education and Science 1969 Report of the Chief Medical Officer, 1966–1968. HMSO, London
Department of Education and Science 1970 Diagnostic and assessment units. Education Survey 9. HMSO, London
Department of Education and Science 1971 Slow learners in secondary schools. Education Survey 15. HMSO, London
Department of Education and Science 1972a Report of the Chief Medical Officer, 1969–1970. HMSO, London
Department of Education and Science 1972b Aspects of special education. Education Survey 17. HMSO, London
Department of Education and Science 1972c The education of the visually handicapped (Vernon Report). HMSO, London
Department of Education and Science 1972d Children with specific reading difficulties. HMSO, London
Department of Education and Science 1973 Special education: a fresh look. Reports on Education 77. HMSO, London
Department of Education and Science 1974a Integrating handicapped children. Education information, Autumn. HMSO, London
Department of Education and Science 1974b Report of the Chief Medical Officer, 1971–1972. HMSO, London
Department of Education and Science 1975 Circular 2/75: The discovery of children requiring special education and the assessment of their needs. HMSO, London
Department of Education and Science 1976 Statistics of education, vol 1. HMSO, London
Department of Health and Social Security 1975 Health Service Circular (Interim Series) 191. Ascertainment of children requiring special education: day release courses for medical officers. HMSO, London
Ewing A W G (ed) 1960 The modern educational treatment of deafness. University Press, Manchester
Fine S 1968 Blind and partially-sighted children. Department of Education and Science: Education survey 4. HMSO, London
Franklin A W, Naidoo S (eds) 1970 Assessment and teaching of dyslexic children. Invalid Children's Aid Association, London
Gastaut H 1964 Enquiry into the education of epileptic children. In: Social Studies in Epilepsy No. 2. British Epilepsy Association, London
Graham P J, Rutter M, Yule W, Pless I B 1967 Childhood asthma: a psychosomatic disorder? British Journal of Preventive and Social Medicine 21: 78–85
Graham P J, Rutter M 1973 Psychiatric disorder in the young adolescent. Proceedings of the Royal Society of Medicine 66: 1226–1229
Grunewald K 1971 The guiding environment: the dynamic of residential living. Paper read at First Regional Conference of the United Kingdom Committee of the World Federation for Mental Health and The National Society for Mentally Handicapped Children, Dublin
Hamblin D H 1975 Residential treatment of maladjusted children. In: Laing A F (ed) Trends in the education of children with special learning needs. Faculty of Education, University College of Swansea
Haskell S 1966 Does squinting matter? Special Education 55: 23–26
Henderson P 1968 The educational problems of myelomeningocele. Hospital Medicine 2: 909–914

Henderson P 1974 Disability in childhood and youth. Oxford University Press, London
Holdsworth L, Whitmore K 1974 A study of children with epilepsy attending ordinary schools. Developmental Medicine and Child Neurology 16: 746–758
Holt K S, Down H, Brand H L 1972 Children's wheelchair clinic. British Medical Journal iv: 651–655
Ingram T T S 1963 Report of the Dysphasia Committee of the Scottish Paediatric Society. Unpublished
Joint Council for the Education of Handicapped Children 1975 Integration or segregation? London
Kershaw J 1973 Handicapped children, 3rd edn. Heinemann, London
Kolvin I, Garside R F, Whitmore K 1975 Action research in child psychology. In: Laing A F (ed) Trends in the education of children with special learning needs. Faculty of Education, University College of Swansea
Kushlick A, Cox G R 1973 The epidemiology of mental handicap. Developmental Medicine and Child Neurology 15: 748–759
Lansdown R 1969 What the research doesn't know. Special Education 58: 20–24
Lansdown R 1970 Day schools for maladjusted children. Association of Workers for Maladjusted Children, London
Lansdown R 1975 Partial sight—partial achievement? Special Education 2: 11–13
Laurence E R 1971 Spina bifida children in school: preliminary report. Developmental Medicine and Child Neurology 13: (Suppl 25) 44–46
Laurence K M, Carter C O, David P A 1968 Major central nervous system malformations in South Wales II: Pregnancy factors, seasonal variation and social class effects. British Journal of Preventive and Social Medicine 22: 212–222
Lenhoff F 1966 Exceptional children. Allen & Unwin, London
Lowden G M, Walker J H 1975 The school health service and the school doctor. In: Bridging in health (Nuffield Provincial Hospitals Trust). Oxford University Press, London
McMichael J K 1971 Handicap: A study of physically handicapped children and their families. Staples Press, London
Maier I 1970 The systematic approach to the treatment of overactive children. The Hester Adrian Research Centre, Manchester
Mannix J B 1972 Survey of children recommended for special education in the ordinary school. Wellbeing (September). West Riding County Council
Marshall A 1967 The abilities and attainments of children leaving junior training centres. London: National Association for Mental Health
Melchior J C 1968 The Danish centre-schools. Developmental Medicine and Child Neurology, 10: 671–673
Miller F J W, Court S D M, Knox E G, Brandon S 1975 The School Years in Newcastle upon Tyne. Oxford University Press, London
Ministry of Education 1952 Report of the Chief Medical Officer, 1950–1951. HMSO, London
Ministry of Education 1954 Circular 276, provision of special schools. HMSO, London
Ministry of Education 1955 Underwood Report: Report of the Committee on Maladjusted Children. HMSO, London
Ministry of Education 1956 Education of the handicapped pupil, 1945–1955. HMSO, London
Ministry of Education 1962 Report of the Chief Medical Officer, 1960–1961. HMSO, London
Ministry of Health 1968 Memorandum on Comprehensive assessment centres. HMSO, London
Minski L, Shepherd M J 1970 Non-communicating children. Butterworth, London
Mitchell R G, Dawson B 1973 Educational and social characteristics of children with asthma. Archives of Disease in Childhood 48: 467–471
Mittler P, Woodward M 1966 Children in hospitals for the subnormal. British Psychological Society Special Report
Naidoo S 1972 Specific dyslexia. Pitman Publishing Co., London
Nash D F E 1969 Teachers—and nursemaids too? Special Education 58: 6–8
National Union of Teachers 1964 The special school: aims, facilities and amenities. London
Nicholls R 1975 Merging their education. Special Education 2: 22–4
Peckham C S, Sheridan M, Butler N R 1972 School attainment of seven-year-old children with hearing difficulties. Developmental Medicine and Child Neurology 14: 592–601
Peirse A 1973 A bold experiment at Bromley. Special Education 62: 12–14
Petrie I 1975 Characteristics and progress of a group of language disordered children with severe receptive difficulties. British Journal of Disorders of Communication 10: 123
Pless I B 1969 Why special education for the physically handicapped pupil? Social and Economic Administration 3: 253–263

Pringle M I K, Fiddes D O 1970 The challenge of thalidomide. Longman, London
Pritchard D G 1963 Education and the handicapped. Routledge & Kegan Paul, London
Rackham K 1975 The role of boarding special schools in the treatment of children with recurrent disabling disorders. Child Care, Health and Development 1: 19–27
Reed M 1971 Audiological services for children. Hearing 26: 36–42
Renfrew C, Murphy K 1964 The child who does not talk. Clinics in Developmental Medicine 13. Heinemann, London
Roe M 1965 Survey into progress of maladjusted pupils. Inner London Education Authority, London
Rose M F 1973 Communication, language and speech for the severely handicapped child. Public Health, London 87: 109–113
Rutter M, Martin J A 1972 (eds) The child with delayed speech. Clinics in Developmental Medicine 43. Heinemann, London
Rutter M, Cox A, Tupling C, Berger M, Yule W 1975 The prevalence of psychiatric disorder. British Journal of Psychiatry 126: 493–509
Rutter M, Graham P, Yules W 1970a A neuropsychiatric study in childhood. Clinics in Developmental Medicine 35/36. Heinemann, London
Rutter M, Tizard J, Whitmore K 1970b Education, health and behaviour. Longman, London
Scottish Education Department, Edinburgh 1944 Report on ascertainment of maladjusted children
Scottish Education Department, Edinburgh 1969 Ascertainment of children with visual handicaps
Scottish Education Department, Edinburgh 1975 The secondary education of physically handicapped children in Scotland
Sheridan M 1962 Comprehensive assessment centres. Monthly Bulletin of the Ministry of Health 21 238–242
Sheridan M 1972 Reported incidence of hearing loss in children of 7 years. Developmental Medicine and Child Neurology 14: 296–303
Sheridan M 1973 Children of seven years with marked speech defects. British Journal of Disorders of Communication 8: 9–16
Smith J M 1970 The treatment of asthmatic children away from home. Public Health 84: 286–290
Smith V H, James F E 1968 Eyes and education. Heinemann, London
Smithells R W 1973 Defects and disabilities of thalidomide children. British Medical Journal i: 269–272
Stores G 1978 School-children with epilepsy at risk for learning and behaviour problems. Developmental Medicine and Child Neurology 20: 502–508
Tew B 1973 SBH: facts, fallacies and future. Special Education 62: 26-31
Tizard J 1964 Community services for the mentally handicapped. Oxford University Press, London
Tizard J 1973 Maladjusted children and the child guidance service. London Educational Review 2, (No. 2): 22–37
Tyrrell S 1975 Some problems of incontinent children attending ordinary schools. Public Health, London 89: 77–80
Varlaam A 1974 Educational attainment and behaviour at school. Greater London Intelligence Quarterly No. 29
Warnock H M (chairman) 1978 Special educational needs: Report of the Committee of Enquiry into the Education of Handicapped Children and Young People. HMSO, London
Watson A 1972 A study of family attitudes to children with diabetes. Community Medicine 128: 122–124
Watson T J 1967 The education of hearing-handicapped children. University Press, London
Watts G K 1972 The education of partially-sighted children. Optician 164: 17–24
Webb L 1967 Children with special needs in the infants' school. Fontana Books, London
Whitmore K 1969 An assessment service for handicapped children. Medical Officer 122: 263–267
Whitmore K 1972 Maladjusted children. Journal of the Association of Educational Psychologists (Suppl)
Wills D 1960 Throw away thy rod. Gollancz, London
Wilson M 1967 The education of brain injured children in the United States of America. Greater London Council, London
Wilson M 1970 Children with cerebral palsy. Department of Education and Science, Education Survey 7. HMSO, London
Wright T, Nicholson J 1973 Physiotherapy for the spastic child: an evaluation. Developmental Medicine and Child Neurology 15: 146–163

Younghusband D, Birchall D, Davie R, Pringle M L K 1970 Living with handicap. National Bureau for Co-operation in Child Care, London

Yule W, Rutter M, Berger M, Thompson J 1974 Over- and under-achievement in reading: distribution in the general population. British Journal of Educational Psychology 44: 1–12

Index

Accident room in hospital, 235
Accidents, epidemiology of, 140
Adolescence, consultants in, 87
   counselling in, 83
   and drugs, 79
   eating problems in, 75
   identity in, 70
   instability in, 53
   neurosis in, 72
   and obesity, 76
   psychosis in, 80
   school refusal in, 74
   self-injury in, 73
   sexual problems in, 76
   social difficulties in, 11
   theoretical model of, 70
   vocational guidance in, 86
Adolescents, assessment of difficulties, 82
   families of, 83
   residential units for, 84
   social difficulties of handicapped, 11
   and society, 83
   suitability of environment, 41
Adoption, 276
After-care, 280
Age-grading of children, 21
Aggression, adolescent, 38
Anorexia nervosa, 75
Area paediatrician, 180
Assessment of social work services needed, 270
Assessment centre, developmental, 241
   educational, 322
   functions of, 252
   in Warnock Report, 294
Assumptions about childhood, 20
Asthma, epidemiology of, 140
Attitudes to disease, 7
Authority, legitimacy of adult, 32
Autistic children, special schools for, 337

Battered babies (*see* Child abuse)
Behaviour disorders in school, 50
Birth-rate, 126
Birth weight and intelligence, 6
Boarding-out of children, 274
Bonding, 64
Breast milk, advantages of, 149
Brotherston Report, 176

Caries, dental, 152
Centre, assessment, 241, 252

Child, definition of, 89
   in family, 48
   handicapped in school, 313
   separation from mother, 272
Child abuse, 9
   epidemiology of, 141
   incidence of, 133
   parents in, 65
Child development, National Study, 129
Child guidance services, 308
Child health, and educational difficulties, 7
   and family life, 8
   malnutrition and, 6
   poverty and, 6
   social factors in, 5
   specialist in, 181
   undergraduate course in, 197
Child Health Associate, 172
Child health care, planning, 161
   programmes, 162
Child health clinics, 189
Child health services, 161
   age range of, 169
   constraints on, 174
   doctors in, 172
   evaluation of, 168
   new professions in, 171
   objectives of, 165
   preventive, 186
   rationale of, 164
   Report of Committee on (*see* Court Report)
   staffing of, 169
Child health visitor, 212
Child-minding, 203
Child psychiatry in hospital, 240
Child-rearing and social class, 38
Childhood, assumptions about, 20
   discovery of, 22
   as an estate, 19
   exploitation of, 25
   meaning of, 33
   morbidity in, 129
   mortality in, 127
   nature of, 27
Children, adoption of, 276
   age-grading of, 21
   at risk, 65
   autistic, special schools for, 337
   with behavioural handicaps, 336
   in care, examination of, 203
   with communication handicaps, 333
   disadvantaged, 61

344 INDEX

Children—contd.
    focuses of concern, 262
    fostering of, 274
    handicapped, 246
    hospital services for, 233
    hospital statistics, 238
    incompetence of, 28
    with learning handicaps, 334
    as marvellous, 20
    with motor handicaps, 329
    residential care of, 277
    roots in the family, 264
    servicing of, 25
    social work services for, 261
    in society, 4
    and the state, 27
    troublesome, 89
    with visual handicaps, 332
Children's Hearings, attitude to children, 29
    conflict of interest, 102
Children's homes, 278
Children's hospital unit, size of, 235
Cleanliness in schools, 306
Clinics, child health, 189
    minor ailments, 308
    paediatric, 28
    special in general practice, 214
    specialist in schools, 308
    under-fives, 174
    well baby, 222
Clinical medical officers, 180
Cohen Committee, 116
Committee on Child Health Services, Report of (see Court Report)
Communicable diseases, care in hospital, 236
    prevalence, 133
Communication, in hospital, 242
    in School Health Service, 295
Communication handicap, 333
Community, role of hospital in, 233
Community child health services (see Child health services)
Community health teams, 230
Community home system, 100
Community medicine, specialist in, 181
Community paediatrics, 3
Community work with children, 43
Compulsory measures of care, 99
Congenital abnormalities in general practice, 217
Congenital malformations, epidemiology of, 138
    prevalence of, 132, 138
Constraints on child health services, 174
Cot deaths, 5
    epidemiology of, 136
    and inadequate mothering, 67
Council, Health Education, 117
Counselling in adolescence, 83
Court, juvenile, attitude to children, 29
Court Report, 176
    district handicap teams, 323
    handicapped children, 251
    hospital care, 237
    recommendations on general practice, 211
    school medical examinations, 301
    staffing of School Health Service, 293
Cruelty, 9

Day nurseries for handicapped children, 258
Deaths, perinatal, 127
Defective mothering, 63
Delinquency, as a process, 94
    role of social worker in, 96
    theories of, 91
    treatment measures, 95
Dental caries, 152
Denver Developmental Screening Test, 194
Depression in teenagers, 60
Deprivation, social, 38
    syndromes of, 64
Deprived areas, studies of, 38
Developmental assessment centres, 241, 252
Developmental delay, 192
Developmental paediatrics, 190
Developmental screening, 192
    ancillary workers and, 194
    in general practice, 223
Disability (see Handicapping disorders)
Disadvantage, social, 39
Disadvantaged children, 61
Discovery of childhood, 22
Disease in childhood, epidemiology of, 126
District handicap team, 323
Divorce rate, 126
Doctors, and the environment, 45
    school, 294
Domiciliary visiting, 190
Drugs, abuse in adolescence, 79
    addiction to, 12
    overdosage in adolescence, 73
    prescribing in general practice, 220
    teenage experimentation with, 52
Dyslexia, 334

Eating problems in adolescence, 75
Education, special, 325
Educational difficulties and child health, 7
Emergencies in general practice, 218
Emotional problems, diagnosis of, 48
    in home setting, 56
    in neighbourhood setting, 54
    in school setting, 50
Emotional stunting, 65
Environment, doctor's role in, 45
    social and physical, 37
Epidemiology, of accidents, 140
    of child abuse, 141
    of congenital malformations, 138
    of disease in infancy and childhood, 126
    of handicapping disorders, 139
    of illegitimacy, 142
    of low birth weight, 137
    of respiratory disease, 140
    of sudden infant death, 136

Epilepsy, prevalence of, 133
Estate, childhood as an, 19
Europe, health education in, 114
Evaluation of child health services, 168
Examination, school medical, 131
Exhibitionism, 78
Expenditure on child health, 174
Exploitation of children, 25

Families, incomplete, 10
  mobile, 203
  nuclear, 23
  problem, 203
  vulnerable, 12
Family, changing needs of, 40
  child in the, 48
  child's roots in the, 264
  faulty interaction in, 93
  with handicapped child, 10
Family doctor (*see* General practitioner)
Family group homes, 278
Family life and child health, 8
Family stress, 9
Feeding of infants, 147
Fertility rate, 126
Fluoridation of water, 153
Foster care, 274

Gastrointestinal disorders in schools, 305
General practice, chronic illness in, 221
  developmental screening in, 223
  emergencies in, 218
  health education in, 227
  home visits in, 212
  hospital referrals from, 214
  immunization programme in, 226
  minor illness in, 219
  morbidity patterns in, 215
  observer variation in, 213
  organization of, 209
  special clinics in, 214
  studies of childhood illness in, 130
  team approach in, 230
  training for, 211
  workload in, 212
General practitioner, in child health service, 178
  and troubled children, 103
General practitioner paediatrician, 212
Glue-sniffing, 79
Group health education, 122
Grouped cottage homes, 278
Growth, measurement in schools, 303

Handicap, classification of, 248
  denial of, 58
  disadvantage of, 61
Handicapped children, 246
  counselling of parents, 254
  detection of, 247
  in general practice, 216
  needs of, 250

parents of, 250
services for, 257
siblings of, 251
social difficulties of, 11
social issues of, 254
teeth of, 153
Handicapped children in school, 278, 313
  classification and numbers, 317
  role of doctor, 323
  special classes, 325
  special schools, 325
Handicapped pupils, categories of, 337
Handicapping disorders, assessment of, 253
  communication, 333
  diagnosis of, 252
  early recognition of, 191
  epidemiology of, 139
  incidence of, 246
  of learning, 334
  of motor function, 329
  prevalence of, 133
  recognition in schools, 320
  and related disorders, 249
  and the school doctor, 309
  of vision, 332
Health authority, co-operation with social services, 198
Health centres, 209
Health education, behavioural basis, 107
  definition and aims, 109
  in general practice, 227
  in groups, 122
  guidelines to needs, 111
  international agencies, 116
  main areas of, 110
  mass media in, 122
  parental needs for, 111
  and parents, 118
  in schools, 119, 307
  targets, 121
  in UK and Europe, 114
Health Education Council, 117
Health records, 199
Health services for children (*see* Child health services)
Health surveillance, 189
  approach to, 201
  programme of, 202
Health visitor, in general practice, 210
  role of, 196
Hearing, screening tests in school, 303
Hearings, children's 29, 102
Hepatitis in schools, 306
High-rise flats, 40
Home, changing environment of, 40
  and emotional stress, 56
Home visits in general practice, 212
Homes, for children, 278
  family group, 278
  grouped cottage, 278
  reception, 279
Homework, children's, 40

346 INDEX

Homosexuality, 77
Hospital, causes of admission to, 131
  communication with, 242
  district general, 235
  functions of, 234
  referral to, 214
  regional children's 237
  role in community, 233
Hospital care, Court Report on, 237
Hospital schools, 258
Hospital services for children, 233
  future of, 243
  organization of, 234
Hospital statistics, 238
Housing, 40
  for handicapped children, 259
Hygiene in schools, 306
Hyperkinetic children, education of, 337
Hypernatraemia, 148
Hypocalcaemia, 148

Illegitimacy, epidemiology of, 142
Illness, chronic in general practice, 221
  management of minor, 219
Immune globulins in milk, 149
Immunization, in general practice, 226
  objectives of, 199
  programmes of, 200
  in schools, 304
Imprinting, 64
Infant feeding, 147
Infant mortality, causes, 128
  epidemiology of, 135
Infection, control in schools, 304
Infectious diseases, care in hospital, 236
  prevalence of, 133
  in schools, 305
Injury, non-accidental (see Child abuse)
Inspections, school medical, 299
Intake, nutritional, 156
Intellectual development and nutrition, 6
Intellectual retardation, 335
Intelligence, and birth weight, 6
  and nutrition, 6
Interactionist theory in delinquency, 95
Intermediate treatment, 97
International Year of the Child, 175

Juvenile delinquency, as a process, 94
  role of social worker in, 96
  theories of, 91
  treatment measures in, 95
Juvenile court, attitude to children, 29
Juvenile justice, balance of interests, 101
  tensions in system, 101

Lactoferrin, 149
Learning disorders, 334
  and the school doctor, 310
Lice in schoolchildren, 306
List D schools, 100

Loneliness in housing estates, 43
Low birth weight, epidemiology of, 137

Malformations, prevalence of, 132, 138
Malnutrition, 6
Marriage, age at, 126
Mass media in health education, 122
Maternal care, quality of, 43
Maternal deprivation, effects of, 272
Measles in schools, 305
Medical auxiliaries, 171
Mental subnormality, 335
Milk, advantages of breast, 149
  dangers of cow's, 148
Mobile families, 203
Mobility, consequences of, 42
Morbidity, in childhood, 129
  in general practice, 130
Mortality in childhood, causes of, 128
  trends in, 127
Mortality in infancy, causes of, 128
  epidemiology of, 135
  trends in, 127
Mortality, perinatal, 134
Mortality rates, trends in, 127
Mother, role of, 43
Mothering, defective, 63
Motor handicap, 329

National Child Development Study, 129
National Health Service, health education in, 117
  integration of, 163
Negative identity in adolescence, 70
Neighbourhood stresses, 54
Neurotic adolescent, 72
Newcastle-upon-Tyne, thousand families in, 129
Non-accidental injury (see Child abuse)
Nurse-practitioners, paediatric, 171
Nursery schools for handicapped children, 257
Nurses, in general practice, 210
  new roles for, 171
Nutrition, of children, 147
  and mental development, 6

Obesity, in adolescence, 76
  in childhood, 151
  in infancy, 151
Objectives of child health service, 165
Occupations concerned with children, 25
Outpatients, children as, 241
Overcrowding, 42
Overdependence, 58
Overprotection, 57

Paediatrician, area, 180
  in child health service, 179
  consultant, 179
  relationship to other professions, 13
Paediatric clinic, 28

Paediatrics, community, 3
  developmental, 190
  preventive, 185
  primary care, 209
  social, 3
Parentcraft, 118
Parents, advice to, 190
  of handicapped children, 250, 254
  and health education, 111, 118
  overprotective, 57
  role in preventive practice, 197
Perinatal deaths, 127
  epidemiology of, 134
Perinatal mortality, survey of, 129
Play, organization of, 44
Playgroups, for handicapped children, 257
  preschool, 44
Poverty and child health, 6
Pregnancy in adolescence, 78
Pressurizing, response to, 59
Preventive paediatrics, 185
  in general practice, 217, 222
  nature of, 187
  scope of, 188
Primary care doctor in child health service, 197
Primary care paediatrics, 209
Problem families, 203
Project systems analysis, 169
Promiscuity, sexual, 78
Psychiatric services for children, 240
Psychosis in adolescence, 80
Psychotherapy in adolescence, 83
Puberty (*see* Adolescence)
Pupils, handicapped, 313
  categories of, 337

Reception homes, 279
Recommended nutritional intakes, 156
Records, health, 199
  in School Health Service, 295
Regional children's hospital, 237
Register, at risk, 195
Registrar-General's classification, 143
Rehousing, effects of, 42
Residential care, 277
  compulsory, 100
Residential nurseries for handicapped children, 258
Residential units for adolescents, 84
Respiratory disease, epidemiology of, 140
Rickets, 154
Risk registers, 195

Scabies in schoolchildren, 307
Schizophrenia, in adolescence, 80
  incipient, 53
School doctors, 294
School health, responsibility for, 173
School Health Service, communications in, 295
  historical development of, 289

legislation and, 291
methods in, 299
objectives of, 290
organization of, 289
records in, 295
relationship to other services, 297
resources and cost of, 296
screening tests in, 302
staff of, 293
School medical inspections, Court Report on, 301
  defects found at, 131
  duration of, 300
  follow-up of, 302
  place of, 299
  purpose of, 300
  results of, 300
  selection for, 301
  special, 302
School refusal in adolescence, 74
Schools, cleanliness in, 306
  control of infection in, 304
  emotional problems in, 50
  health education in, 119
  in hospitals, 258
  List D, 100
  outbreaks of infection in, 305
  special, 325
  specialist staff of, 328
Screening, developmental, 192, 223
Screening tests in School Health Service, 302
Self-injury in adolescence, 73
Separation of mother from child, 272
Service, school health (*see* School Health Service)
Services, child guidance, 308
  social work, 261
Sexual problems in adolescence, 76
Sexuality, inverted, 78
Siblings of handicapped children, 251
Slum clearance, 42
Social class, and child-rearing, 38
  classification by occupation, 143
  effects of, 38
Social deprivation, effects of, 38
Social difficulties of handicapped child, 11
Social disadvantage, 39
Social environment and child development, 37
Social factors in child health, 5
Social paediatrics, 3
Social work services, assessment of need, 270
  for children, 261
  co-operation with health services, 198
  legislation and organization of, 267
  problems of, 280
Social worker and juvenile delinquency, 96
Socialization, 37
Society, children in, 4
  focus on the child in, 266
Solvent abuse, 79
Special care baby units in hospital, 236
Special classes for handicapped children, 325

INDEX

Special education, 325
Special schools for handicapped children, 325
Specialists, in child health, 181
  in community medicine, 181
Staff, of School Health Service, 293
  specialist in schools, 328
Statistics, inpatient, 240
  outpatient, 241
Still-birth, 127
Stress on the family, 9
Stunting, emotional, 65
Stycar test, 194
Sudden infant death, 5
  epidemiology of, 136
Supervision orders, 99

Team, multi-disciplinary in general practice, 230
Teenage depression, 60
Teeth, caries of, 152
  and fluoride, 153
  of handicapped children, 153
Tensions in juvenile justice system, 101
Thousand families study in Newcastle-upon-Tyne, 129

Training, for general practice, 211
  for School Health Service, 293
Transsexuality, 79
Transvestism, 79
Troubled children and the family doctor, 103
Troublesome children, 89
Tuberculosis in schools, 306

Under-fives clinic, 174
Undergraduate teaching in child health, 197
United Kingdom, health education in, 114

Vision, screening tests in schools, 302
Visual handicap, 332
Vitamin D deficiency, 154
Vocational guidance for adolescents, 86
Vulnerable families, 6

Warnock Report, and assessment centres, 294
  and special education, 318
  and universal education, 8
Welfare state and child health, 161
Well baby clinic, 222
Woodside system of developmental screening, 226

Youth Service Bureau (USA), 98